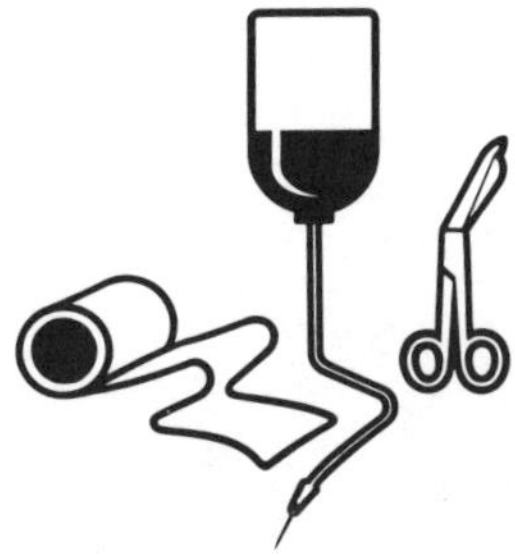

medical nursing for animal health technicians

FIRST EDITION

EDITED BY
PAUL W. PRATT, VMD

American Veterinary Publications, Inc.
5782 Thornwood Drive, Goleta, CA 93117-3896

Library of Congress Catalog Card No. 84-72184

ISBN 0-939674-13-0

PRINTED IN THE UNITED STATES OF AMERICA

preface

"Observation more than books, experience rather than persons, are the prime educators."
A. B. Alcott

As a squeaky-clean young associate in my first job in a busy small animal practice, I overflowed with knowledge of the complexities of veterinary medicine. However, I had very few *practical* skills. In that regard, I am forever indebted to the AHT in that practice who taught me the basics of medical nursing.

With great modesty and a minimum of sarcasm, she taught me how to bandage a foot so the bandage stayed on for days rather than minutes, how to clean ears without general anesthesia and a vacuum unit, and how to catheterize even the smallest veins without making a sieve of the animal's cephalic or jugular vein. In short, she taught me to use my hands as well as my head.

Medical nursing is the heart of an AHT's duties; without such skills, AHTs severely limit their contributions to their patients and employers. Though this book is no substitute for actual experience in working with animals under clinical or field conditions, it supplies enough information to enable even AHTs new to the field to quickly become an integral, productive part of a practice, the veterinarian's "right-hand man" (person?).

We are grateful to our group of 16 authors, who contributed the essence of their years of experience in caring for animals. We also thank the many instructors in AHT programs for their excellent suggestions in developing the content of this book.

Paul W. Pratt, VMD
Editor

authors

Wilbur A. Aanes, DVM, MS
Professor
College of Veterinary Medicine
Colorado State University
Fort Collins, CO 80523

Ray Allen, Jr.
General Manager
Silver Creek Ranch
2500 East Valley Road
Montecito, CA 93108

Colin C. Bullmore, DVM
Carmichael Animal Hospital
5536 Marconi Ave.
Carmichael, CA 95608

Thomas P. Colville, DVM
Associate Professor
Department of Veterinary Science
North Dakota State University
Fargo, ND 58105

Karl Faler, BS
SW 110 McKenzie
Pullman, WA 99163

Kate Faler, DVM, MS
SW 110 McKenzie
Pullman, WA 99163

Richard B. Ford, DVM, MS
Associate Professor, Internal Medicine
School of Veterinary Medicine
North Carolina State University
Raleigh, NC 27606

Cynthia S. Intravartolo, RVT
Berwyn Veterinary Associates
2845 S. Harlem Ave.
Berwyn, IL 60402

Kristine A. Kazmierczak, RVT
Department of Small Animal Clinics
College of Veterinary Medicine
Purdue University
West Lafayette, IN 47907

Linda R. Krcatovich, LVT
Food Animal Technician
Veterinary Clinical Center
Michigan State University
East Lansing, MI 48824

Jennifer S. Krish, AAS
Large Animal Hospital Supervisory Technician
School of Veterinary Medicine
North Carolina State University
Raleigh, NC 27606

Charles R. Kuhn, MS
2445 Sycamore Glen Drive
Sparks, NV 89431

Ann M. Lamar, LVT
Senior Equine Technician
Veterinary Clinical Center
Michigan State University
East Lansing, MI 48824

Jan Rasmussen, RVT
Parkwise Animal Hospital
1800 West Irving Park Road
Schaumburg, IL 60172

Steven D. Van Camp, DVM
Diplomate, American College of Theriogenologists
Assistant Professor
School of Veterinary Medicine
North Carolina State University
Raleigh, NC 27606

John T. Vaughan, DVM
Dean
School of Veterinary Medicine
Auburn University
Auburn, AL 36849

contents

3. SUPPORTIVE CARE

4. TREATMENT TECHNICS FOR SMALL ANIMALS

5. TREATMENT TECHNICS FOR HORSES

6. TREATMENT TECHNICS FOR FOOD ANIMALS

L.R. Krcatovich

7. THERIOGENOLOGY

S.D. Van Camp & J.S. Krish

1

first aid

T.P. COLVILLE

GENERAL CONSIDERATIONS

First aid is the emergency care and treatment of a patient with an injury or sudden illness before full medical and surgical care is available. The primary objectives of first aid are to keep the animal alive until it can be seen by the veterinarian and to make the animal comfortable.[1]

Legal and Ethical Considerations

A great deal can be done to help an animal in an emergency situation by a technician knowledgeable in first aid technics. Prompt first aid often means the difference between life and death for a badly injured or severely ill animal.

In providing first aid to an animal in the absence of the veterinarian, however, a technician must be careful not to overstep his or her legal and ethical limitations. What an animal health technician is legally entitled to do varies with the laws of each state. In general, the offering of a diagnosis, prescription of medication, and performance of what could be construed, even loosely, as surgery without the supervision and/or advice of a veterinarian should be scrupulously avoided. This precludes potential legal difficulties for the individual and his or her employer should an inappropriate and/or unsuccessful treatment be administered. It also maximizes the animal's chances of recovery by preventing the potentially disastrous effects of a misdiagnosis under the pressure of an emergency situation. Finally it allows one to avoid undertaking procedures or administering medications with which one is not thoroughly familiar and for which one is not, by training and experience, completely qualified.

When an animal health technician is confronted with a medical emergency and the veterinarian is not immediately available, it is far better to apply basic first aid principles designed to improve the animal's chances of survival than to undertake drastic actions that could make the situation worse. Keeping a cool head and applying a logical system of first aid priorities can save the lives of many severely ill or injured animals.

Transport of Injured Animals

The basic principle of transporting an injured animal is to get it to a veterinarian as quickly as possible without making its injury any worse or causing any injuries to the people trying to help it. This usually can be accomplished by taking a moment to think about how the injured animal can most safely be transported before attempting to move it.

Injured or severely ill animals are often in pain and may act irrationally. Avoiding personal injury, therefore, must be an important concern of anyone attempting to attend to such an animal. Taking such precautions as applying a gauze, rope or necktie muzzle to a dog, handling a small dog or cat through a towel or blanket, and avoiding the powerful hooves of an injured large animal indirectly benefits the animal while maintaining human safety.

Often an animal's condition can be stabilized somewhat before attempted transport. This can take the form of such things as controlling severe hemorrhage, applying a temporary splint to a fracture, or hosing down a victim of heatstroke. Talking over the telephone with a person who has an injured animal often allows advice to be given on how best to handle the animal for transport to the clinic.

Large animals can usually only be transported in a trailer or truck. Some advance planning, though, can often make a great deal of difference in the animal's condition on arrival at the veterinary clinic. The animal should be well bedded for cushioning if it is recumbent, and adequately restrained with ropes and/or panels, etc, to prevent further injury during transport.

Small animals may be carefully carried in the arms or in a box or basket if their injuries and/or dispositions allow it. Others, such as those suspected of having spinal injuries, extensive trauma, or those that are unconscious, can best be transported on a blanket, or, preferably, on something stiff, such as a board or even on a wooden or screen door. If necessary the animal can be secured to the makeshift stretcher with belts or ropes to help ensure minimal movement during transport.

Initial Examination and Management

There usually is not time to obtain a detailed history or perform a thorough physical examination when presented with an acutely injured or ill animal. Often the situation dictates that first aid treatment for obvious life-threatening conditions be carried out as the animal is being examined for further, less obvious and urgent injuries.

In an emergency situation, an animal must be examined quickly and decisions made logically on how best to carry out the basic objectives of first aid. The most serious, life-threatening conditions must be considered before attention is turned to other matters. It must be kept in mind that emergency patients are not just a fractured leg or a large burn but entire animals whose overall well-being must be the overriding concern in rendering first aid.

Priorities

Stay Calm: In an emergency situation there is a natural tendency to become excited and try to do everything at once, or possibly to panic and become incapable of doing anything useful. To aid a severely injured or ill animal one must maintain a clear head and be able to think logically in assessing the situation and formulating a treatment plan.

Notify the Veterinarian as Soon as Possible: First aid is of great benefit to the patient and may well save its life, but it should receive the more complete care that only a veterinarian can provide.

Ensure Your Own Safety: Be certain that the animal is adequately restrained through use of such equipment as muzzles, leashes, blankets and towels in the case of small animals, or ropes, squeeze chutes and stocks in the case of large animals.

Stop Hemorrhage: Although minor bleeding can be temporarily ignored, major hemorrhage should be controlled with pressure or tourniquets.

Ensure Adequate Respiration: Clear the airway of debris, fluid, etc. Intubate the trachea if necessary.

Treat for Shock If Necessary

Proceed with Further Examination and First Aid Treatment

Equipment and Supplies

The needs for first aid equipment and supplies vary from clinic to clinic, but the following list includes items that can be very useful if readily available:

Baking soda
Bandaging materials (gauze pads, roll cotton, roll gauze, tape)
Blankets, towels
10% dextrose
Endotracheal tubes, various sizes
Examination gloves
Forceps for removing foreign bodies
Hydrogen peroxide
Ice
Lemon juice or vinegar
Oxygen
Sterile, isotonic saline
Stethoscope
Stomach tubes, various sizes
Table salt
Thermometer
Tourniquet
Towel clamps
Water-soluble lubricant

Species Considerations

Because various animal species are cared for in veterinary hospitals, it is important that each animal be evaluated in the context of what is normal and/or desirable for its species. For example, a healthy horse may lose a liter of blood without severe consequences, while the loss of a few drops of blood can be fatal for a parakeet.

The methods for handling animals, particularly in an emergency situation, must be appropriate for the species. Large animals, such as horses and cattle, usually cannot be restrained by strictly manual means due to their strength and size. Squeeze chutes and stocks are often needed, along with ropes and halters. Small animals, such as dogs and cats, can usually be restrained manually, although muzzles, towels, blankets and leashes are often needed.

The safety of the personnel working on an animal, as well as that of the animal itself, must be an important consideration in any procedure undertaken. The steps necessary to ensure safety and to facilitate efficiency must be carefully planned and executed, and be appropriate for the species being treated.

FIRST AID FOR SPECIFIC CONDITIONS

Shock

Summary

Shock

Signs

1. Weakness and/or unconsciousness
2. Pale mucous membranes
3. Cool skin and extremities
4. Rapid heart rate
5. Weak pulse
6. Shallow, rapid breathing
7. Poor capillary refill

First Aid

1. Maintain respiration
2. Control bleeding
3. Keep warm
4. Position with the head lowered
5. Monitor pulse and administer CPR, if necessary

The term "shock" is used to describe a very complex and dangerous clinical syndrome generally characterized by an inadequate perfusion of tissues with blood by the cardiovascular system, resulting in cellular hypoxia. If uncorrected, this hypoxia can lead to cell death, which, on a massive scale, can have disastrous and frequently fatal consequences.

Cause

There are many potential causes of shock, including:

Decreased blood volume, usually resulting from a severe loss of blood or plasma. This usually results from serious hemorrhage, which can be either external and readily apparent or internal and more difficult to ascertain, or from severe loss of fluids from such serious external lesions as extensive burns.

Severe stress, either physical or psychological. Such things as extensive traumatic injuries and severe pain can be inciting causes of shock.

Infection with certain toxin-producing bacteria. Some of these bacterial toxins affect blood vessels, causing blood to "pool" in parts of the circulatory system and a consequent precipitous drop in blood pressure.

Abnormal cardiac function. Conditions that seriously interfere with the normal pumping action of the heart, such as severe heart failure, myocarditis, cardiomyopathy and severe arrhythmias, can cause shock.

Pathophysiology

When there is any considerable drop in blood pressure, the body attempts to compensate and maintain circulatory function. Peripheral arteries and veins constrict and the heart rate and force of contraction increase. The cardiac output is redistributed in an attempt to maintain the blood supply to the brain and heart at the expense of the peripheral circulation. Blood flow to peripheral areas, such as the skin, muscles, intestines and kidneys, is decreased, with resulting hypoxia of these tissues. Anaerobic cellular metabolism, resulting from this hypoxia, produces increased amounts of lactic acid, upsetting the delicate acid-base balance of the body and resulting in acidosis. Damage to organs, such as the intestines and kidneys, can be severe.

If the blood supply to the brain begins to fail, changes in the level of consciousness are seen, ranging from excitement to unconsciousness.

Clinical Signs

The signs of shock are related to the body's attempts to maintain cardiovascular function through changes in cardiac function and redistribution of the cardiac output to the vital organs. Signs of shock include:

1. Weakness and/or unconsciousness.
2. Pale mucous membranes. This can best be evaluated at the gingivae, conjunctivae and the inner aspect of the vulva or prepuce.
3. Coolness of the skin and extremities.
4. Increased heart rate.
5. Weak pulse.
6. Shallow, rapid breathing.
7. Poor capillary refill. Apply sufficient pressure to an unpigmented area of the gingivae with a finger to cause the area to turn white. Upon releasing the pressure, the pink color should return within 1-2 seconds. A refill time any longer than 2 seconds indicates poor peripheral circulation.

First Aid

Maintain respiration by keeping respiratory passages clear, administering oxygen if possible, and giving artificial respiration if needed. Impaired respiration contributes to the already hypoxic state of the animal.

Control bleeding to help prevent further decrease in the circulating blood volume and oxygen-carrying capacity.

Keep the animal warm with blankets, towels and hot water bottles (wrapped in towels to prevent burning).

Position the animal with the head slightly lower than the rest of the body to help maintain blood supply to the brain.

Monitor the pulse. If cardiac arrest occurs, administer cardiopulmonary resuscitation.

Cardiac Arrest

Summary
Cardiac Arrest

Signs

1. Unconsciousness
2. Lack of respiration
3. Lack of pulse
4. Lack of heartbeat

First Aid

1. Artificial respiration (15-20/minute)
2. Cardiac massage (60/minute)

Cardiac arrest is the cessation of effective heart function. It usually occurs as either ventricular fibrillation, in which the heart "quivers" randomly, or asystole, in which it goes "limp" and stops all activity. In either case the circulation of blood stops, which deprives the tissues, especially the brain, of needed oxygen. This hypoxic brain damage is generally reversible if circulation can be restored within 3-4 minutes.[2] After this period, irreversible brain damage is likely to have occurred. Even if circulation can then be restored, the animal's behavior and/or function will probably not return to normal.

It is vital to *act immediately* in a case of cardiac arrest if there is to be any chance of recovery.

Clinical Signs

Clinical signs of cardiac arrest include unconsciousness, lack of respiration, lack of pulse and lack of a detectable heartbeat.

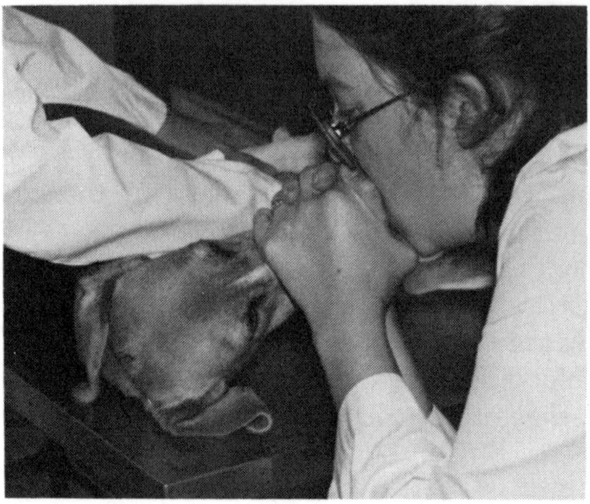

Fig 1. Artificial respiration is given by cupping the hands around the muzzle and blowing into the nares.

Cardiopulmonary Resuscitation

Without special equipment, cardiopulmonary resuscitation (CPR) is not usually effective in large animals, such as horses and cattle, due to their size. This discussion, therefore, deals with CPR technics applicable to animals small enough for effective CPR to be carried out by 1 or 2 people without special equipment (dogs and cats primarily).

Cardiopulmonary resuscitation consists of artificial respiration and external cardiac massage. The basic etiology of irreversible brain damage due to cardiac arrest is cerebral hypoxia. Reestablishing circulation does little or no good if the blood being circulated is not adequately oxygenated. In addition, without adequate ventilation, carbon dioxide levels in the blood rise rapidly and the animal becomes severely acidotic, further compounding the problem. Establishing adequate ventilation through artificial respiration is vital to effective CPR.

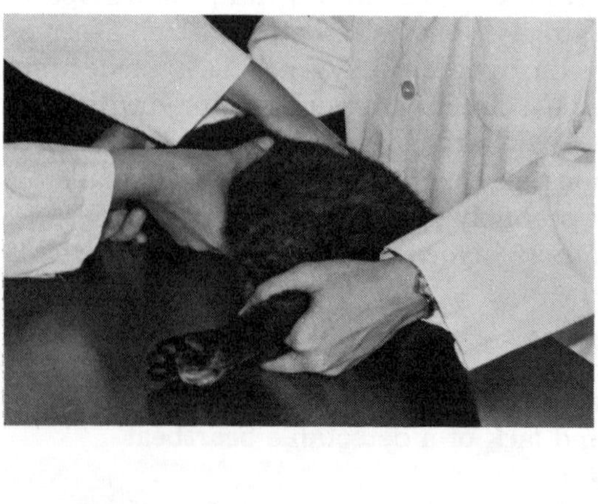

Fig 2. External cardiac massage is applied to cats or other small animals by compressing the chest between the fingers and thumb.

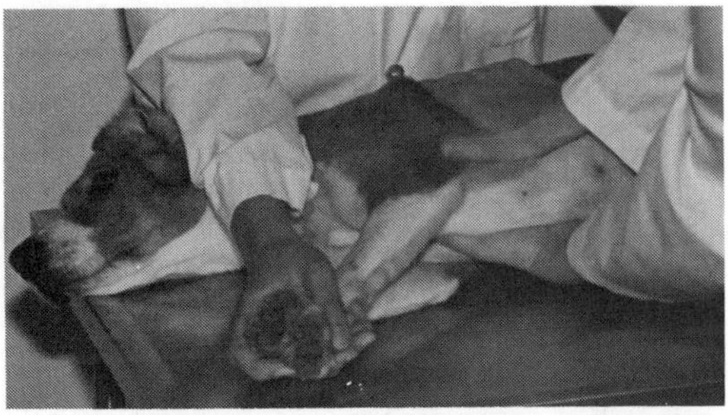

Fig 3. External cardiac massage is applied to a medium-sized dog by compressing the animal's chest between the hands.

To perform artificial respiration, intubate the animal with an endotracheal tube, if possible. Inflate the cuff (if present), and artificially ventilate the animal at a rate of 15-20 breaths/minute by blowing into the end of the tube, using an Ambu resuscitation bag, or connecting the tube to an inhalant anesthesia machine with the anesthetic vaporizer turned off and, with pure oxygen flowing, compressing the rebreathing bag. If endotracheal intubation is impossible, cup your hands tightly around the muzzle and ventilate by blowing into the nose 15-20 times/minute (Fig 1).

Regardless of what technic of artificial respiration is applied, after inflating the lungs for each breath, remove *all* pressure *completely* and allow the lungs to deflate passively before administering the next breath. This release of pressure is important for adequate respiratory gas exchange and to allow effective return of blood to the heart via the large veins in the thorax.

Because the valves of the heart allow a one-way flow of blood only, if the heart can be compressed rhythmically by applying pressure to the thorax over the heart, the valves will ensure that blood flows in the appropriate direction. This is the principle of external cardiac massage.

The heart is most efficiently compressed from side to side since this is the narrowest dimension of the thorax in most dogs and cats. With the animal in lateral recumbency and the foreleg in a position as though the animal were standing, compression is applied to the area of the thorax underlying the elbow. In very small animals the chest can be compressed between the fingers and thumb of one hand (Fig 2). In medium-sized animals compression can be accomplished with one hand on each side of the thorax (Fig 3). In larger animals compression is best applied from the top by compressing the chest between the hands and the tabletop or floor (Fig 4). Compress for a count of 2 and release for a count of 1, at a rate of 60 compressions/minute. The effectiveness of cardiac massage can be evaluated

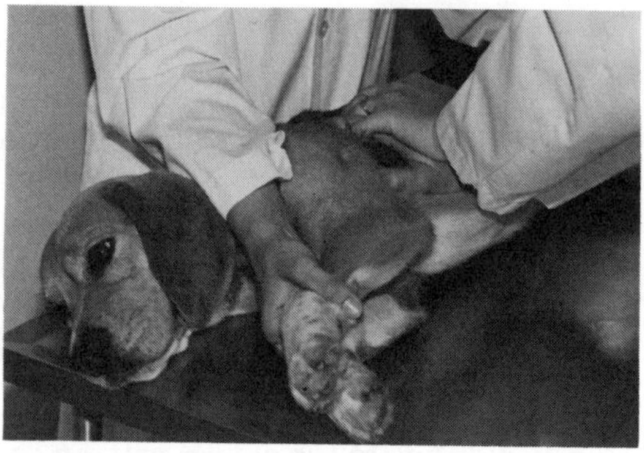

Fig 4. External cardiac massage is applied to larger animals by compressing the chest between the tabletop and hands.

by having someone else palpate for a pulse wave during each chest compression.

The ratio of respirations to chest compressions should be about 1 respiration to each 4 chest compressions. Check periodically to see if a spontaneous heartbeat and breathing have resumed. If they have not, continue CPR until a veterinarian can examine the animal.

Hemorrhage

Summary
Hemorrhage

Signs

1. Arterial blood (bright red, spurts rhythmically)
2. Venous blood (dark red, flows freely without spurting)
3. Capillary blood (oozes into wound without much pressure)

First Aid

1. Apply pressure
2. Apply a tourniquet if necessary
3. Treat for shock if necessary

Cause

Hemorrhage, the escape of blood from damaged blood vessels, can cause serious problems. Profuse hemorrhage can decrease the circulating blood volume sufficiently to cause shock. Hemorrhage that is not severe enough to cause shock may still cause tissue hypoxia, which can stress the animal and may compound other concurrent problems. Even mild hemorrhage can delay wound healing and contribute to development of infection, since blood is an excellent bacterial growth medium.

Hemorrhage can occur from individual blood vessels or from groups of vessels. Hemorrhage can occur from arteries (generally the most serious source), veins and/or capillaries (generally the least serious source). Arterial bleeding is characterized by bright-red blood that spurts under considerable pressure in time with the pulse. Blood escaping from veins is dark red and flows freely without spurting. Capillary blood oozes into a wound without much pressure.

First Aid

The arrest of hemorrhage is called hemostasis. First aid hemostasis is usually accomplished by applying pressure directly to the hemorrhaging area or by applying a tourniquet to slow the flow of blood through hemorrhaging vessels.

Pressure can be applied by direct digital pressure or by use of a pressure bandage. Direct digital pressure is very effective and involves placing a clean cloth over the wound and applying manual pressure. If no cloth is available, effective pressure can be applied directly with the fingers.

A pressure bandage is a bandage firmly applied over a clean cloth on the wound. It must not, however, be applied so tightly as to cause damage due to impaired circulation. Incorporating something bulky, such as a small gauze roll, rolled-up gauze sponges or crumbled pieces of cloth or paper, into the bandage over the wound helps apply direct pressure to the hemorrhaging area (Figs 5, 6).

A tourniquet, which can be a commercially available rubber or fabric one or just such an item as roll gauze, a necktie or belt, can temporarily help reduce bleeding from an extremity while a pressure bandage is applied. It can also be helpful in combination with pressure for very serious bleeding. It should be applied proximal to the wound

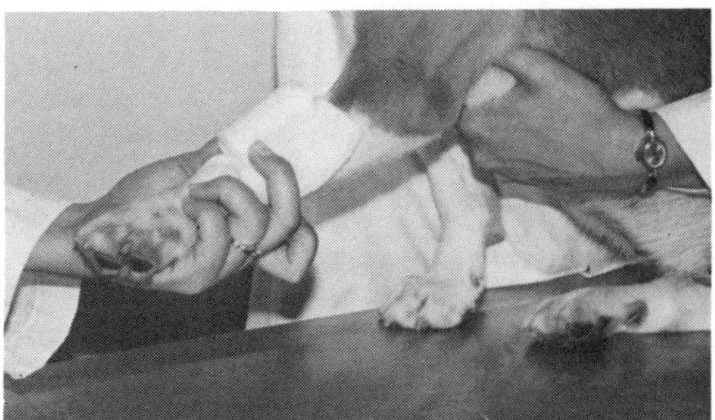

Fig 5. A pressure bandage can be applied by placing a small gauze roll over a gauze sponge.

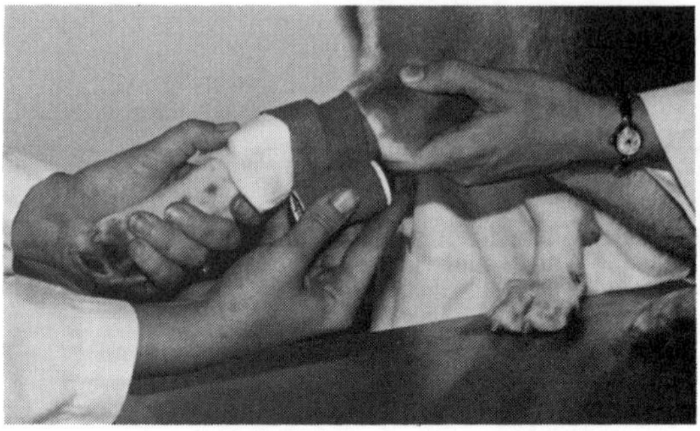

Fig 6. Elastic wrap is applied over the gauze roll to complete the pressure bandage.

to help control arterial hemorrhage or distal to the wound for venous hemorrhage.

Although a tourniquet can be a great aid in hemostasis if used properly, it also can cause serious damage if improperly applied. It should be applied tightly enough to slow or stop the hemorrhage but loosely enough so that a finger can easily be slipped beneath it. Slowly release the tourniquet for one minute every 10 minutes and do not reapply it unless it is still necessary.

Open Wounds

Summary
Open Wounds

Signs

1. Abrasion = surface scraped off
2. Incision = clean cut
3. Laceration = tissues torn
4. Puncture = small opening in surface

First Aid

1. Control hemorrhage
2. Treat for shock, if necessary
3. Protect the wound

Cause

Open wounds are injuries involving interruption in the surface of the skin or mucous membranes. The major types of open wounds include abrasions, incisions, lacerations and punctures.

In abrasions, the skin or mucous membrane is "scraped" off. Although they may be painful, abrasions usually are not very serious unless they are extensive, very deep or involve vital structures.

Incisions are clean cuts made by sharp objects, such as pieces of glass or metal. Depending on their size, depth and location, incisions can be serious due to infection and/or damage to underlying structures.

Lacerations have ragged, irregular edges and can be serious for the same reasons as incisions. The amount of tissue trauma can be greater with lacerations than with incisions, which can add to their seriousness.

Punctures are made by pointed objects, such as nails, teeth and projectiles. They usually appear as relatively small openings in the skin, but the damage beneath the surface can be quite extensive. Unless they are known to be shallow and small, punctures should be considered potentially very serious.

First Aid

First aid for wounds, in priority order, is to control hemorrhage, treat for shock, if necessary, and prevent further trauma and/or contamination of the wound. A cold compress applied to a fairly fresh wound can help control hemorrhage, prevent or reduce swelling, and help reduce pain. Self-trauma can be prevented by adequate restraint and use of such devices as muzzles and Elizabethan collars on small animals, and neck cradles or cross-ties on large animals. The wound can be protected with a sterile, or at least clean, dressing secured with gauze and/or tape.

Penetrating Foreign Bodies

Cause

Penetrating foreign bodies are objects that have penetrated the skin and are still present. They may include such objects as needles, fishhooks, porcupine quills and splinters. The damage caused by external foreign bodies may be purely superficial and limited to the skin, or may extend to deeper structures and tissues. For this reason, all penetrating foreign bodies should be considered potentially serious.

First Aid

The general principle of first aid for penetrating foreign bodies is to remove the object if it can be done *easily* without causing further trauma or pain, and treat the wound appropriately. If, however, the object cannot be easily removed, or if removing it would cause further trauma (*eg,* barb on a fishhook), it is best to leave it in place and try to keep the animal as comfortable as possible until the veterinarian can examine it. Anesthesia and surgery may be necessary for its removal.

Objects that penetrate very deeply, particularly into the abdomen or thorax, generally should be left in place, if possible, until the veterinarian can examine the animal. Thorough evaluation of vital structures in the vicinity of the foreign body may be necessary before it can be safely removed.

Fractures

Summary
Fractures

Signs

1. Pain
2. Swelling
3. Diminished function
4. Abnormal angulation or movement
5. Crepitus

First Aid

1. Handle gently
2. Cover and protect wounds
3. Control hemorrhage and treat for shock, if necessary
4. Apply a temporary splint, if possible

Fractures, or broken bones, can be classified according to many criteria. The simplest classifications, from a first aid standpoint, are according to the extent of the fracture and the integrity of the skin over the fracture site.

If the bone is not completely fractured, it is called an *incomplete (greenstick) fracture.* A *complete fracture* separates the bone into 2 or more segments. A *comminuted fracture* is one in which the bone is separated into more than 2 segments. In *simple (closed) fractures,* the overlying skin is intact. In a *compound (open) fracture,* the bone protrudes through the overlying skin.

Clinical Signs

The signs of a fracture can vary and depend on the location and extent of the fracture, the temperament of the animal, and the presence and extent of other injuries. Common fracture signs include: pain at or near the injury site; swelling and bruising at or near the injury site; decreased or absent function of the affected part (*eg,* inability to bear weight on a fractured leg); abnormal angulation and/or movement of the affected part; and crepitus, *ie,* a grating sensation when the broken ends of a bone rub together. *Do not deliberately test for crepitus* as it causes pain and may cause further injury.

First Aid

The main objectives of first aid for fractures are to prevent further injury and to make the animal more comfortable. An animal with a fracture is in severe pain, and the sharp ends of the fracture fragments can cause considerable damage to the surrounding tissues. Handle an affected animal gently, do not move it any more than is absolutely necessary, and use proper restraint to prevent personal injury. Control any serious hemorrhage and treat for shock if necessary. Cover and protect any serious wounds, particularly in the case of compound (open) fractures.

Many fractures, particularly those in the lower (distal) part of a limb, can be effectively stabilized with a temporary splint. This can decrease movement and prevent further trauma at the fracture site. An effective temporary splint can be made from virtually any reasonably stiff material, such as rolled-up magazines or newspapers and pieces of wood or cardboard.

To apply a temporary splint, pad the leg with such material as cotton or cloth, place the splint material against or around the leg, and secure it with tape, strips of cloth, rope or string. Try to immobilize the joints above and below the fracture site with the splint.

Another even more effective temporary splint is a modified Robert Jones bandage. In addition to stabilizing the fracture site, this type of splint helps reduce or prevent the swelling that often contributes to the pain of a fracture and that makes subsequent reduction of the fracture by the veterinarian more difficult. It is applied by wrapping many layers of roll cotton around the leg (large animals may require several rolls) and then compressing the roll cotton with an elastic wrap (Figs 7-12).

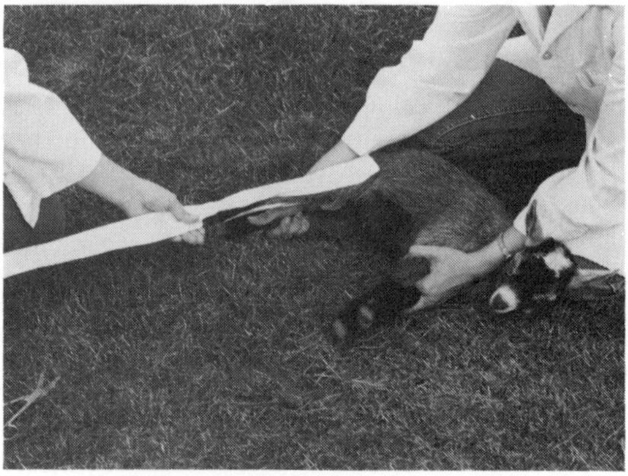

Fig 7. To apply a Robert Jones bandage, adhesive tape is put on the medial and lateral surfaces of the affected limb, with the pieces of tape joining distad at a distance about equal to the length of the leg.

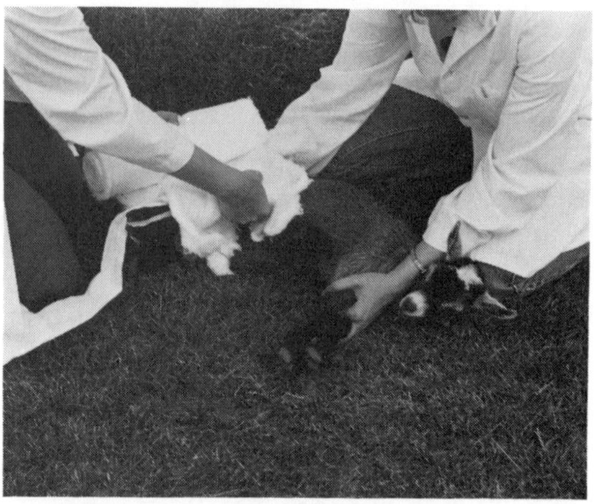

Fig 8. Roll cotton is unrolled and the paper removed. Then, the taped leg is wrapped with the roll cotton.

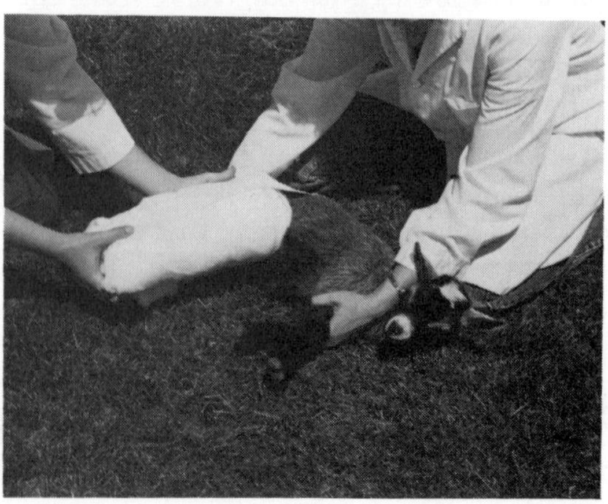

Fig 9. After the roll cotton is applied, the tape stirrup is reflected up over the cotton.

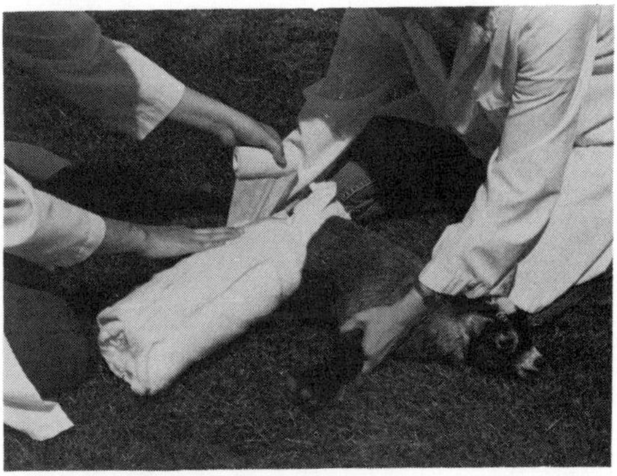

Fig 10. Elastic wrap is firmly applied over the roll cotton and reflected tape stirrup.

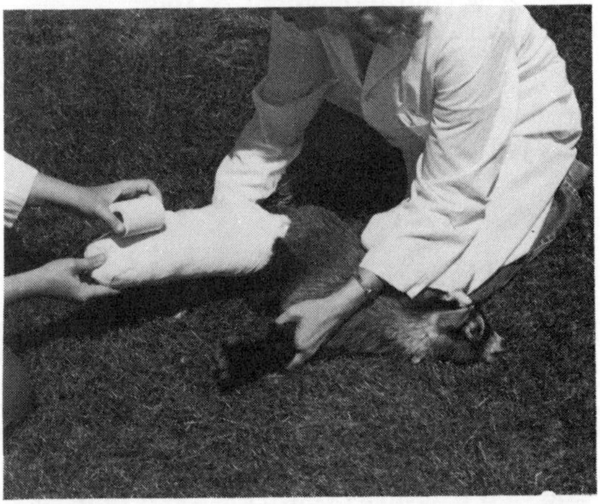

Fig 11. The elastic wrap is then covered with adhesive tape.

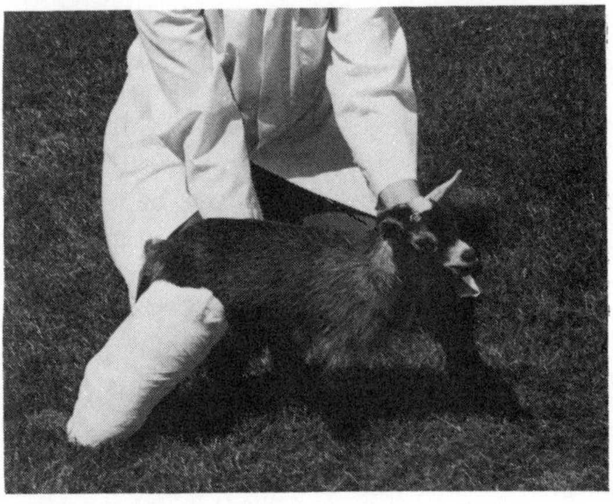

Fig 12. Completed Robert Jones bandage.

Dislocations

Summary
Dislocations

Signs

1. Pain
2. Swelling
3. Abnormal joint function
4. Abnormal joint position or angulation
5. Apparent shortening of limb

First Aid

1. Control hemorrhage and treat for shock, if necessary
2. Avoid movement of joint

A dislocation is a displacement of a bone from its normal position in a joint, usually as a result of trauma.

Clinical Signs

The signs of a dislocation, like those of a fracture, can be quite variable, but include: pain, particularly when the joint is moved; swelling around the dislocated joint; abnormal or absent function of the affected joint; abnormal angulation of the leg at the affected joint (This differs from that due to a fracture in that abnormal angulation due to a fracture occurs *between* joints.); and apparent shortening of the limb.

First Aid

First aid for dislocations is mainly symptomatic since their reduction usually requires general anesthesia due to the pain involved and the muscle spasms that must be overcome. An animal with a dislocated joint may be in severe pain and so should be handled carefully, gently and with adequate restraint to ensure personal safety. Control any serious hemorrhage and treat for shock, if necessary. Avoid movement of the affected joint as much as possible, and keep the animal quiet and as comfortable as possible.

Head Injuries

Summary
Head Injuries

Signs
1. Altered level of consciousness
2. Abnormal vision
3. Abnormal pupil size and pupillary response
4. Abnormal posture and movement
5. Abnormal respiration
6. Hemorrhage from the ear canals

First Aid
1. Keep animal quiet and observe for changes in status
2. Maintain respiration
3. Control hemorrhage and treat for shock, if necessary
4. Treat any serious wounds
5. Administer CPR, if necessary

Cause

Since the head is a particularly vital and vulnerable part of the body, cranial trauma frequently has more serious consequences than equivalent trauma to other parts of the body. Head injuries may include bruises, wounds, hemorrhage or fractures.

Cranial trauma can be very serious because of the extreme fragility of the brain. Being rigidly encased in bone, the traumatized brain tissue has no room to expand. Depressed cranial fractures and intracranial hemorrhage, bruising and edema cause the brain to swell, resulting in increased intracranial pressure. The severity of the damage depends on its site and extent. Even seemingly mild brain trauma can be life threatening.

Clinical Signs

Signs of brain damage may be very obvious or subtle. Severe brain damage can result in instant death, while very slight damage can cause very slight functional and/or behavioral changes.

A variety of clinical signs may be observed in brain-damaged animals.[3] The level of consciousness may range from normal alertness to coma. Initial consciousness followed by a lapse into unconsciousness usually indicates severe injury. Brain damage may result in blindness or altered pupillary function and/or size. Pupils that are abnormal on initial examination and that become normal on subsequent examination indicate a favorable prognosis. Abnormal ocular findings include miosis (pupillary constriction), mydriasis (pupillary dilation), anisocoria (asymmetric pupillary size), lack of response to light or dark, and nystagmus (horizontal, vertical or circular movement of the globes).

Brain damage may also cause a head tilt, inability to stand or walk normally, partial or complete paralysis, altered muscle tone (flaccidity or rigidity) and convulsions. Abnormal respiration in the absence of respiratory tract lesions indicates possible damage to the respiratory control center in the brainstem. Hemorrhage from the external ear canals is another indication of severe cranial trauma.

First Aid

First aid for cranial injuries is directed toward preventing further damage and maintaining vital functions. The animal should be kept quiet and comfortable, and observed closely for changes in status. Respiration should be watched closely and the trachea intubated if necessary. Control serious hemorrhage, treat serious wounds, treat for shock if necessary, and be prepared to administer CPR, if necessary.

Spinal Injuries

Summary
Spinal Injuries

Signs

1. Pain in neck or back
2. Weakness of limbs
3. Paralysis of limbs
4. Anesthesia of limbs

First Aid

1. Avoid movement of spine
2. Maintain respiration
3. Control serious hemorrhage and treat for shock, if necessary

Cause

Most serious spinal injuries are due to trauma or degeneration of intervertebral disks. Traumatic injuries usually involve fractures or dislocations of vertebrae, with associated damage to the spinal cord. Degenerated intervertebral disks can herniate dorsad to compress the spinal cord.

The severity of spinal injuries is often related to the type and severity of clinical signs exhibited. Pain and/or weakness generally indicate less serious damage than do anesthesia and/or paralysis.

Clinical Signs

Clinical signs seen with spinal injuries depend on the location, nature and severity of the damage. Typical signs of spinal trauma include pain, weakness, paralysis and loss of feeling in the limbs.

Spinal injuries can cause pain, usually in the neck and/or back region. If able, the animal walks gingerly, with the back and neck kept rigid. Weakness may be evident in the rear legs and perhaps in the front legs also. The animal may not be able to support itself.

Any paralysis usually affects the rear legs but may also affect the front legs. The muscles of the paralyzed legs may be rigid or, more commonly, flaccid.

Any anesthesia usually affects the rear legs but may also involve the front legs. There is a complete absence of pain perception when a painful stimulus, such as pinching a toe, is applied to the foot.

First Aid

First aid for spinal injuries is aimed mainly at preventing further trauma to the spinal cord. Animals with suspected spinal injuries should be kept quiet and moved as little as possible. A spinal injury is always serious, but as long as the spinal cord is maintained intact, the situation is not hopeless. The animal should be transported with as little movement of the spine as possible. If possible, the animal should be carried on something rigid, such as a board. General first aid care should be given to other injuries, such as hemorrhage, extensive wounds or shock.

Convulsions

Summary

Convulsions

Signs

1. Muscle twitches
2. Collapse
3. Uncontrolled shivering, paddling and thrashing

First Aid

1. Keep the environment quiet
2. Prevent the animal from injuring itself

Cause

Convulsions, also called seizures, epileptic seizures and fits, result from abnormal brain activity that causes involuntary contractions of skeletal muscles, which may be localized or generalized.

Potential causes of convulsions include epilepsy, toxicities (as from lead, antifreeze, insecticides, rodenticides), such infections as distemper and toxoplasmosis, CNS tumors, such metabolic disturbances as diabetes mellitus, and such developmental conditions as hydrocephalus.

Convulsions may have several forms. Focal seizures involve only a limited area of the body. Grand mal convulsions involve the entire body. The petit mal or psychomotor type, if recognized at all, is seen as a period of apparent confusion or inattentiveness.

Clinical Signs

The signs of convulsions depend on their type and severity. Some affected animals may show altered behavior that signals a convulsion is about to begin. This can take many forms, such as licking the lips, twitching of the muscles and restlessness. The convulsion itself usually begins with involuntary muscle twitches and contractions. The animal may apparently lose consciousness, collapse, paddle, shiver, twitch, and shake. Convulsions usually last from a few seconds to a few minutes, and the animal may appear dazed and disoriented for a time immediately after a convulsion. Prolonged, continuous convulsions are called status epilepticus and can be very dangerous for the animal.

Seizures cannot be shortened by first aid; they have to run their course. They can, however, be prolonged by continued stimulation from bright lights, loud noises or rough handling. It is important to remember that brief convulsions are not, in themselves, usually harmful to the animal. However, the animal may be injured by falling or thrashing about.

First Aid

First aid should, therefore, be aimed at 2 main areas. *Keep the environment as quiet as possible* to avoid prolonging an otherwise brief seizure. *Keep the animal from injuring itself.* Be sure it is on the floor or ground, and remove furniture and other objects it might knock over on itself. After the seizure has run its course, quietly and calmly reassure the animal as it emerges from the postseizure period of disorientation.

Epistaxis

Summary
Epistaxis

Signs

1. Hemorrhage from the nose

First Aid

1. Keep animal calm
2. Apply ice packs over nasal passages
3. Elevate the nose
4. Treat for shock, if necessary

Cause

Epistaxis, or hemorrhage from the nose, can have many potential causes. Such things as trauma, severe exercise (especially in horses), nasal tumors, blood clotting disorders, and violent sneezing can cause an episode of epistaxis.

Epistaxis of relatively short duration is not usually a serious problem. Prolonged epistaxis, however, can be serious. Severe blood loss can result in anemia, hypoxia and shock, and respiration can be impaired due to partial obstruction of the respiratory passages and aspiration of blood into the lungs.

First Aid

First aid for epistaxis is aimed at getting blood to clot at the source of the hemorrhage. The animal should be kept as quiet as possible since rapid, excited breathing decreases the chances of a clot forming. Ice packs placed over the nasal passages can help hasten clot formation, as can elevation of the nose. Treat for shock, if necessary.

Respiratory Obstructions

Summary
Respiratory Obstructions

Signs

1. Gagging or choking
2. Difficult breathing
3. Cyanosis
4. Unconsciousness

First Aid

1. Keep animal calm
2. Remove any pharyngeal foreign bodies
3. If necessary, compress chest forcefully a few times
4. Pass an endotracheal tube if possible and/or necessary
5. Administer oxygen
6. Give artificial respiration, if necessary

Cause

The causes of respiratory obstruction vary and include foreign bodies (bones, balls, toys, food), trauma to the nasal passages, pharynx, larynx or trachea, tumors, infection, allergic reactions and inhaled irritants.

Clinical Signs

The signs of a respiratory obstruction are related to impairment of normal gaseous exchange and include gagging or choking, dyspnea (difficult breathing), cyanosis (mucous membranes turn dark purplish blue) and unconsciousness.

First Aid

First aid for respiratory obstruction is directed at reducing the body's need for oxygen and increasing the rate of gaseous exchange. The animal should be kept as cool, calm and quiet as possible to minimize its need for oxygen and heat elimination. Check for foreign bodies in the pharynx by pulling the tongue forward and examining visually or manually. If a foreign body cannot be removed manually or with forceps, compressing the chest forcefully a few times may expel it. Do this by placing the animal in lateral recumbency and compressing the thorax with the hands from above or with the hands on either side of the chest. Repeat as necessary.

Administration of oxygen to an animal with impaired respiration can be life saving. An inhalant anesthesia machine, with the vaporizer turned off, can be used with a face mask or endotracheal tube.

If the animal is unconscious, keep its tongue pulled forward to open up the pharynx, and pass an endotracheal tube, if possible. Give artificial respiration, if necessary.

Rib Fractures

Summary
Rib Fractures

Signs
1. Painful respiration
2. Pain and crepitus at fracture site
3. Flail chest

First Aid
1. Keep the animal calm and quiet
2. Administer oxygen
3. Stabilize flail chest with a towel clamp

Clinical Signs

Clinical signs include painful respiration, pain and crepitus at the fracture site, and flail chest. The last occurs when multiple rib fractures produce a "floating" segment of the chest wall that moves paradoxically, *ie,* in on inspiration and out on expiration, and interferes with proper expansion of the lung.

First Aid

First aid for rib fractures is aimed at increasing the efficiency of respiration. The animal should be kept as calm and quiet as possible. Administer oxygen if necessary and possible. If flail chest is present, stabilize the floating segment by grasping its central portion with a towel clamp and applying traction outward (abaxially).

Diaphragmatic Hernia

Summary
Diaphragmatic Hernia

Signs

1. Difficult breathing
2. Muffled heart and lung sounds
3. Peristaltic sounds in the chest

First Aid

2. Keep the animal quiet and calm
2. Elevate the cranial end of the animal
3. Administer oxygen, if necessary
4. Give artificial respiration, if necessary
5. Treat for shock, if necessary

Cause

A diaphragmatic hernia is a tear in the diaphragm that allows protrusion of abdominal viscera into the thorax. It may be congenital or, more commonly, traumatic.

Clinical Signs

The signs of a diaphragmatic hernia are related to the pressure of the herniated abdominal contents on the lungs, which prevents their normal expansion. The severity of the signs depends on the site and size of the diaphragmatic tear, the amount of abdominal viscera present in the chest, and the activity of the animal. The condition of an affected animal can change very rapidly as abdominal organs move in or out of the thorax.

Typical signs include dyspnea (difficult breathing), peristaltic sounds and muffled heart and lung sounds on thoracic auscultation. The degree of dyspnea depends on the extent of abdominal organ displacement into the thorax. Severe dyspnea may lead to cyanosis and collapse.

First Aid

First aid for diaphragmatic hernias is aimed at maintaining respiratory function and preventing more abdominal viscera from slipping into the thorax. The animal should be kept as calm and quiet as possible. Elevate the cranial end of the animal to help prevent additional abdominal contents from slipping into the chest. Administer oxygen if the animal becomes cyanotic or loses consciousness. Give artificial respiration if necessary, and treat for shock if necessary.

Bloat in Ruminants

Summary

Bloat

Signs
1. Abdominal distension
2. Labored breathing
3. Anorexia
4. Decreased or no eructation
5. Possible cyanosis
6. Possible collapse

First Aid
1. Keep the animal quiet
2. Pass a large stomach tube, if possible

Cause

Bloat in ruminants is an excessive accumulation of gas, which may be free or trapped in a foamy froth, in the rumen. Mild bloat is not an emergency, but severe bloat causes a great deal of discomfort and interferes with respiration through pressure on the diaphragm that interferes with normal expansion of the lungs. Severe bloat can be fatal.

Clinical Signs

The signs of bloat in ruminants include abdominal distension, labored breathing, anorexia, decreased or no eructation, cyanosis and collapse.[4]

First aid for bloat is aimed at diminishing the body's oxygen needs and attempting to remove the gas from the rumen. Keep the animal as calm and quiet as possible. Pass a large, well-lubricated stomach tube, if possible, to relieve the pressure. However, this may not be very effective in cases of frothy bloat.

Gastric Dilation in Dogs

Summary
Gastric Dilation

Signs
1. Abdominal distension
2. Difficult breathing
3. Possible cyanosis
4. Possible shock

First Aid
1. Keep the animal calm and quiet
2. Pass a stomach tube, if possible
3. Administer oxygen, if possible
4. Treat for shock, if necessary

Cause

Gastric dilation in dogs is the canine equivalent of bloat in ruminants. The stomach rapidly distends with gas and may undergo volvulus (torsion). The distended stomach compresses the posterior vena cava, decreasing venous return to the heart and applies pressure to the diaphragm, compromising respiration. The animal can become rapidly acidotic and hypoxic, which lead to shock and possible death.

Clinical Signs

The signs of gastric dilation in dogs are very similar to those of bloat in ruminants and include abdominal distension, dyspnea (difficult breathing), cyanosis and shock.

First Aid

First aid for gastric dilation is aimed primarily at minimizing the animal's oxygen needs and attempting to relieve distension. Keep the animal as calm and quiet as possible. If possible, pass a well-lubricated stomach tube to relieve the pressure. If gastric torsion is present, it may not be possible to pass the tube into the stomach, so do not force it. Administer oxygen, if possible, and treat for shock, if necessary.

GI Foreign Bodies

Cause

Gastrointestinal foreign bodies consist of virtually anything other than food, water or medication swallowed by an animal. Metal, cloth, wood, bones, rubber, etc, may be ingested accidentally during feeding (large animals), play and/or chewing (small animals).

The dangers with GI foreign bodies include gastrointestinal perforation, laceration, abrasion or partial or complete obstruction. Because many foreign bodies, even sharp ones such as needles, pass harmlessly through the GI tract without causing any difficulties, ingestion of a foreign body without subsequent clinical signs of difficulty (vomiting, abdominal pain, etc.) does not necessarily constitute an emergency situation.

A common foreign body in cats is a string or thread that becomes looped around the base of the tongue and trails down the esophagus into the GI tract. The intestine attempts to move the firmly anchored string, resulting in plication (accordion pleating) and possible intestinal laceration and/or necrosis.

First Aid

First aid for GI foreign bodies is primarily symptomatic. *Do not* attempt to make an animal vomit up a foreign body as this would likely cause more damage and trauma than leaving the foreign body where it originally lodged. Some foreign bodies in the mouth or pharynx can be removed easily without causing further damage.

If a string or thread is found looped around the base of the tongue in a cat, *do not attempt to pull it out* as this may severely damage the GI tract. Instead, carefully cut the string or thread, and observe the animal closely.[3] The string may pass through the tract uneventfully once it is cut or, if the obstruction persists, surgery may be necessary.

Rectal Prolapse

Summary
Rectal Prolapse

Signs

1. Reddish mass protruding from the anus
2. Straining

First Aid

1. Lubricate well and replace, if possible
2. Keep prolapsed tissue moist
3. Apply hypertonic solution, if possible

Cause

A rectal prolapse is an eversion of the rectum through the anus. It occurs most frequently in young animals due to excessive straining to defecate.

Dangers with a rectal prolapse include drying and necrosis of the exposed, everted rectal mucosa and swelling of the prolapsed mass due to impairment of its venous return. Arteries continue to pump blood into the prolapsed mass, but pressure at the anus may partially occlude veins draining blood from the mass.

Clinical Signs

The prolapsed mass appears as a reddish mass protruding from the anus, frequently accompanied by severe straining. It may be quite small and round or quite large and long, resembling a long sausage.

First Aid

First aid for a rectal prolapse is aimed at either replacing the prolapsed mass or, if this is not possible, protecting the exposed mass from trauma and drying. Small, recent prolapses may be replaced without much difficulty. Gently clean the mass with warm water, if necessary, lubricate it well, and apply gentle, constant pressure to replace it. If the mass cannot be easily replaced, keep it moist and protected by surrounding it with gauze sponges or cloth moistened with isotonic saline (or tap water if saline is not available). Use of a hypertonic solution, such as 10% dextrose, instead of saline, not only prevents drying but also osmotically decreases the swelling.

External Hernias

Cause

A hernia is protrusion of an organ or tissue through an abnormal opening. Abdominal hernias are most common and consist of abdominal contents that protrude through an opening in the abdominal musculature, covered only by skin. Hernias may be congenital or due to trauma and/or weakened tissues. Most are visible externally.

The main dangers with hernias are that the herniated tissues, especially if they include portions of the GI tract, may become strangulated at the hernial opening, and that herniated tissues may be exposed if the skin over them is broken.

Incisional hernias occur at the site of a disrupted surgical incision. Inguinal hernias occur in the inguinal region (groin), usually through the inguinal ring. Perineal hernias occur in the perineal region, beside the anus. Umbilical hernias occur at the umbilicus, on the ventral midline.

A hernia usually appears as a soft, "doughy" swelling. It may be reducible, in which case the contents can be easily pushed back through the hernial opening, or irreducible, in which case the contents cannot be easily replaced.

First Aid

First aid for reducible hernias consists of replacing the contents and bandaging the area for support to prevent its immediate recurrence. In the case of irreducible hernias, keep the animal quiet and prevent it from traumatizing the hernia.

Paraphimosis

Summary
Paraphimosis

Signs

1. An abnormally sustained penile erection

First aid

1. Gently clean, if necessary
2. Apply icepacks if severely swollen or traumatized
3. Lubricate well and advance prepuce over penis
4. If not reducible, protect and keep moist
5. Apply hypertonic solution, if possible

Cause

Paraphimosis is an inability of the engorged penis to retract back into the prepuce following erection. It usually occurs after coitus and is recognized as a sustained erection after the penis should have retracted back into the prepuce.

First Aid

First aid for paraphimosis is aimed at protecting the exposed penis and attempting to replace it into the prepuce. Gently clean the penis if necessary. If it is severely swollen (edematous) and/or traumatized, cold packs may be helpful in reducing swelling before attempting to replace it. Lubricate the penis well, evert the preputial opening somewhat, and gently advance the prepuce craniad over the penis. If the prepuce cannot be easily advanced over the well-lubricated penis, keep the penis moist by surrounding it with gauze sponges or cloth moistened with isotonic saline (or water, if saline is not available). Use of a hypertonic solution, such as 10% dextrose, can help reduce swelling osmotically.

Uterine Prolapse

Summary
Uterine Prolapse

Signs

1. A reddish mass protruding from the vulva

First Aid

1. If prolapse is small, attempt replacement by gently cleaning, lubricating and applying pressure
2. If not replaceable, keep moist and protect
3. Apply hypertonic solution if possible

Cause

A uterine prolapse is an eversion of the uterus through the vaginal opening. It usually occurs shortly after parturition. Dangers with a uterine prolapse include swelling of the prolapsed tissues due to impaired venous return, and drying and necrosis of the exposed uterine mucosa.

Clinical Signs

A prolapsed uterus appears as a reddish mass protruding from the vulva. It can be small or very large.

First Aid

First aid for a uterine prolapse is aimed at replacing the uterus or, if that is not possible, protecting it. If the prolapse is small, replacement can be attempted by gently cleaning the exposed mucosa, if necessary, lubricating it well, and applying constant, gentle pressure. If the prolapse is large or replacement is unsuccessful, keep the exposed tissues clean and moist (use isotonic saline or water or a hypertonic solution such as 10% dextrose), and prevent self-trauma.

Dystocia

Parturition, or the birth process, can be divided into 3 normal stages.

The first stage of labor consists of uterine contractions and dilation of the cervix. The dam acts restless and uncomfortable.

The second stage of labor consists of the actual delivery of the fetus. The dam's intermittent, forceful abdominal contractions increase in frequency up to expulsion of the animal.

The third stage of labor consists of delivery of the placenta. This usually occurs almost immediately after the birth of small animals but may take several hours in large animals.

Dystocia, or difficult labor, can be maternal or fetal in origin. Causes of maternal dystocias include abnormalities of the pelvis that narrow the birth canal, weak uterine contractions, uterine torsion and psychologic disturbances. Causes of fetal dystocia include a large fetus, twinning and malpositioning.

In many cases, particularly in companion animals, more aid is given during parturition than is needed. This can actually produce dystocias due to maternal distraction by unnecessary human participation. The vast majority of births occur with no problems and no need of human intervention.

It is beyond the scope of this discussion to describe all of the potential problems that can occur during parturition and the steps necessary to resolve them, but there are certain general principles related to helping with the birth process once the decision to intervene has been made.

Cleanliness

Anything that touches the neonate or is inserted into the dam's birth canal should be sterile or very clean. The environment in which the birth is taking place should be as clean as possible.

Lubrication

Use sterile aqueous lubricant liberally to aid extraction of the fetus and prevent injury to the dam's birth canal.

Traction

If traction is necessary to help with the delivery, it should be applied only to the legs and *not* to the head, if possible. The slippery neonate should be grasped with cloths, towels or gauze sponges and pulled gently and steadily. Work *with* the dam, not against her, by pulling when she has a contraction.

Care of Neonates

If placental membranes cover the face of the neonate and the dam does not quickly remove them, do so manually. Allow the dam to clean up the neonate and stimulate respiration if she will. If she is not so inclined, it may be necessary to clear the neonate's nose and mouth of fluids and rub it gently but vigorously with a soft towel or cloth to stimulate respiration. If breathing does not begin shortly, give artificial respiration.

Burns

Summary
Burns

Signs
1. Minor burns indicated by reddened skin and blisters
2. Major burns indicated by edematous or charred skin

First Aid
1. Keep animal quiet and prevent self-trauma
2. Irrigate chemical burns
3. Apply cold compresses
4. Monitor vital signs and treat for shock, if necessary

Cause

Burns can have many possible causes, including friction or abrasion, as from being dragged by a car, flames, contact with a hot object, chemical burns, radiation (sunburn) and electricity, as from chewing on electrical cords or lightning strike.

Burns can be classified several different ways, but, for the purposes of first aid, they can be conveniently divided into minor (superficial) burns and major (deep) burns.

Minor burns, although painful, are not generally life threatening, and recovery is usually rapid unless they are very extensive.

Major burns cause extensive tissue destruction that extends down into, and even through, the deepest layers of skin. In addition to the extensive tissue damage itself, with its attendant pain and healing problems, complications can result due to the loss of the protective skin covering and subsequent inflammation in the exposed tissues. These include extensive fluid, electrolyte and protein loss, shock due to fluid, electrolyte and protein imabalances, and infection that begins locally and can spread systemically.[5]

Clinical Signs

The signs of the 2 main categories of burns differ mainly in the appearance of the affected skin. Minor burns are painful, the skin is reddened (this may be difficult to see if the haircoat is heavy and/or the skin is darkly pigmented), blisters may be present, and the hair may be singed but still firmly attached. Major burns are also painful, and the skin may be edematous, charred or entirely destroyed. If major burns are extensive the animal is usually reluctant to move.

First Aid

First aid for burns is aimed at preventing further damage, and helping reduce pain. Keep the animal quiet and prevent self-trauma. Apply cold compresses to help lessen pain and inflammation. If it will be some time before the animal can be seen by a veterinarian, apply either a sterile (or at least clean) dry dressing or one moistened with sterile isotonic saline. Do not apply oily dressings to burns. Monitor vital signs, and treat for shock, if necessary.

If the burn is from a corrosive chemical, irrigate the wound well with sterile isotonic saline, or plain tap water if saline is not available, to dilute and wash away the corrosive material.

Frostbite

Summary
Frostbite

Signs

1. History of exposure to severe cold
2. Affected tissues may be reddened, pale or scaly

First Aid

1. Warm the affected area rapidly in lukewarm water, then dry it
2. Prevent self-trauma

Frostbite is the freezing of tissues, usually in extremities such as the ears, tail and limbs.

Clinical Signs

The signs of frostbite can be quite variable, but usually the history of exposure to severe cold is helpful. Frostbitten tissues may be reddened or pale, and may be scaly.

First Aid

First aid for frostbite is aimed at warming the affected tissue and minimizing tissue trauma. Do not rub or massage the frozen tissues and do not apply snow or ice.[2] Warm the affected area rapidly in lukewarm water.[6] Immerse the area or use warm moist towels that are changed frequently, then gently dry the area after it is warmed. Finally, prevent self-trauma by the animal.

Heatstroke

Summary
Heatstroke

Signs

1. Elevated rectal temperature
2. Weakness
3. Collapse
4. Rapid pulse
5. Bright-red mucous membranes
6. Shock

First Aid

1. Cool the animal
2. Monitor the rectal temperature and stop treatment as temperature approaches normal
3. Treat for shock, if necessary

Cause

Heatstroke, or hyperthermia, is an excessive elevation of the body temperature due to high environmental temperatures. The condition frequently is accompanied by stress of some kind. Usually the animal has been confined in an area with a high ambient temperature, such as a dog in an automobile with the windows rolled up on a hot, sunny day, or an animal confined outdoors on a hot day with no access to shade and/or water.[7]

Clinical Signs

Most of the signs of heatstroke are nonspecific. A history of exposure to high environmental temperatures is helpful in determining if an animal is affected. Typical signs include elevated rectal temperature (generally to 105-110 F), weakness, collapse, rapid pulse, bright-red mucous membranes (may turn pale as the animal goes into shock), and shock.

First Aid

First aid for heatstroke is aimed at quickly reducing the animal's core temperature. The first consideration is how best to cool the animal. It should be taken out of the sun and, if possible, immersed in or sprayed with cool water. Treat for shock, if necessary. Take the rectal temperature every 5 minutes, and stop treatment as the temperature approaches normal. In very severe or unresponsive cases, cold-water enemas may be useful, but they obviate use of the rectal temperature to monitor progress. Once the rectal temperature is back to near normal, dry the animal off to prevent hypothermia.

Hypothermia

Summary
Hypothermia

Signs

1. Subnormal body temperature
2. Shivering
3. Decreased pulse rate
4. Weakness
5. Unconsciousness
6. Shock

First Aid

1. Warm the animal
2. Monitor the rectal temperature and stop treatment as the temperature approaches normal
3. Treat for shock, if necessary

Cause

Hypothermia is an abnormal lowering of the body temperature, usually resulting from exposure to low environmental temperatures or drugs that interfere with normal body temperature regulation, such as anesthetics and some tranquilizers.

Clinical Signs

Many of the signs of hypothermia are nonspecific. A history of exposure to low environmental temperatures or to drugs that interfere with normal body temperature regulation is helpful in determining if an animal is affected. Typical signs include subnormal rectal temperature ($<95°$ F), shivering (may be inhibited by some drugs), decreased pulse rate, weakness, unconsciousness and shock.

First Aid

First aid for hypothermia is aimed at rewarming the animal, done with warm-water baths, blankets or towels, recirculating water blankets, hot-water bottles (wrapped to prevent burning), or careful use of electric heaters. Be careful not to burn the animal. Monitor the rectal temperature and stop treating as the temperature approaches normal. Treat for shock if necessary.

Eye Injuries

General First Aid Principles

Because the eyes are such delicate and vital structures, the aim of first aid for eye injuries is to prevent further damage to the area. This can be accomplished by adhering to some general first aid principles.

Do not attempt to overtreat ocular injuries, as this may cause more damage. Do not force the eyelids open to examine the eye. Cold compresses, gently applied, may help relieve pain and reduce swelling and inflammation. If a bandage is to be applied to protect an injured eye, apply a bandage to the normal eye also since movement of the uncovered normal eye causes unwanted movement of the injured eye. Finally, do not apply pressure to an injured eye. The eye can easily be ruptured if the sclera and/or cornea are weakened.

First Aid for Eyelid Injuries

The most frequent eyelid injuries are contusions and/or lacerations. The most effective first aid for these is to control hemorrhage with direct pressure or cold compresses, bandage for protection, if necessary, and prevent self-trauma.

First Aid for Injuries to the Globe

Subconjunctival hemorrhage is a common result of head trauma. It looks rather bad but is usually not a serious problem in itself and seldom requires any treatment. However, it should be a signal to look for other ocular lesions.

Chemical irritants can cause severe eye damage. Affected eyes should be irrigated with sterile isotonic saline or plain water, as soon as possible, for 10-15 minutes.

Abrasions, contusions and lacerations of the globe are among the most serious ocular injuries. First aid is aimed at stopping hemorrhage, preventing swelling, preventing further damage and relieving pain. Gentle application of cold compresses is helpful but application of pressure to the damaged eye must be avoided. The eye can be irrigated to remove foreign material, if necessary, and bandaged for protection. Prevent self-trauma by the animal.

Ocular Foreign Bodies

Summary
Ocular Foreign Bodies

Signs
1. Grossly visible foreign bodies in the eye
2. Blepharospasm
3. Rubbing at eyes
4. Swollen eyelids

First Aid
1. Remove superficial foreign bodies, if possible
2. Do not remove foreign bodies protruding from the eyeball
3. Control hemorrhage and swelling, if necessary
4. Protect the eye

Cause
Ocular foreign bodies may consist of virtually any foreign material, such as wood, metal, stone, dust and plastic. They may be the primary cause of an eye injury or may be secondary. They may be beneath the eyelids but external to the globe itself, protruding from the globe, or entirely within the globe.

Clinical Signs
The signs of an ocular foreign body are largely nonspecific unless the foreign body is grossly visible. They include blepharospasm (eyelids clamped shut; do not force the eyelids open), rubbing or pawing at the eyes, and swollen eyelids.

First Aid
First aid for ocular foreign bodies depends mainly on their position. Foreign bodies external to the globe may be removed, if possible, by irrigating with sterile isotonic saline or with a sterile cotton swab. If the foreign body cannot be easily removed, leave it alone and protect the eye from self-trauma.

Foreign bodies protruding from the globe should *not* be removed as this may result in collapse of the globe. Protect the eye from further damage and do not apply any pressure to the globe. Foreign bodies within the globe should not be disturbed. Protect the eye from further damage, control hemorrhage and swelling with cold compresses, if necessary, and do not apply any pressure to the globe.

Proptosis

Summary
Proptosis

Signs

1. Globe protruding from the socket

First Aid

1. Do not try to force the globe back into the socket
2. Keep the eye moist
3. Protect the eye from further trauma

Cause

Proptosis is the displacement of the globe out of the socket. The eyelids then close behind the displaced globe, preventing its return. It occurs most commonly in brachycephalic breeds, such as Pugs, Pekingese and Bulldogs, as a result of trauma. It is very serious since, without attention, the proptosed globe may swell and rapidly dry out, resulting in permanent damage and blindness.

Clinical Signs

A proptosed globe is very obvious as it protrudes prominently from the socket.

First Aid

First aid for a proptosed eye is aimed at keeping the globe moist and preventing further damage until it can be replaced in the socket. Do not attempt to force the globe back into the socket. The lids, which are closed behind it, usually prevent replacement; further damage to the eye may result from any applied pressure.

The globe should be kept moist by applying cold fluids directly, or soaking gauze sponges and gently applying them to the globe. Sterile isotonic saline or a hypertonic solution, such as 10% dextrose, which can help reduce swelling osmotically, should be used. If neither of these is available, tap water can be used. Keep the animal quiet and protect the globe from further trauma.

Suspected Poisoning

Cause

Animals can be poisoned by any of a multitude of potentially toxic substances. The source may be poisonous plants or toxic chemicals used or stored near the animal, such as pesticides, paints, cleaning compounds, petroleum products or antifreeze.

Clinical Signs

Very few poisons produce distinctive signs. Most cause such nonspecific signs as excitability or depression, weakness, incoordination, salivation, vomiting and/or diarrhea, abdominal pain, convulsions and shock.

Poison Control Centers

A large number of government-sponsored Poison Control/Information Centers are located throughout the US and Canada. They can provide up-to-date information on poisons and appropriate treatment. The telephone number of the nearest center should be listed in the local telephone directory or can be obtained by contacting the nearest human hospital.[8]

First Aid

First aid for suspected poisonings is aimed at maintaining vital functions and decreasing the effects of the poison by removing it from the animal's system, diluting it or neutralizing it with an appropriate antidote.

It is important to identify the source of the poison, if possible. Toxic chemicals frequently have antidotes or first aid procedures listed on their labels. Get as much information from the owner as possible. If possible, have them bring the suspected poison, in the original package if it is a chemical, in with the patient.

If the animal is conscious and able to swallow, an attempt can be made to induce vomiting, if indicated. Unless the poison is a corrosive substance, such as a strong acid, alkali or petroleum product, induce vomiting in small animals with a teaspoon of table salt (NaCl) placed on the back of the tongue or a teaspoon (5 ml) of hydrogen peroxide given PO every 5 minutes. If acids have been swallowed, give bases, such as sodium bicarbonate (baking soda) and water PO. For alkalis, give acids, such as lemon juice or vinegar and water PO. For petroleum products and other corrosive substances, give water or milk PO to dilute the poison in the GI tract.

If the animal is unconscious, convulsing or in shock, give symptomatic first aid as needed.

References

1. Firth, in Catcott: Animal Health Technology. 2nd ed. American Veterinary Publications, Santa Barbara, 1977.
2. Burkholder: Emergency Care and First Aid for Small Animals. Creative Infomatics, Aspen, CO 1979.
3. Kirk and Bistner: Handbook of Veterinary Procedures and Emergency Treatment. 3rd ed. WB Saunders, Philadelphia, 1981.
4. Siegmund: The Merck Veterinary Manual. 5th ed. Merck, Rahway, NJ, 1979.
5. Farrow, in Kirk: Current Veterinary Therapy VI. WB Saunders, Philadelphia, 1977.
6. Dieterich, in Kirk: Current Veterinary Therapy VI. WB Saunders, Philadelphia, 1977.
7. Schall, in Kirk: Current Veterinary Therapy VI. WB Saunders, Philadelphia, 1977.
8. Oehme, in Kirk: Current Veterinary Therapy VI. WB Saunders, Philadelphia, 1977.

2

general patient management

C.C. BULLMORE & C.R. KUHN

General patient management involves several related areas, including admissions, medical records, physical examination, patient handling and hospital care. The chapter is subdivided into small and large animal sections to make clear some fundamental differences between these 2 groups of animals from the standpoint of the technician. A small section on medical calculations is also included.

ADMISSION OF SMALL ANIMAL PATIENTS

Initial Client Contact

The telephone conversation is usually the client's first contact with the veterinary hospital. Good client-hospital relations are critical at this stage. The potential client can be won or lost before the patient has even seen the doctor.

Answering the telephone constitutes an overlap of duties between the receptionist and technician. It may be necessary for the AHT to schedule appointments or to assist a client in determining if a veterinary examination is needed. Most clients do not realize that the veterinarian cannot talk to everyone who calls about their pet. Often they are equally ignorant of the training of the technician and that you are qualified to help answer their questions about animal health. Tactfully inform them that the doctor is with a patient, seeing a client, or in surgery and cannot be interrupted at this time. Avoid the phrase, "The doctor is busy." The assumption on the part of the client might be that if the doctor is too busy, he or she should call another veterinarian. Explain that as a well-trained technician you can assist them.

Scheduling appointments at first glance seems very routine. There are some major points that should be noted, however. Most veterinarians take about 15 minutes per office visit or about 4 calls per hour. The basic information needed to schedule a visit includes: client's full name; pet's name and breed; reason for visit; telephone number where client can be reached during the daytime; and regular or new client? With this information the receptionist can have the medical record pulled before the client walks in the door. Being able to greet the pet by name is good public relations. Having the record ready is a time saver and helps project an image of efficiency.

The client's full name and animal's name are needed to avoid pulling the wrong record. Knowing the breed of the pet can have a bearing on the amount of time needed for the appointment. (Practitioners often need more time with birds and exotic pets and charge more for these office visits than for dogs or cats.)

The reason for the visit is important in using time most economically. A complicated (and more time consuming) case should be scheduled adjacent to a simple call, such as a vaccination. Thus, if the first appointment takes more than the allotted time, part of that time can be made up with a routine vaccination call scheduled next. If an infectious disease is suspected, it can be of benefit to schedule the pet when fewer other animals would be exposed, such as during the slowest part of the day or the last call before lunch. With coughing listed as the major reason for the visit, a technician can explain that it would be best for the pet to wait outside or in the car until the doctor is ready. Other clients appreciate not having their animal exposed to one that may have a contagious disease.

Being able to reach the client by telephone can be very helpful if an emergency arises. Prolonged surgery or an unexpected emergency case may require rescheduling of their appointment. A new client can be advised to come a few minutes early to fill out the information needed for a medical record. Realizing that this client has never previously been to your hospital can save much frustration in looking for a medical record that has not yet been made. Being prepared by having the record ready and knowing why the pet is scheduled for a visit can help the doctor greatly in budgeting valuable time.

There are always a few people who do not realize they need an appointment to see the doctor. Many of these clients would not dream of walking in unannounced to their hairstylist. But then, Fifi just needs a shot and her ears checked, not a facial, manicure, shampoo, wash and set. Grin and bear it. Try to fit these people in between scheduled appointments, but let them know that a wait is to be expected and that an appointment is required for future visits. Take regularly scheduled appointments first if they are on time for their visits.

When genuine emergencies are involved, a rapid assessment is needed to determine the seriousness of the problem (see Chapter 1). Breathing difficulty, bleeding, poisonings, shock or convulsions should take priority, regardless of scheduling. The medical record can be pulled after the patient has been given an emergency examination to determine the need for immediate life-saving measures. Often the owner's level of concern for the pet's condition is not matched by the results of the examination. Some clients are overly concerned and can exaggerate or misread clinical signs. When a genuine emergency exists, efficient action on the part of the technician is required.

If the pet is to be admitted to the hospital for treatment or observation, some form of identification (ID) is needed. A cage card, including the date of admission, name of owner and patient, can be attached to the animal's cage or run. Some hospitals use an ID neck band that can be typed or marked with a waterproof marker to avoid possible confusion if the pet were moved without also moving the appropriate cage card.

History

A proper diagnosis can depend as much on a history as it does on the findings of the physical examination. On a routine visit, some history is volunteered by the client to the receptionist or technician. Important pieces of information often are not explained by the client because they were not recognized as relevant to the current problem. Eliciting a good history from a client is an art that can be learned by a technician to save time for the doctor and help avoid errors of omission that could be costly for both the client and patient by delaying proper diagnosis.

Questions should be asked without prejudice. A totally different answer can be obtained to a question, depending upon how that question is asked. Try not to put words in the client's mouth. If asked, "Has your cat been drinking a lot of water lately?", it is easiest for a client to say, "yes" or "no." But if asked, "Has your cat's water consumption increased, decreased, or remained unchanged, or can you tell?", the owner may admit that 3 cats drink out of the same bowl and he or she cannot be sure what this cat's water consumption has been. Ask the question that offers alternatives, including "I don't know." It may be necessary to ask the same question more than once but in a different manner.

The history should begin with the basic complaint. What was it that caused the owner to be concerned enough to seek professional help? How long has the problem been present? In what order did the signs appear? (Which came first, the vomiting or the diarrhea?) Has the owner given any medication or tried to treat the problem? What effect did this have, if any? Has the pet had this problem before? If so, when? What was done for the problem at that time? What previous illnesses or accidents has this animal had? Some of these questions may not seem relevant to the client (or the technician), but the answers to these questions could supply the missing piece of data needed to determine a diagnosis.

More generalized questions should be asked after the initial complaint has been investigated. Where does this pet live: indoors, outdoors or both in and out? What part of the country is the animal from? Some diseases have a definite geographic distribution. What type of diet is fed: dry, canned, semimoist packets or table food? What brands are offered most often? Is the pet eating normally? Are bowel movements regular and normal in color and consistency? (Does the owner know what the bowel movement habits of this pet are?) Has the owner seen any evidence of vomiting? Are the urinary habits normal? When were the last vaccines given and for what diseases? Many owners reply, "The shots are up to date," but often they do not know what "up to date" really means. Get specific dates and types of vaccinations given or assume that they are overdue.

Are any other pets in the household healthy? Does this pet have any contact with other animals? Has the patient been boarded in a kennel or groomed by a professional groomer in the last 30 days? Contact with other animals may be a significant factor. Has this animal been exposed to any toxic substances? Remember to consider garden and household products, as well as garbage containers, plants, medication and foreign objects. All of this information can be useful in establishing a list of possible diagnoses.

When dealing with a genuine emergency, maintenance of life functions is primary. Some basic information is needed, but obtaining a detailed history must be postponed until emergency medical care has been rendered. More reliable responses to questions can be obtained after the owner has had time to calm down. The one major exception regards suspected poisoning cases. Exposure to any toxic substances must be discussed with the client immediately. Did the client observe the pet eating or drinking a poisonous substance? Has the owner used any snail bait, fertilizer, herbicides, insecticides, etc, that the pet could have contacted? If possible, the container of any suspected intoxicant should be brought to the hospital with the patient. First aid instructions often can be found on the box or bottle, along with the chemical ingredients of the contents. With this information, the local poison control center can help by providing specific recommendations for treatment.

SMALL ANIMAL MEDICAL RECORDS

Until recently, most veterinarians in private practice have kept medical records on a card index system filed alphabetically in a set of small drawers, each about the size of a shoe box. The cards may be 3x5 or 5x7 inches and contain all of the medical information on one or more pets over a several-year period. The disadvantages of this record system are obvious. Lack of space discourages proper recording of detailed information. Cramped writing and numerous abbreviations become routine, making interpretation of the entries very difficult for another veterinarian treating the same animal. Ancillary information, such as laboratory results, may have to be filed separately. To obtain the complete record on a patient means going to 2 or more places, which is time consuming and increases the chance of a misfile. Changing addresses on the cards is inconvenient. Outdated files cannot be easily identified for removal to update the system. The only advantages to this system are that it is very inexpensive and records can be stored in a minimum amount of space.

Another type of record is the single sheet, with medical information on one side and the financial record for that client on the other. This style uses a sheet that is 11x6¾ inches, with the owner's last

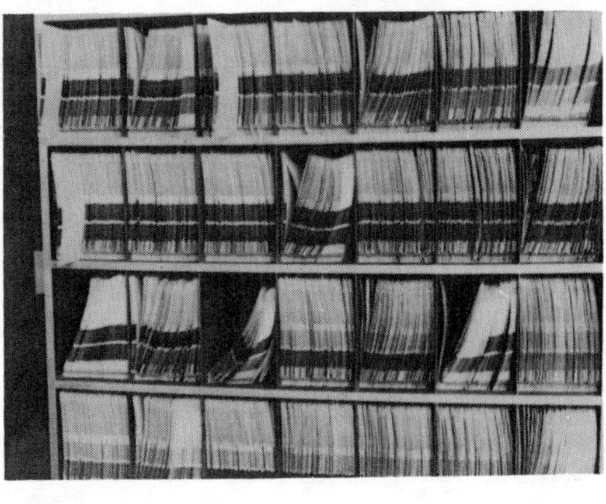

Fig 1. A color-coded file folder system.

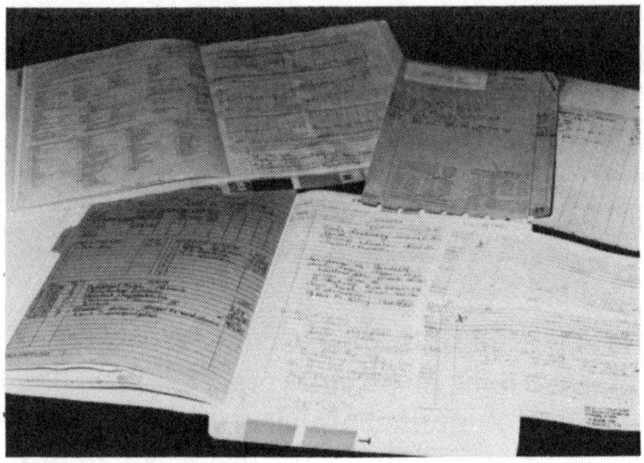

Fig 2. File folder records (upper and lower left) compared to the single-sheet record (upper right) and 5x7-inch card records (lower right).

name placed in the top right-hand corner. The records are stored by rows in a large bin, with the name visible by partially overlapping each sheet. When a sheet is removed, a gap appears in the sequence of files, thus helping to eliminate misfiling. On the reverse side of the page are several columns designed to classify the client charges by category (surgery, radiology, medication, etc), and indicate amount paid and balance due. This is superior to the card system because it offers more space and a record of all financial transactions. However, there are still space and filing limitations for adding laboratory data sheets and the need for more detailed record keeping, as would be required for lengthy hospitalization.

A good medical record system uses a file folder with the capacity to handle 8½x11-inch sheets. These files can be color coded, using bands on the edge of the folder to represent letters of the alphabet or a numeric code system that can be individualized to the size of the practice (Figs 1, 2). Misfiling is minimized by color coding, since an error stands out clearly. Each pet can have a separate section of the folder, divided by a card, to avoid confusion if the client has several animals. Year bands can be used to allow periodic culling of old files to keep the system updated. The record system should be scanned annually and any file with a 3-year-old band should be considered inactive and removed. The important advantage to this filing method is that more space is available for detailed record keeping on each patient. Laboratory results, radiology and surgical reports, previous medical records, and letters can all be placed in the folder for easy retrieval.

A medical record, regardless of the style employed, must contain the following information to meet legal standards and the requirements of the practice code:

1. Client's name, home address and telephone number.
2. Work address and telephone number (not required but very useful).
3. Name and full description of the animal (species, breed, sex, neutering status, birthdate, color).
4. Medical information
   a) Dates of hospital visits or periods of custody of the animal.
   b) History of the animal's condition, including reason for visit.
   c) Physical examination findings and diagnosis.
   d) Treatment and medication used (with complete directions).
   e) Results of laboratory tests, radiographs, etc.
   f) Progress and disposition of the case.

Medical record requirements vary among states. The above outline should be sufficient to meet most standards. In addition to these requirements, some states recommend keeping a separate surgical log, containing the date of surgery, client and patient name, type of surgery performed, and surgeon's name. This record can prevent confusion regarding the particulars of any surgery performed by

REGISTRATION FORM

PLEASE PRINT DATE ______

NAME ______ (LAST / FIRST / MIDDLE INITIAL) SPOUSE ______

ADDRESS ______ (STREET) CITY ______ ZIP CODE ______ HOME PHONE ______

OCCUPATION ______ WORK PHONE ______

EMPLOYER ______ ADDRESS ______ CITY ______ ZIP ______

SPOUSE'S EMPLOYER ______ ADDRESS ______ CITY ______ ZIP ______

REFERRED BY ______

PROFESSIONAL FEES ARE TO BE PAID AT THE TIME THEY ARE RENDERED. PLEASE CIRCLE YOUR PREFERRED METHOD OF PAYMENT

CASH CHECK

SIGNATURE OF OWNER ______

SIGNATURE OF PERSON PRESENTING THIS PET FOR TREATMENT IF OTHER THAN OWNER ______

SPECIES ______ BREED ______ COLOR ______

PET'S NAME ______ SEX ______ ALTERED: YES[ ] NO [ ] BIRTH DATE ______ (MONTH DAY YEAR)

DATE OF LAST VACCINATION ______ TYPE ______ WHERE ______

______ TYPE ______ WHERE ______

CREDIT REFERENCES ______

DRIVER'S LICENSE NO. ______

Fig 3. Registration form suitable for use in file folder record system.

CARMICHAEL ANIMAL HOSPITAL

Registration

Client Information

Owner's Name and Address	Last	First		Middle
	Street	City	State	Zip
Referred By	Yellow Pages ☐	Relative or Friend ☐	Name ______	
Phone and Emergency Numbers	Home Phone	Husband Work Phone	Wife Work Phone	Emergency Phone
Method of Payment	Cash ☐ Check ☐	Mastercard ☐ Visa ☐	D.L. # ______	

Patient Information

Pet's Name ______ Breed ______

Sex ______ Date of Birth ______

Pet Obtained From? Breeder ☐ Pet Store ☐ Neighbor☐ Other☐

Has your pet been spayed (females) or neutered (males)?

Yes ☐ No ☐ If so, when? ______

Has your pet been vaccinated? Yes ☐ No ☐ If so, when? ______

For what? ______

What is your pets diet? Dry ☐ Canned ☐ Semi-moist ☐ Table food ☐

Are there other pets in the household? Yes ☐ No ☐

If so, what kind? ______

Is your pet currently taking medication? Yes ☐ No ☐

If so, what kind? ______

Does your pet suffer from any allergies? Yes ☐ No ☐

If so, what kind? ______

Do you have any problems with its behavior? If so, check below:

Housebreaking ☐ Biting ☐ Disobeying ☐ Running off☐

Fighting ☐ Disturbing neighbors ☐ Other ☐ ______

A DEPOSIT IS REQUIRED ON ALL HOSPITALIZED PATIENTS, BALANCE TO BE PAID UPON DISCHARGE. MASTERCARD, AND VISA SERVICE AVAILABLE.

Signature of owner or responsible party ______ *Date* ______

Fig 4. A detailed registration form includes some of the animal's history.

that hospital. In California, a radiology log is also required to record dates, exposure factors and patient information for every film made.

The file folder medical records system allows each hospital to design its own sheets. One simple alternative would use only 3 basic forms: registration, history and worksheet. The first page of the record would be a client registration form, filled out by every new client on the initial visit and updated when current information

CARMICHAEL ANIMAL HOSPITAL

CLIENT:			PATIENT:	
SPECIES:	BREED:	SEX M M/C F F/S	BIRTHDATE:	COLOR:

D.H.L.-P.											
RABIES											
PARVOVIRUS											
F.V.R.-C.-P.											
DENTISTRY											
FECALS											
WORMING											

SURGICAL PROCEDURES		DATE
1		
2		
3		
4		
5		
6		
7		
8		

RADIOGRAPHIC PROCEDURES		DATE
1		
2		
3		
4		
5		
6		
7		
8		

DATE ENTERED	PROBLEM NO.	PROBLEM	DATE RESOLVED

DRUG SENSITIVITIES	

Fig 5. The medical/surgical summary sheet provides space for a detailed history of the animal's previous medical problems on one page.

changed, such as a new address or telephone number (Fig 3). Credit information, including driver's license number and employment data, can also be included on this sheet. A more complex registration form includes basic questions about the pet as an aid in establishing a history (Fig 4).

Following the registration form is a medical-surgical summary sheet, with a complete description of the patient at the top (Figs 5, 6). Background information can be tabulated, including vaccination

BRENTWOOD PET CLINIC
MEDICAL–SURGICAL SUMMARY

Client's name ________ Animal's name ________ Birth Date ________

Sex ________ Breed ________ Color ________ Referred by ________

DHL-P											
Rabies											
FVR-C-P											
FECALS											
DENTISTRY											
WORMING											

ACUTE SELF-LIMITED (TEMPORARY) PROBLEMS

Prob. No.	PROBLEM	Dates of Occurance									
		1	2	3	4	5	6	7	8	9	10
A											
B											
C											
D											
E											
F											
G											
H											
I											
J											
K											
L											
M											
N											

MAJOR PROBLEM LIST

Prob. No.	PROBLEM—Active	Date Entered	Date Resolved
1			
2			
3			
4			
5			
6			
7			
8			
9			
10			

RADIOGRAPHIC PROCEDURES	Date
1.	
2.	
3.	
4.	
5.	
6.	
7.	
8.	
9.	

SURGICAL PROCEDURES	Date
A.	
B.	
C.	
D.	
E.	
F.	
G.	

DRUG SENSITIVITIES

1.
2.
3.
4.
5.

Fig 6. Another style of medical/surgical summary sheet provides space for information on previous major and minor medical problems, radiographic results and any drug idiosyncrasies.

dates, heartworm tests, fecals, previous surgeries and radiographic studies, as well as long-term medical problems. This allows the doctor or technician to become familiar with a patient's previous history quickly, without need to leaf through many pages of written records.

The bulk of the medical record is the worksheet, which contains information on the current problem, answers to history questions, phy-

Table 1. Centrigrade (Celsius) and Fahrenheit Temperature Equivalents

Centigrade (C)	Fahrenheit (F)
36.0	96.8
36.5	97.7
37.0	98.6
37.5	99.5
38.0	100.4
38.2	100.8
38.4	101.1
38.6	101.5
38.8	101.8
39.0	102.2
39.2	102.6
39.4	102.9
39.6	103.3
39.8	103.6
40.0	104.0
40.2	104.4
40.4	104.7
40.6	105.1
40.8	105.4
41.0	105.8
41.2	106.2
41.4	106.5
41.6	106.8
41.8	107.1
42.0	107.5

Table 2. Common Cage Card Abbreviations

Appetite	App	Urination	Urine
none	0	none	0
ate small portion	⊖	normal	+
ate half meal	⊖	large volume	+ +
ate full meal	⊕	bloody urine	BU
Bowel Movements	BM	Vomiting	Vomit
none	0	none	0
normal stool	+	vomited once	+
soft stool	S	vomited twice	+ +
diarrhea	D	bloody vomitus	BV
bloody diarrhea	BD		

sical examination findings, laboratory test results, diagnoses, treatments, and daily progress notes. The worksheet is essentially a simple, lined page with space for the date, remarks, and charges in a column at the edge.

For hospitalized patients, some basic information is recorded in the medical record by the AHT each day before the veterinarian examines the patient. Included should be the temperature, pulse rate and respiratory rate. The temperature may be recorded in Fahrenheit or Celsius (Table 1). The pulse and respiratory rates should be record-

Owner: Patient:

DATE	APP	BM	URINE	VOMIT	INSTRUCTIONS

Fig 7. This cage card has columns in which information on an animal's appetite, bowel movements, urination and any vomiting is recorded daily.

ed in beats and breaths per minute, respectively. Also of value is information on appetite, urination, bowel movements and any vomiting. A code system can be used for the last items and the information recorded on the patient's cage card by the person cleaning and feeding that patient each morning (Table 2). A cage card is large enough to record this data for several days if used properly (Fig 7).

PHYSICAL EXAMINATION OF SMALL ANIMALS

Vital Signs

Before a patient is examined by the doctor, a brief history should be obtained and the vital signs checked by the technician and recorded in the medical record, regardless of the reason for the visit. Many problems may be detected by performing these basic tasks on all patients, even apparently healthy ones. Normal rectal temperature and pulse and respiratory rates (TPR) for dogs and cats are listed in Table 3. Be sure that the thermometer has been shaken down and reads no higher than 96 F before rectal insertion. Using lubrication and a slight rotational movement, the thermometer is gently inserted about 2 inches and held in place for 2 minutes for a reliable reading. After the thermometer is removed and wiped off, the temperature obtained is recorded. Storing the thermometer in an antiseptic solution helps avoid cross-contamination between patients.

Table 3. Normal Temperatures, Pulse Rates and Respiratory Rates for Cats and Dogs

	Cats	Puppies	Adult Dogs	Toy Breeds
Rectal temperature				
F	100.5-102.5	100.5-102.5	100.5-102.5	100.5-102.5
C	38.0-39.1	38.0-39.1	38.0-39.1	38.0-39.1
Pulse rate (/min)	110-130	70-220	70-180	70-220
Respiratory rate (/min)	20-30	15-40	10-30	15-40

The pulse is taken at the femoral artery, inside the thigh, or by palpating the heart in smaller animals. A stethoscope can be helpful in recording heart rates in obese animals. Respiratory rates can be taken by observation, or by placing a hand on the thorax. Pulse and respiratory rates should be recorded as the number counted in one minute. With practice, counting for 10-15 seconds and then multiplying by 6 or 4, respectively, speeds up this procedure.

General Assessment

When first looking at an animal from a distance, you should note its general condition and attitude. The dog or cat may be of normal weight, underweight or obese. Its disposition could be friendly, nervous, placid or aggressive. Careful observation can alert an AHT to possible danger in the handling of a patient. Take the time to look from a distance first. Get a feeling for the pet's overall appearance and temperament before you proceed with the physical examination.

Physical Examination

Animals may be examined in several ways. I prefer the front-to-back system. Starting with the nose, I examine the animal anatomically, finishing with the rear feet and tail. For the purpose of teaching, however, an organ system approach is best. After mastering the basic technic, pick the method of examination that you feel confident in using.

Vital signs are checked initially, followed by obtaining an accurate body weight to the nearest pound if over 25-30 lb, or the nearest ounce if under 25 lb. Some technicians prefer the metric system of weight; however, most of us are more comfortable using pounds and ounces. Accurate weights are essential in the medical record for calculating doses and to assess weight loss or gain in subsequent visits.

In a routine physical examination there are 9 areas to consider in the organ system approach. Use your senses to describe the findings.

Sight, smell and touch (palpation) are all important. Describe the location, appearance, and size of any abnormalities. Do not make diagnoses; simply record what is seen. Avoid drawing conclusions as to why the problem exists.

1. *The Skin:* Is the haircoat shiny and glossy or dry and brittle? Are there areas of hair thinning or hair loss (alopecia)? Does the dog or cat have a scratching or itching problem (pruritus)? Are there skin lesions? Are there red, inflamed areas (erythema)? Does the animal have fleas, ticks or lice? Do you detect an abnormal odor to the skin? If the patient tolerates handling, be sure to feel every part of its surface. A long coat can hide significant lesions.

2. *Eyes and Ears:* Can the patient see and hear? Owners sometimes state that the pet has a problem seeing or hearing; however, clients are often unaware of these problems until they are pointed out. Moving an object before an animal's eyes and noting if it tracks the object with its eyes is a good test of vision. Be careful not to create a current of air by moving a large object, such as the hand, too quickly and close to the face, as this air movement can be detected by the pet and misinterpreted by an examiner as visual perception. Tossing a cotton ball in the air usually elicits a response in a normal patient without causing any artifactual errors.

What do the eyes look like? Are they both open? Is there an ocular discharge or evidence of tearing (lacrimation)? Chronic overflow of tears (epiphora) is common in small breeds of dogs and leaves a reddish-brown discoloration of the hair in the corners of the eyes. Is the white of the eye (sclera) reddened or discolored? Are the pink mucous membranes that surround the eye (conjunctivae) pale, normal or irritated? Is the cornea clear and shiny? Are both pupils of equal size? Do they respond to light by constriction? Does the pupil appear black? Is there a grayish-blue haziness or white opacity (cataract) in the pupil? Is the third eyelid (nictitating membrane) partially protruding over the eye?

Do the ears have an odor? Are they clean or filled with exudate? Is any ear discharge wet, dry, dark, creamy, bloody, etc? Does the animal show any head shaking behavior? Are the ears painful when handled? Does the ear flap (pinna) have any discolorations or swellings? Does the animal respond to sound?

3. *Musculoskeletal System:* Watch the animal walk to detect any lameness problem. Stand in front of the patient and, using one hand on each limb, gradually move from the shoulders down past the elbows and wrist (carpus) to the digits. Asymmetry of the limbs can be detected more easily when comparing the left and right sides

simultaneously. Do the same for the rear legs by standing behind the animal and palpating the limbs from the hips down past the stifles to the tarsus and toes. Palpate the thorax and trunk to check for lumps or pain. Gently flex and extend each joint of all 4 legs, checking for smoothness of motion, swelling, pain or muscle wasting (atrophy). It may be necessary to place the dog or cat on its side while examining the joints of the proximal limbs (Fig 13).

4. *Respiratory System:* Is there a nasal discharge from one or both nostrils? Is sneezing or coughing evident? Palpate the larynx and trachea gently. Does tracheal manipulation elicit an exaggerated cough response? Are the respirations shallow or deep in nature? Auscultate the lungs, beginning with the large airways (trachea and bronchi) in the cranial portion of the thorax and moving to the central thorax to listen to the intermediate airways. Finish with the smallest airways (bronchioles) in the caudal portion of the thorax. In normal animals, respiratory sounds are heard only during inspiration and the very first part of expiration. The majority of expiration is thus silent. To properly auscultate the chest, a quiet room is essential. Politely request that everyone stop talking for a few minutes. Hold the dog's mouth closed to prevent panting. Respiratory sounds are faint and require practice to discern.

5. *Cardiovascular System:* Initially check the color of the oral mucous membranes. Do not be misled by the presence of brown or black pigment, sometimes found in the gums (gingivae) of some animals. Look for a bright, healthy pink color that indicates good perfusion. Chow Chow dogs have dark blue-black pigment in the gums, lips and tongue. To the novice this may appear abnormal. Capillary refill time (CRT) is tested by pressing on the gum above the canine tooth with a finger, quickly releasing the pressure and timing how long it takes for reappearance of a pink color in the blanched area. Normal CRT is 1-2 seconds. A pale gum color or prolonged CRT indicates anemia or a circulatory disturbance. The femoral pulse rate has already been counted while checking vital signs. Its character should be described as strong, weak or irregular. Further descriptions of the pulse character may be made by the doctor.

The next step is auscultation of the heart. Begin in the pulmonic area, on the left side of the chest at the third intercostal space, ventrad toward the sternum. The aortic area is located in the fourth intercostal space at the costochondral junction (area where rib bone and cartilage join). The mitral area is located in the ventral fifth intercostal space, near the sternum. The last area of cardiac auscultation is in the tricuspid area, on the right side of the thorax at the fourth in-

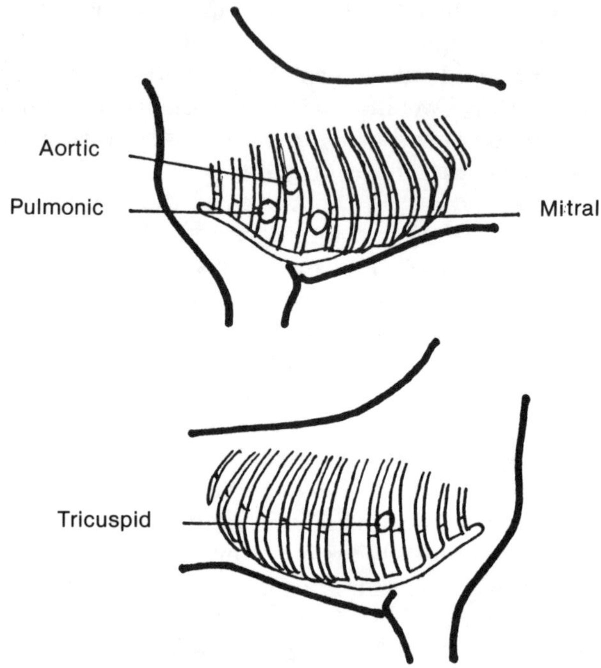

Fig 8. Areas for auscultation over the heart valves.

tercostal space, near the costochondral junction. At each of these points, the valve that corresponds to the name of the area can be heard most distinctly (Fig 8). The normal heart sound should consist of 2 separate beats, with a silent interval between them: LUB DUB, LUB DUB, LUB DUB, etc. Any additional sounds, or blurring together the first and second sounds constitute a heart murmur. When evaluating the heart, it is important to check the heart rate and compare it to the pulse rate palpated at the femoral artery. The pulse rate can be lower than the heart rate (pulse deficit) in certain medical conditions.

6. *Gastrointestinal System:* Begin at the mouth by examining the teeth. A brownish discoloration of the teeth, known as calculus, may be seen in some middle-aged and older pets. This material can cause the gums to recede, resulting in premature loosening and loss of the teeth (periodontal disease). Inflammation of the gums (gingivitis) is indicated by a reddening along the gum line and usually is secondary to the presence of dental calculus.

Is the tongue symmetric? Can the animal swallow normally? Is there a problem with drooling or excessive salivation?

Palpation of the abdomen is useful in assessing the stomach, intestinal tract, liver and spleen. A distended stomach or painful loops of bowel may be evident; palpation can elicit a reaction from the patient. Some tenderness may be expected with any normal animal as a result of nervousness. Extreme tenderness or crying can indicate pain and a possible abdominal disturbance. Gas, fluid or normal stools can be palpated in the intestinal tract after some practice. The liver margin may be palpable in slender dogs and most cats, protruding just caudal to the rib cage. In large dogs or obese animals the liver may not be felt. The spleen, a flat, tongue-shaped organ in the mid-abdomen, is not usually palpable unless enlarged due to disease or use of certain drugs. Any masses that cannot be identified should be noted on the record. Tumors of the spleen, liver or intestinal tract may be detected early by skillful abdominal palpation. Be gentle when examining the abdomen, particularly if pregnancy is a possibility. If you encounter an animal that vigorously resists abdominal palpation, by tensing the abdominal muscles, it is better to skip that part of the examination and notify the doctor than to traumatize the animal by attempted palpation.

Examine the anus to determine if the anal sacs, on either side of the anus, are distended or if any irritation or abnormal lumps are present. A digital rectal examination, using a lubricated glove, can be used to detect prostatic enlargement or displacement in male animals. This type of examination may be helpful in assessing the character of the stool and can also be used to aid in expressing distended anal sacs.

7. *Reproductive and Urinary Systems:* Examination of the reproductive system of male animals should be begun at the penis. In the dog, gently retract the prepuce and examine for irritation on the surface of the penis. A certain small amount of thick, greenish discharge is present in all normal male dogs. Excessive licking or irritation of the prepuce may be evidenced by redness or pain on examination. Next, examine the scrotum. Is the scrotal skin irritated, thickened or discolored? Palpate each testis individually. Are they symmetric and uniform in size and shape? Is there pain on examination of the scrotum or testes? Testicular asymmetry, a disparity in testicular size, may indicate a testicular tumor, atrophy, or previous infection.

In female animals, begin the reproductive tract examination at the vulva. Is there a vulvar discharge? Describe the quantity and appearance of any discharge found. Is there swelling of the labia, indi-

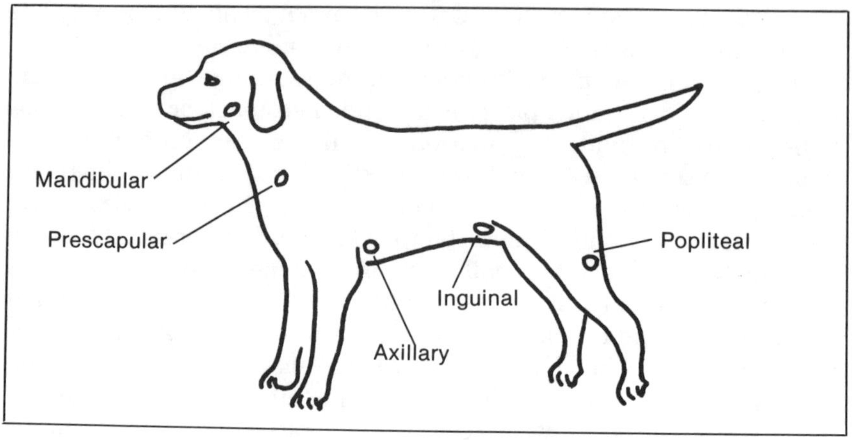

Fig 9. Normally palpable lymph nodes on the dog.

cative of estrus or infection? The internal reproductive tract of non-pregnant females is usually not palpable. Observing a scar or palpating steel sutures in the abdominal wall can indicate that the animal has been spayed. Lack of such a scar or palpable sutures does not rule out a previous spay operation. Careful palpation of the mammary glands is important, especially in older bitches. Examine each gland and nipple individually, progressing from the most cranial gland, caudad. Small cystic growths or nodules may not be visible but may be evident on careful, systematic palpation.

When palpating the caudal abdomen, the full or partially full urinary bladder may be evident as a smooth-surfaced, egg-shaped structure that slips easily between the fingers and thumb when felt. If urine has recently been voided or only a small amount is present, the bladder may not be palpable. Pain on palpation of the urinary bladder, especially in male cats, may indicate an infection or obstruction. Bladder stones (calculi) may be palpable with practice. Though in cats both kidneys are palpable behind the rib cage, ventral to the spine, only the left kidney may be felt in dogs. The cat's greater flexibility permits a more complete abdominal examination.

8. *Lymph Nodes:* The mandibular lymph nodes are palpable at the angle of the jaw as firm ovoid masses. The prescapular nodes are located cranial to the shoulder blades. Obesity may prevent palpation of these lymph nodes. The axillary lymph nodes, located in the "underarm" area, and the inguinal lymph nodes, located in the groin, are not palpable unless they are pathologically enlarged. The popliteal lymph nodes are palpable in normal animals caudal to the knee (Fig 9).

As all of the lymph nodes commonly examined are symmetric from one side of the animal to the other, an enlargement on one side can indicate inflammation or infection in the area drained by that node. Pain upon palpation of the nodes should be recorded. Generalized enlargement of all lymph nodes can occur in some infectious diseases and lymphosarcoma.

9. *Nervous System:* When first examining the animal, determine if the gait and mental attitude are normal. Is there lameness? Does the animal have a stumbling or uncoordinated gait (ataxia)? Is the animal bright and alert or is there evidence of mental depression, listlessness and lethargy? Injury to the brain or cranial nerves may manifest itself as a head tilt or nystagmus. Nystagmus is the involuntary, rapid horizontal or vertical movement of the eyeballs. Aimless wandering in circles or head pressing against a wall or other objects also indicates brain injury.

Pain, weakness or paralysis of the forelegs or rear legs may indicate spinal cord damage. These patients should be examined with extreme care to prevent injury to the examiner and further injury to the patient by manipulation. Pain sensation in each limb may be tested by pinching the toes with the fingers or small hemostats. The normal response is withdrawal of the limb *and* an indication that the patient felt the pinch by turning the head, curling the lip or crying. Simple withdrawal of the limb, without conscious recognition by the patient, can be a spinal reflex and thus, not a true test of whether the animal has sensation or not.

Check the anus to determine the presence of normal tone. An open, flaccid anal sphincter indicates lower spinal cord damage. Can the patient urinate? Is the urinary bladder overdistended and easily expressed upon palpation? Does urine flow just in response to gravity and not due to a conscious effort by the patient? Both of these situations could indicate neurologic bladder damage.

A peripheral nerve injury may be manifested as failure to respond when one limb is stimulated by a pinch or as lameness. The patellar tendon (kneejerk) reflex can be elicited in normal animals by sharply tapping the patellar tendon with the handle of a pair of scissors and watching the response. This reflex may be difficult to determine in a nervous or tense patient. An intact patellar reflex does not necessarily mean the spinal cord is intact, as the reflex remains intact even if the cord is severed completely anywhere cranial to the midlumbar cord.

Proper neurologic examination requires a veterinarian's training but the above basic examination can alert the AHT to the presence of gross neurologic deficits.

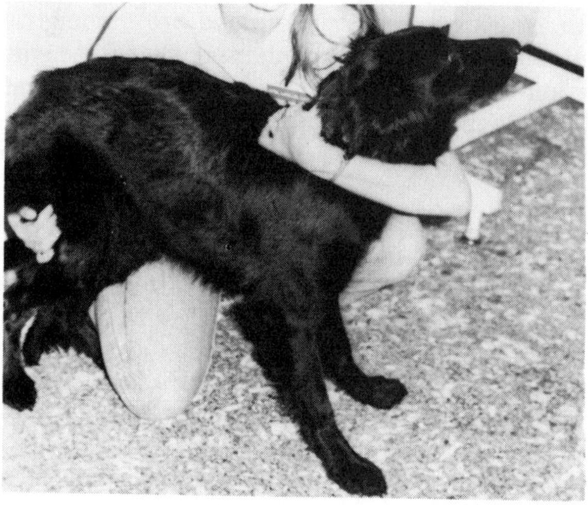

Fig 10. Dogs can be safely lifted with one arm around the neck and the other beneath the rear legs.

HANDLING AND RESTRAINT OF SMALL ANIMALS

Dogs

It is a good idea to require all clients to have their dogs on a leash upon admission to the veterinary hospital. Surprisingly, many owners fail to realize the importance of this simple safety precaution. Watching the animal enter the reception room and observing its responses enable the AHT to assess the personality of the pet in advance of direct contact. Some dogs that are normal at home can become very nervous or even vicious in a veterinary hospital. The owner may volunteer the information that the dog has bitten a handler previously. Do not rely upon the client to give you advance warning that an animal is belligerent.

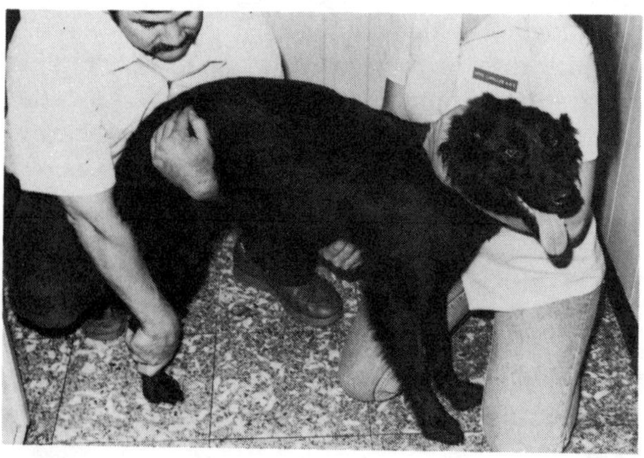

Fig 11. Two people may lift a large or injured dog, with one handling the forequarters and the other the rear.

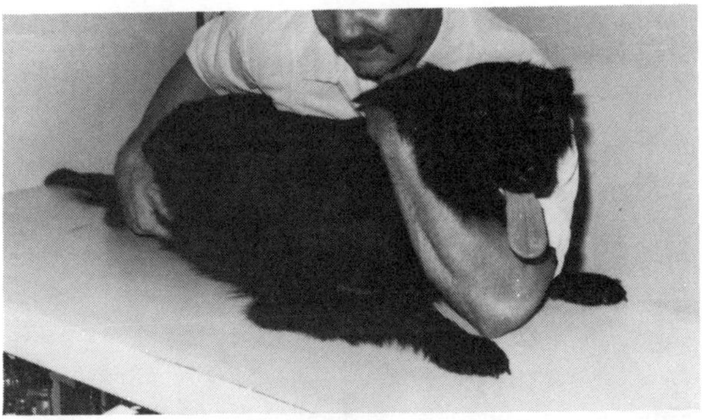

Fig 12. Standard restraint position for examination of a dog.

A small dog (under 40 lb) can be easily lifted by placing one arm around the animal's neck to control the head and using the second arm to scoop up the rear end (Fig 10). An alternative to scooping the animal around the rear legs is to place the arm under the abdomen, cranial to the rear legs, and lift the dog beneath the abdomen. If an abdominal injury or pregnancy is suspected, this second method of lifting should be avoided. For a larger dog, a 2-person lift allows better control and less strain for the technician (Fig 11).

Examination tables are smooth surfaced to prevent animals from attaining a good grip that may make holding a pet more difficult. The technician should be on the opposite side of the examining table from the veterinarian. The dog should be standing or in normal sternal recumbency, with the forelegs stretched out in front. The head must be controlled at all times. For nervous animals, a hugging grip, with the arm around the neck, allows the best control. The second arm can be placed around the abdomen and thorax, stabilizing the animal against the technician's body (Fig 12). Having the owner stand in

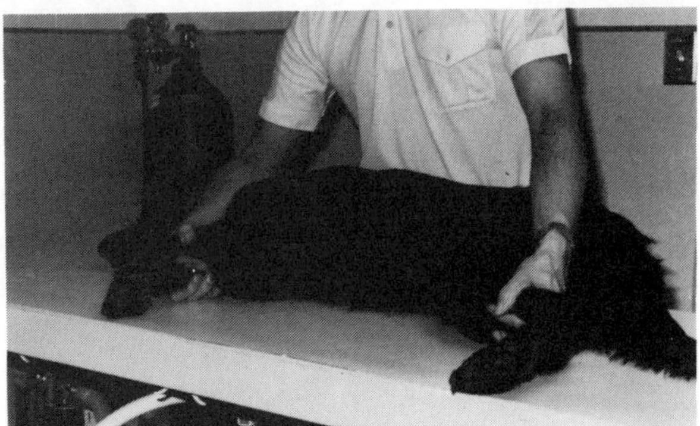

Fig 13. Dog kept in lateral recumbency for IM injection or electrocardiography.

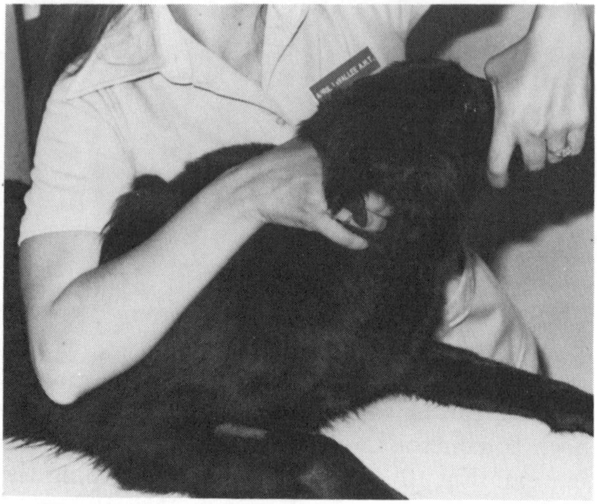

Fig 14. Restraint for ear examination limits head movement.

front of their pet, where he or she can be clearly seen, is often an advantage, as frequently the animal attempts to turn and look at the owner. An easy-going, friendly animal can be examined with minimal restraint since no painful procedures are anticipated in a routine physical examination.

To restrain a dog on its side, the forelegs are held in one hand with the middle finger separating the legs (Fig 13). The second hand holds the rear legs in a similar manner. The dog should be positioned with the legs held away from the handler and perpendicular to its body. Using one elbow to hold the dog's neck on the table prevents raising

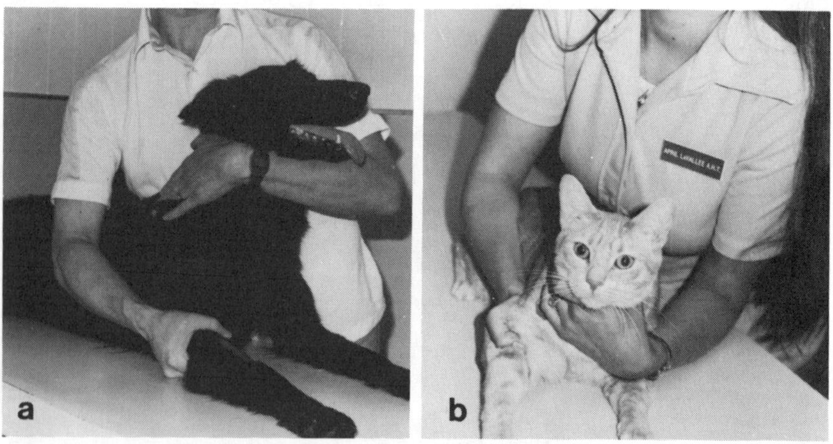

Fig 15. Restraint for IV injection of the cephalic vein in the dog (a) and cat (b).

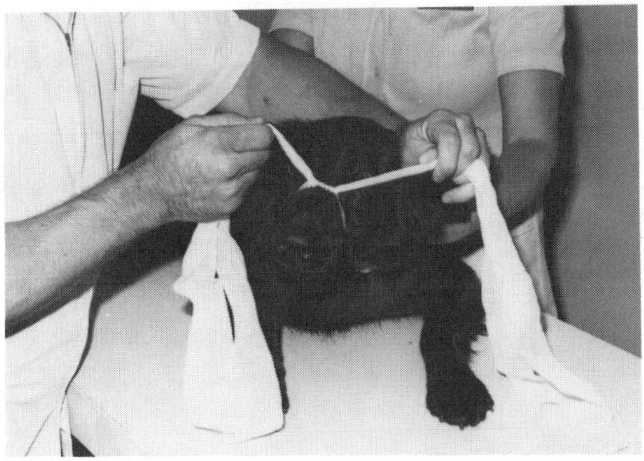

Fig 16. The first loop of a gauze muzzle is tied over the bridge of the nose, while the assistant steadies and points the dog's head toward the operator. The ends of the tie are looped under the chin and pulled behind the dog's head.

the head. The other elbow can be used to press down on the dog's rear quarters. For large dogs, only the lower limb of each pair must be gripped, as it is the lower limb the dog uses to right itself from a prone position. This restraint position is useful when examining the joints, making an ECG and giving some types of injections.

For an ear examination, one hand is placed on the muzzle and the second behind the skull, with the elbow holding the animal's chest and trunk into the technician's body (Fig 14). Such a position prevents gross movement of the head when the ear is being examined with an otoscope. With exceptionally painful ear conditions, sedation may be required to allow a full examination.

For administration of IM and SC injections, the normal restraint position is adequate, hugging the head with one arm and controlling

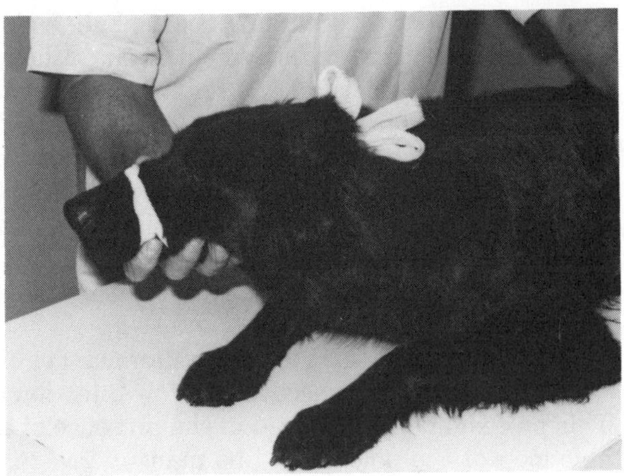

Fig 17. After the ends are looped under the chin and pulled behind the head, they are tied in a bow for easy removal, avoiding pinching the ears.

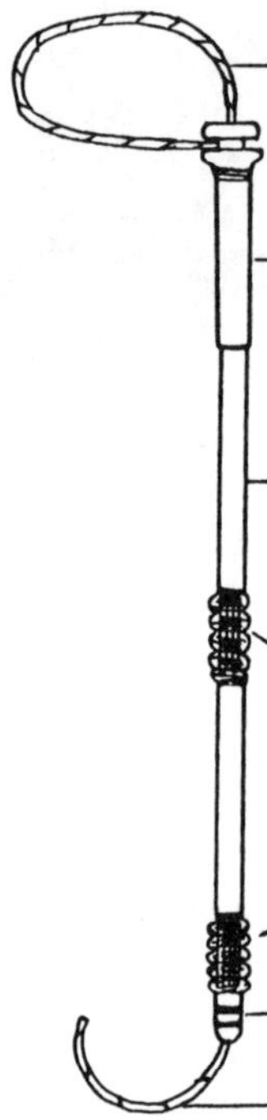

Fig 18. A well-constructed restraint pole or "come along."

the torso with the other (Fig 12). For IV injections, the animal handler must control the head with one arm while extending the foreleg with steady pressure and occluding the cephalic vein (Fig 15).

Animals that are excessively nervous, reluctant or downright belligerent may require a muzzle for the safety of the handler. A muzzle can be fashioned from nonstretch gauze and tied over the nose, crossed beneath the chin and then tied in a bow behind the head (Figs 16, 17). It is important to explain to the pet owner that it is easy for the dog to breathe through the nose while the mouth is tied closed. This is not a painful or uncomfortable procedure for the dog, but it may be misinterpreted by the client as unnecessary or even cruel unless properly explained in advance.

For the patient that is totally unmanageable, a restraint pole or "come along" may be needed to allow injection of a sedative (Fig 18). This pole should not be used in the presence of the client. The adjustable loop of the pole should be maneuvered to include the head and one front leg of the small dog and then tightened down to prevent escape. Incorporation of one front leg in the noose prevents inadvertent strangulation of the patient due to struggling that may overtighten the loop. This device should be released as soon as possible after the injection is completed. The patient should be allowed to calm down and feel the full effect of the medication before the examination is begun.

For an IM injection,an alternative to the restraint pole is to thread the dog's leash through the cage bars. By pulling the head against the bars, a rear leg can be safely grasped and the injection made. If a dog is known to be difficult to handle, tranquilizers may be dispensed for the owner to administer before the animal is admitted to the hospital. Tranquilization may not be advisable if it jeopardizes the dog's health or masks signs of illness.

Moving slowly and calmly and avoiding unnecessary noise enable an animal handler and veterinarian to examine most animals. If a dog is reluctant to follow the handler on a leash when taken into the hospital, it helps to have the owner leave first. When the client is out of sight, most dogs follow the handler with little problem. Some animals do not respond to gentle handling and may require more physical restraint or use of tranquilizers. These animals may be strays that have had little human contact or may be excessively fearful, maladjusted pets that only do well with their owners, in familiar surround-

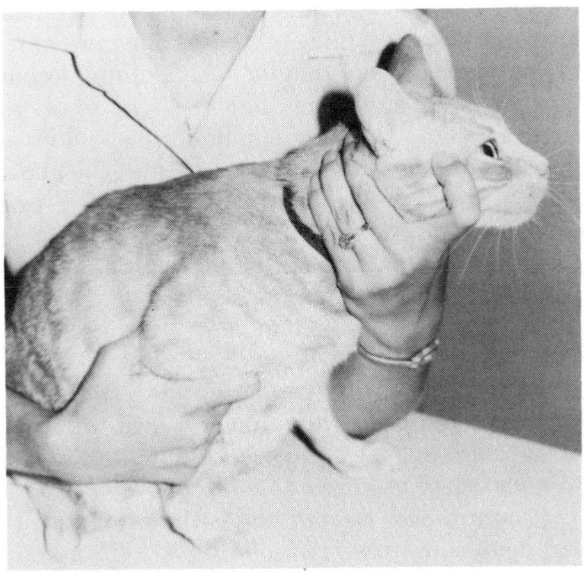

Fig 19. Restraint of a cat for ear examination or treatment.

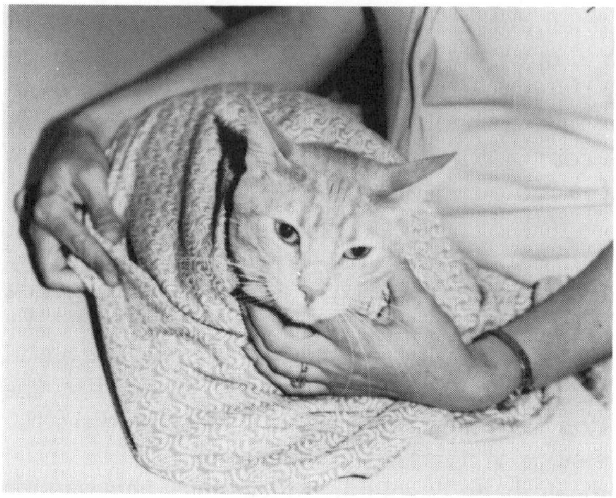

Fig 20. Wrapping the cat in a towel allows easy pill administration and manipulation of the head.

ings. Others may be genuinely in pain and only reacting instinctively when handled by strangers in an unfamiliar environment.

Cats

Bringing the cat to the veterinary hospital in a cardboard box or other suitable carrier is highly recommended, as this prevents altercations between pets in the waiting room, as well as preventing injury to the owner. Examining a cat that has already been made nervous by a dog in the waiting room can be difficult. Minimal restraint is the most successful way to examine most cats. Giving injections or taking blood samples is more challenging because of the smaller size, flexibility and agility of cats.

To examine the ears, the handler should use one hand under the chin and neck and the other to restrain the forelegs (Fig 19). Very nervous cats may be wrapped in a large, thick towel, with just the head exposed (Fig 20).

A towel can also be used to pick up a difficult cat by throwing it completely over the animal, then scooping it up. Particularly aggressive, biting cats can be handled with thick leather gloves that have a wide cuff to protect the lower forearm. It is far safer to sedate these patients than to attempt to examine a frightened animal. Cats do not respond to physical restraint or a firm tone of voice as well as dogs. Struggling with a fractious cat can lead to injury that could be avoided with use of a sedative.

Cats are best carried under the arm, with the fingers separating and controlling the forelegs (Fig 21). The elbow is used to hold the

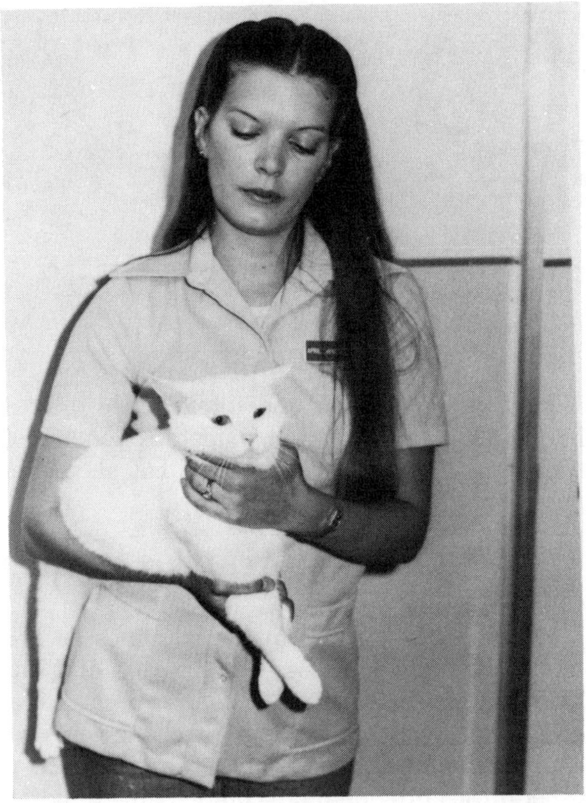

Fig 21. The forelegs of the cat are controlled and the body supported by one arm, while the other remains free to manipulate the head or open doors.

cat's body against the waist and hips of the handler. The free hand can then be used for opening doors or controlling the head as necessary. Carriers should be used whenever possible when admitting or discharging patients from hospital wards.

It is considered reasonable to hold a cat by the scruff of the neck, using the loose skin, only when no other means of restraint is possible. Holding the cat at arm's length prevents injury to the handler and does not harm the patient if done properly. It is preferable not to use this form of handling in view of the client, as it is commonly misinterpreted as cruel. Under no circumstances should a *dog* be picked up from the ground using the loose skin over the neck and back area, as such handling is unnecessarily painful for dogs.

Subcutaneous injections are usually not painful and require minimal restraint. The handler may simply distract the cat's attention by scratching or petting while the injection is made. More restraint is needed for an IM injection. With the cat in lateral

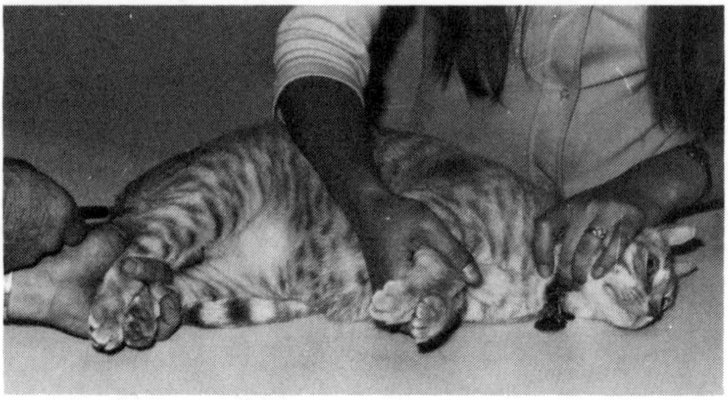

Fig 22. Cat held in lateral recumbency for IM injection.

recumbency, the head and forelegs are fully controlled using both hands. The rear legs are managed by the person giving the injection (Fig 22). After the injection, the cat should be released quickly to avoid unnecessary struggling.

HOSPITALIZATION OF SMALL ANIMALS

Observation

The veterinarian normally examines all hospitalized patients at least once daily to assess the progress of treatment. The technician may be responsible for the animal's cleanliness, feeding, watering and, most important, noting any changes in its condition. The technician is in a unique position to observe each patient because these other duties provide more contact time to notice behavioral changes. A good observer makes notes on significant events, such as passage of urine or feces, eating, drinking, vomiting, coughing and any change in attitude. Notations can be made on cage cards or in the medical record under daily progress notes.

Feeding and Watering

Feeding and watering the animals is a basic duty performed by the kennel person or technicians, depending on the hospital. Ideally, each cage should contain a metal ring to support a stainless-steel bowl so it cannot be tipped over by the animal. The bowl should be washed and properly disinfected daily. Fresh water should always be available for hospitalized pets unless specifically prohibited by the doctor in charge of the case. Some doctors use the abbreviation *NPO, nothing per os* or nothing by mouth, for those patients.

Feeding schedules vary for different types of patients. Normal puppies and kittens should be fed every 6-8 hours, while most adult animals are only fed once or twice daily. Typically, all patients allowed food are fed early in the morning to determine if their appetites are good before the morning examination and treatment. Paper disposable dishes are becoming popular because they are sanitary, light to carry, noiseless and do not require washing. Animals scheduled for surgery or blood tests that day should not be fed. Patients undergoing general anesthesia should not be fed because of the danger of vomiting and subsequent inhalation of the vomitus. Aspiration pneumonia is a serious postanesthetic complication. Feeding may affect the results of blood tests and make proper interpretation difficult. Vomiting patients should not be fed until examined by the doctor.

Sanitation

After moving the animal and before cleaning the cage, check to see if any samples of stool, urine or vomitus have been requested in the medical record or on the cage card. Place the appropriate samples in sealed containers and refrigerate. Mark the cage card to indicate appetite, bowel movement, urine, etc, and then remove the cage papers and clean the cage. The best cages are stainless steel or fiberglass and do not have square corners or pitted surfaces. Spray all surfaces with a standard disinfectant solution, (*eg,* Roccal-D: Winthrop, Nolvasan: Fort Dodge) and wipe off, including the ceiling of the cage. Remove the water bowl and replace it with a clean one. Wash down the cage bars to remove feces, urine and saliva. Add new cage papers, if they are used, and move to the next patient. Remember when moving an animal to also move the cage card to avoid misidentification.

Temperature Control

Patients recovering from surgery or suffering from hypothermia may need an artificial source of heat. Warm water circulating pads provide a uniformly warm, but not overly hot, surface on which a sick animal can rest. With this type of pad, electrical shock is very unlikely, dangerous hot spots do not develop, and the animal will not become overheated. The disadvantages include the relatively high cost and vulnerability to damage by teeth and claws. Standard electrical heating pads must be wrapped in a towel and checked regularly for signs of wear or cord fraying. Overheating and burns are possible from improperly maintained electrical heating pads or improper use, such as allowing an animal to lie on a hot pad, unattended, for hours.

An incubator is ideal for puppies and kittens. Used human pediatric incubators are often available from medical equipment dealers. An oxygen tank and vaporizer may be added to the incubator to provide an intensive care unit for smaller patients (Fig 23). Hot-

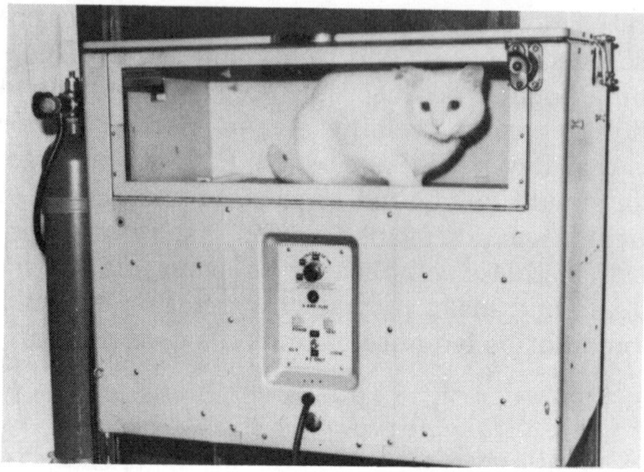

Fig 23. Pediatric incubator converted to a small intensive care unit by addition of an oxygen tank and vaporizer.

water bottles can be used to warm a puppy or kitten if care is taken to avoid burns.

Recumbent Patients

Decubitus ulcers (bed sores) are uncommon in small animals because few of our patients are recumbent long enough to develop pressure sores. Most patients that do not show signs of recovery in a few days are euthanized. Human convalescent patients may develop such sores due to prolonged bed rest. Proper padding of the cage floor is important to keep recumbent patients comfortable. (See section on large animals in this chapter.)

Any patient that is in lateral recumbency while recovering from anesthesia or immobilized by a splint should be gently rolled to its opposite side at least hourly to help prevent circulatory problems. When a patient is forced to remain on one side for a prolonged period, blood tends to pool in the dependent limbs and organs. The pulmonary air spaces (alveoli) tend to collapse due to the effect of gravity in the dependent lung lobes. As a result, the lower lung has more blood but less open alveoli, while the upper lung has less blood and more open alveoli. This is known as a mismatching of perfusion and ventilation. By frequently turning the patient and encouraging deep breathing with an occasional vigorous rub, circulatory compromise can be prevented.

In recumbent patients with an indwelling urinary catheter, the catheter can be hooked up to a used IV infusion set taped into an empty IV bottle placed on the floor. This simple system allows continual urine flow by gravity, measures the amount produced, and keeps the patient dry. An alternative approach, if the volume of urine produced need not be recorded, is to place the patient on a grate elevated ½-1 inch off the cage floor. Grates are often used with feline patients being treated for urethral obstruction with an indwelling urinary catheter.

Collars

When urinary or IV catheters, splints, bandages or sutures are used, there is a danger of self-trauma or destruction of the device by chewing or licking. To prevent such occurrences, an Elizabethan collar can be used (Fig 24). Some felines are able to reach over such collars if they are not fitted properly. Plastic Elizabethan collars, fastened with snaps, may be purchased, or collars can be made from corrugated cardboard and taped around the animal's neck. These devices discourage dogs and cats from licking sutures, chewing bandages or splints, and pulling out catheters. Several brands of distasteful sprays and creams also are available to stop chewing or licking. Intravenous catheters rarely are licked or chewed excessively by animals if they are properly inserted and are not painful. They must be checked frequently for the presence of tissue swelling or infection that may initiate self-trauma. The few animals that continually try to chew out a catheter, despite all restraint devices, should be tranquilized if their health permits.

Patient Discharge

While the primary purpose of a veterinary hospital does not involve grooming pets, appearances do count. Before any hospitalized

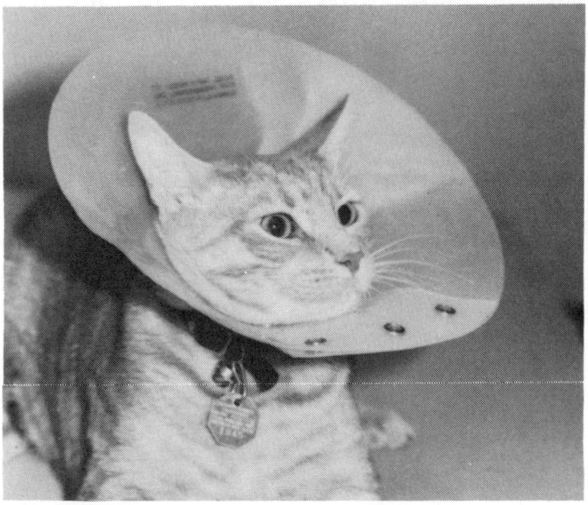

Fig 24. Plastic Elizabethan collar prevents self-mutilation.

patient is discharged, it should be brushed and checked to see if it is clean. Any pet confined to a cage is likely to develop an odor that is objectionable to the owner. If the animal's condition permits, the animal should be bathed, dried and combed out. Wipe the eyes free from any discharge, clip the nails as needed, remove any bandages from previous IV injection or catheter sites and use a scented spray to lightly touch up the coat when dry. Never send an animal home with fleas. These small steps are always appreciated by clients. Try to ensure that the pet looks healthier, is cleaner, and smells better than when it arrived.

Isolation

A well-designed isolation facility in a veterinary hospital has a separate entrance for pets with suspected contagious diseases. Patients admitted to the hospital for a possible infectious disease should be taken directly to isolation and assumed to be contagious until proven otherwise. The medical record should be marked to indicate the location of this patient. Hospitals not having a completely separate isolation area can help reduce the danger of contamination by keeping surrounding cages empty, moving the patient as little as possible, and disinfecting instruments and washing one's hands after handling the animal. Table 4 contains a list of common infectious diseases of cats and dogs.

The isolation facility must have an area for cages, runs, a sink, a treatment table and medical supplies. A separate ventilation system is desirable. A clean smock should be worn and left in the isolation unit when duties are completed. This simple procedure helps prevent exposure of other patients to contamination from clothing. Hands should always be washed between patients, especially those with an infectious disease. Using disposable gloves when handling animals

Table 4. Common Infectious Diseases of Dogs and Cats, Necessitating Isolation

Dogs	Cats
Canine distemper	Feline panleukopenia (distemper)
Canine infectious hepatitis	Toxoplasmosis
Leptospirosis	Feline leukemia virus infection
Parainfluenza and other respiratory infections	Upper respiratory infections
Canine parvovirus enteritis	Feline infectious peritonitis
Sarcoptic mange	Notoedric mange
Dermatomycosis (ringworm)	Dermatomycosis (ringworm)

with fungal skin diseases and scabies is recommended. A surgical mask is probably not routinely needed but is recommended in rabies suspects and in birds with psittacosis, both zoonoses that can be transmitted by inhalation of aerosolized organisms.

Care should be taken in handling soiled cage papers as saliva, blood, urine and feces may contain infectious organisms. All staff members working in the isolation unit must adhere to these basic sanitation procedures if they are to effectively prevent the spread of disease. Clients should be informed that a recovered pet may shed the infectious agent for several days or weeks. When discharged from the hospital, these pets should have limited contact with other animals for a reasonable period, according to the doctor's instructions.

IDENTIFICATION OF SMALL ANIMALS

Cage cards and ID bands have already been mentioned. It must be emphasized that if a hospitalized patient is moved, the appropriate cage card must follow the animal. In large facilities, a more complete animal description may be required to avoid identification errors.

All pet owners should be encouraged to buy personalized name tags for their pet's collar that include name, address and telephone number. Collars may be removed and returned to the owner upon admission of the pet to the hospital as a safety precaution, as a collar buckle or tag can become entangled in the cage bars or kennel fencing, resulting in strangulation. Such an accident could result in a negligence suit against the veterinary hospital. Also, loss of a collar, leash, favorite toy or blanket in the kennel or hospital ward environment can upset the client. It is best not to take any such items into the hospital when a patient is admitted for any reason.

Dog licenses are another form of identification. The licensing of dogs is a method of ensuring proper vaccination against rabies. When a pet is vaccinated for rabies, the client usually is issued a rabies tag listing the hospital name, address and a serial number. A log is kept at the hospital to allow identification of any lost animal if the tag number is known. This extra service fosters good relations with clients, as many lost pets can be reunited with their owners with a simple telephone call.

Pet health insurance is now available in several states and promises to become more widespread in future years. Proper identification of an insured animal is required to avoid insurance fraud. Some companies are issuing ID tags with a complex code of letters and numbers to avoid the problem of an owner switching tags from an insured animal to another that is not insured. The encoded data on the tag includes policy number, type of coverage, and a complete animal description.

Tattooing

Tattooing is becoming more popular as a method of identification in dogs and occasionally in cats. Its main advantage is that it is permanent. It is also slightly more costly than other identification methods and causes some minor discomfort for the animal during the procedure. Dogs may be tattooed inside the pinna or on the inner thigh. Veterinarians, dog clubs or breeders may provide this service, using a numbering system to identify the pet. Some owners request that their telephone number or driver's license number be used for identification purposes. Some national registry organizations use the owner's social security number for a more recognizable and uniformly identifiable code system. However, obtaining an owner's name from only the social security number can be very difficult.

There are 2 basic types of tattoo equipment: the vibrator tattooer and the tattoo clamp. The vibrator type uses 4-10 fine needles that vibrate at high speed and implant the tattoo ink into the outer layer of skin with minimal discomfort. The area to be tattooed should be shaved and gently cleansed before the procedure. Tranquilization may be needed due to the noise produced by the vibrating unit.

The jaws of the tattoo clamp are designed to accommodate several inserts that consist of pins arranged in letters and numbers. These pins pierce the skin of the ear when clamped, leaving tiny holes that are then filled by gently massaging tattoo ink into the area. These tattoo markings are not easily removed and can last the lifetime of the pet. In young animals the tattoo markings expand as the pet grows. Black ink is used for most skin types. Green ink is available for darkly pigmented skin that may obscure a black tattoo.

MEDICAL CALCULATIONS

Systems of Measurement

There are 3 general units of measurement: length, weight and volume. Various systems have been developed to express these measures in standard units, and each system has a unit for measuring length, weight and volume.

The systems of measurement include the metric, apothecary, avoirdupois, troy and imperial. The first 3 will be discussed briefly to provide a basic understanding of terms used commonly in medical calculations.

Table 5. Metric Prefixes and Their Numeric Equivalents

Prefix	Numeric Equivalent
kilo-	1000 or 1×10^3
deci-	0.1 or 1×10^{-1}
centi-	0.01 or 1×10^{-2}
milli-	0.001 or 1×10^{-3}
micro-	0.000001 or 1×10^{-6}

Metric System

The units of measurement in the metric (decimal) system are the meter (length), gram (weight) and liter (volume). These basic units are then subdivided to form new units, which are multiples of 10 of the original unit, thus the term decimal system. There is a trend to use this system exclusively and internationally for measurement.

The metric system is based on a system of prefixes added to the basic unit to form these new measures. Once the 3 basic units and the prefixes have been learned, the system is the same whether one is measuring length, weight or volume. Table 5 lists the prefixes used in the metric system, along with their corresponding numeric equivalents. Thus, the prefix kilo- in front of a basic unit, such as a meter, means 1000. A kilometer is then 1000 meters. Similarly, centi- means 1/100 and thus a centimeter is one-hundredth of a meter. The metric system was originally designed in terms of the meter, the units for weight (gram) and volume (liter) were derived from it.

After an object or characteristic has been measured, the results must be recorded, making sure to include the unit of measurement. Knowing that something is 10 has no value unless we know that it is 10 centimeters (cm), 10 liters (L), or 10 kilograms (kg).

To illustrate use of metric system terminology, the weighing of a dog might be used as an example. If the dog weighs 12,400 g, the weight can be expressed as 12.4 kg because 12,400 g x 1 kg/1000 g = 12.4 kg. The general rule is to express the measurement in the largest appropriate unit, maintaining a whole number if possible. For example, if the object weighed only 950 g, the weight would not be recorded as 0.95 kg but as 950 g. In the same manner, it is generally preferable to report the length of an object as 17.2 cm rather than as 0.172 m, though both numbers indicate the same length.

In summary, the basic units of measurement in the metric system are the meter, liter and gram. The prefixes attached to each of these units indicate a part or multiple of that unit. Thus, 1 gram = 10 decigrams, 100 centigrams, 1000 milligrams, or 1,000,000 micrograms. By using these prefixes and their decimal equivalents, one can

Table 6. Avoirdupois Units for Length, Weight and Volume

Length:	12 inches (in) = 1 foot (ft)
	3 ft = 1 yard (yd) = 36 in
	5280 ft = 1 mile (mi) = 1760 yd
Weight:	437.5 grains (gr) = 1 ounce (oz)
	16 oz = 1 pound (lb = 7000 gr
Volume:	16 oz = 1 pint (pt)
	2 pt = 1 quart (qt) = 32 fluid ounces (fl oz)
	4 qt = 1 gallon (gal) = 8 pt

convert grams to kilograms by dividing by 1000 (1000 g = 1 kg), meters to centimeters by multiplying by 100 (1 m = 100 cm), or liters to milliliters by multiplying by 1000 (1000 ml = 1 L).

Avoirdupois System

This is the most commonly used measurement system in the US. The units of measuring length are the inch, foot, yard and mile. Measurements of weight are the grain, ounce and pound. Fluid ounce, pint, quart and gallon are measurements of volume.

The principal advantage of the metric system over the avoirdupois system is the ease of conversion from one unit to another within a given measurement. That is the km, cm and mm are all multiples of 10 of the meter. As illustrated in Table 6, the conversion of avoirdupois units is not as convenient.

Apothecary System

Although the apothecary system is not commonly used today, the dosage of many drugs, such as morphine, aspirin, atropine, phenobarbital and nitroglycerine, is still expressed in apothecary units. With some modifications, the system is very similar to the avoirdupois system.

The apothecary system of weights consists of grains, scruples, drams, ounces and pounds (Table 7). The grain in the apothecary system is exactly the same value in the avoirdupois system.

Volume in the apothecary system is measured in the same manner as in the avoirdupois system, with the addition of minims and drams. The units for length are the same as in the avoirdupois system.

The major difference between the apothecary and avoirdupois systems is the additional units in the apothecary system. It is important to keep in mind, however, the differences in the number of ounces that comprise a pound. Using the appropriate abbreviations for each system prevents confusion as to which system was used.

Table 7. Apothecary Units for Weight and Volume

Weight:	20 grains (gr) = 1 scruple
	3 scruples = 1 dram = 60 gr
	8 drams = 1 oz = 24 scruples
	12 oz = 1 lb = 96 oz
Volume:	60 minims = 1 fluid dram
	8 fluid drams = 1 fl oz
	16 fl oz = 1 pt
	2 pt = 1 qt
	4 qt = 1 gal

Conversion Between Systems

It may be necessary to convert values from one measuring system to another. The process of conversion is exactly the same as in converting between different units of measurement within the same system. The following is a general procedure for conversion:

Step 1: Find the appropriate conversion table and value.
Step 2: Multiply the original value by the appropriate conversion factor.
Step 3: Report the results in the new units.

Because the grain is an equivalent weight, the inch an equivalent length, and the fluid ounce an equivalent volume in the apothecary and avoirdupois systems, only one conversion is given: 15.4 gr = 1 g; 1 in = 2.54 cm; 1 fl oz = 29.6 ml.

An example is the conversion of 10 mg/kg to the appropriate mg/lb (avoir). As the conversion factor is grams, the dosage must first be converted from mg/kg to mg/g:

Step 1: 1000 g = 1 kg
Step 2: 10 mg/kg × 1 kg/1000 g = 10 mg/1000 g = 1 mg/100 g
Step 3: Dosage is 1 mg/100 g

The next conversion is from mg/g to mg/gr:

Step 1: 15.4 gr = 1 g
Step 2: 1 mg/100 g × 1 g/15.4 gr = 1 mg/1540 gr
Step 3: Dosage is 1 mg/1540 gr

Finally, to convert mg/gr to mg/lb

Step 1: 7000 gr = 1 lb
Step 2: 1 mg/1540 gr × 7000 gr/lb = 7000 mg/1540 lb = 4.55 mg/lb
Step 3: Dosage is 4.55 mg/lb

An alternative to this long procedure involves applying the information that 2.2 lb = 1 kg. If this conversion had been used in the previous example, only 3 steps would be involved:

Table 8. Metric, Apothecary and Avoirdupois Equivalents for Weight, Length and Volume

Weight:	1 mg = 1/60 gr
	15 mg = 1/4 gr
	30 mg = 1/2 gr
	60 mg = 1 gr
	1000 mg = 1 g
	1000 g = 1 kg
	2.2 lb = 1 kg
	1 oz = 28 g
	8 oz = 1/2 lb = 227 g
	16 oz = 1 lb = 454 g
Length:	1 mm = 0.04 in
	10 mm = 1 cm = 0.4 in
	1 in = 2.54 cm
Volume:	1 ml = 1 cubic centimeter (cc)
	100 ml = 1 deciliter (dl)
	1000 ml = 10 dl = 1 liter (L)
	1 tsp = 5 ml
	1 tbsp = 15 ml
	1 fl oz = 30 ml
	8 fl oz = 250 ml = 1 cup
	16 fl oz = 500 ml = 2 cups = 1 pt
	32 fl oz = 1000 ml = 4 cups = 1 qt
	1 gal = 4000 ml = 4 qt = 8 pt

Step 1: 2.2 lb = 1 kg
Step 2: 10 mg/kg × 1 kg/2.2 lb = 4.55 mg/lb
Step 3: Dosage is 4.55 mg/lb

Prescriptions sometimes are written in what are referred to as household equivalents, such as the teaspoon, tablespoon and glassful. Their metric and avoirdupois (apothecary) equivalents are as follows:

1 teaspoon (tsp) = 5 ml
1 tablespoon (tbsp) = 15 ml = ½ fl oz
1 glassful = 240 ml = 8 fl oz

Table 8 contains the equivalents for the metric, apothecary and avoirdupois measurements of length, weight and volume.

Calculating Drug Dosages

Before medication is given by mouth or injection, 4 basic facts must be known: the patient's weight; the required dosage; the concentration of the medication; and the frequency of administration. The weight of the patient is already known from the physical examination and is in the medical record in pounds or kilograms. The dosage of most commonly used drugs and their frequency of administration are found in standard reference texts and in the drug's package insert. The dosage may differ from one species to another. The concentration of the drug is found on the container, in mg or gr for tablets and capsules and mg/ml for oral liquids and injectables.

To calculate the amount of drug to be given, multiply the patient's weight by the dosage from the reference source, *eg,* 15 lb × 10 mg/lb = 150 mg. If the medication comes in 100-, 200-, and 500-mg tablets, the amount of drug, divided by the size of the tablet, equals the number of tablets to be given, *eg,* 150 mg/100-mg tablet = 1.5 tablets.

To calculate the amount of medication to be injected, multiply the patient's weight by the drug's dosage and divide by the drug's concentration, *eg,*

$$\frac{15 \text{ lb} \times 10 \text{ mg/lb}}{100 \text{ mg/ml}} = 1.5 \text{ ml.}$$

It may be necessary to change the concentration of a liquid medication by diluting it with sterile water to enable more accurate dosing. A good example is ketamine HCl (Ketaset: Bristol), which comes in a concentration of 100 mg/ml. In anesthetizing small birds with ketamine HCl, it is important to dilute the drug to avoid overdosage.

Problem: Dilute a sample of ketamine HCl by a factor of 10.

Solution: Ketamine HCl is 100 mg/ml. If diluted by a factor of 10, the final concentration would be 10 mg/ml. Take 1 ml of ketamine and add 9 ml water. The 100 mg of drug has been diluted to a total volume of 10 ml. The new concentration is then:

$$\frac{100 \text{ mg}}{10 \text{ ml}} = 10 \text{ mg/ml}$$

When dealing with percentage problems, remember that percent means parts per hundred, *eg,* 10% equals 10 parts per 100 parts. In the metric system, percent of solution equals grams of solute (substance dissolved) per 100 ml solvent (liquid base). For example, a 5% solution of drug A contains 5 g drug A in 100 ml water (or other vehicle).

Sodium thiamylal (Bio-Tal: Bio-Ceutic) is a short-acting barbiturate anesthetic for IV use that is stored in powder form and requires reconstitution in sterile water for use. To prepare this solution, 2 basic facts are required:

1. What amount of drug is in the bottle?
2. What percent concentration is desired for use?

The amount of drug in the bottle is recorded on the label. The percent concentration desired may be 5%, 4% or 2%, depending on the intended use. To mix a 5% solution, take 5 g drug (solute) and add 100 ml water (solvent), *ie,*

$$5\% = \frac{5 \text{ g drug}}{100 \text{ ml water}}$$

Problem: To mix a 4% solution in a bottle that contains 5 g of drug, how much water is required?

Solution: Remembering 4% = 4 g/100 ml, a simple proportion equation can be set up:

$$\frac{4 \text{ g}}{100 \text{ ml}} = \frac{5 \text{ g}}{X}$$

where X = number of ml water needed for a 4% solution. Solving for X, X = 125 ml.

To mix a 2% solution in the same bottle containing 5 g of powder, 2% = 2 g/100 ml. Therefore:

$$\frac{2 \text{ g}}{100 \text{ ml}} = \frac{5 \text{ g}}{X}$$

Solving for X, X = 250 ml.

On occasion it is necessary to mix a more dilute solution from a concentrated mixture. An example is found in mixing a 5% or 10% solution of dextrose for IV administration.

Problem: How much 50% dextrose is required to make a liter of 10% dextrose?

Solution: 50% means 50 g/100 ml and 10% means 10 g/100 ml. In a liter of 10% dextrose there are 100 g dextrose, *ie,* 10 g/100 ml × 1000 ml = 100 g. Therefore 100 g dextrose would equal 200 ml 50% dextrose, *ie,*

$$\frac{50 \text{ g}}{100 \text{ ml}} = \frac{100 \text{ g}}{X}$$

Solving for X, X = 200 ml 50% dextrose. To make this solution, add 200 ml 50% dextrose to 800 ml sterile water. The resulting liter contains 10% dextrose.

Sample Problems

Using the sample chart below, answer the following problems for these hypothetical medications. The answers follow the last problem.

1. How much chloraplex is required for one injection for a 10-lb Dachshund?
2. If asked to give desoxythane to a 60-lb German Shepherd, how many tablets and what size would you use?
3. A 5-lb cat needs a 2-week supply of avitrollin. How many tablets and of what size would you dispense?

Drug	Dosage: Dog	Cat	How Supplied
Avitrollin	5 mg/lb PO BID	10 mg/lb PO BID	50-, 100-, 200-mg tabs
Betamide	not used	20 mg/lb IM TID	50 mg/ml
Chloraplex	50 mg/lb IV QID	25 mg/lb IV QID	100 mg/ml
Desoxythane	4 mg/10 lb PO SID	not used	8-, 16-, 32-mg tabs
Episol	½ gr/5 lb IM TID	½ gr/5 lb IM TID	1 gr/ml

PO = per os (by mouth)
IM = intramuscular
IV = intravenous

SID = once daily (every 24 hr)
BID = every 12 hr
TID = every 8 hr
QID = every 6 hr

4. The patient in question 3 also needs an injection of betamide. In preparing the injection, how much medication would you withdraw from the vial into the syringe?
5. A 30-lb Corgi is hospitalized and requires Episol injections for 2 days. The doctor wants to know if one 10-ml vial of medication is enough to properly treat the dog for both days? If more medication is needed, how many more 10-ml vials must be purchased?

Answers to Problems

1. Patient's weight × dosage for dog = amount of medication:

$$10 \text{ lb} \times 50 \text{ mg/lb} = 500 \text{ mg}$$

$$\frac{\text{amount of medication}}{\text{Concentration}} = \text{volume of injection;}$$

$$\frac{500\text{mg}}{100 \text{ mg/ml}} = 5 \text{ ml}$$

2. Patient's weight × dosage for dog = amount of medication: 60 lb × 4 mg/10 lb = 240 mg/10 lb = 24 mg

$$\frac{\text{amount of medication}}{\text{size of tablet}} = \text{number of tablets;}$$

24 mg/8-mg tablet = 3 tablets
24 mg/16-mg tablet = 1½ tablets
24 mg/32-mg tablet = ¾ tablet

All 3 answers are correct. The choice of which size tablet to administer rests with the AHT and may be influenced by the number of each tablet size available.

3. Using same 2 formulas above with the values plugged in:
   5 lb × 10 mg/lb = 50 mg
   $$\frac{50 \text{ mg}}{50 \text{ mg per tablet}} = 1 \text{ tablet}$$
   If other-sized tablets are used, it requires splitting the tablets into halves or quarters, which is not desirable. One 50-mg tablet given twice daily for 2 weeks:
   1 tab × 2/day × 14 days = 28 tabs.
4. Using 2 basic formulas:
   5 lb × 20 mg/lb = 100 mg
   $$\frac{100 \text{ mg}}{50 \text{ mg/ml}} = 2 \text{ ml}$$
5. Using 2 basic formulas:
   30 lb × ½ gr/5 lb = 15 gr/5 = 3 gr
   $$\frac{3 \text{ gr}}{1 \text{ gr/ml}} = 3 \text{ ml per dose to be given}$$
   As this drug is given TID, 3 injections are needed per day of hospitalization. Therefore, 3 ml/injection × 3 injections/day × 2 days = 18 ml.
   Since one vial contains only 10 ml of drug, there is not enough medication to treat the dog both days. Another vial is required to have enough for both days of treatment.

ADMISSION OF LARGE ANIMAL PATIENTS

Initial Presentation

The introduction to a large animal patient almost always begins by telephone contact. The job of the AHT is to determine the immediate presenting complaint and the urgency with which the problem should be treated. Determining the reason for the call or the seriousness of the injury or current morbid state is the first objective. Many horse owners overstate the urgency with which their animal should be attended. Also, "poor doers" on a ranch may be on their last legs but can recover with immediate and proper care.

Admission of large animals to the hospital, or treatment in the field, requires owner registration and compiling of patient information. Owner registration entails collection of the owner's personal data, including place of residence and business, registered ranch or farm name, if any, source of referral, any insurance policy number for the animal and means of payment. Client records may be indexed by alphabet, zip code, date of last visit or whatever means the veterinarian and office staff find most effective (see Small Animal Medical Records).

Clients presenting large animals at the hospital or clinic should be handled with patience and courtesy. Horses should be quietly unloaded with the help of the owners to minimize the animal's anxiety. Untie the horse through the escape door first, toss the rope over its neck, open the back door and drop the backbar or chain. Have an assistant or the owner stand at the door to guide the horse down the ramp and grab the lead rope. Speak quietly and always approach the animal at an angle, never from behind. Once the horse is unloaded, circle the horse out of kicking range and lead it to a convenient spot for ease of examination. Tie the horse with a slip knot in the lead rope, never by the bridle reins, to a secure post, avoiding fence rails or gates. Be calm and confident. A nervous handler creates a nervous horse, resulting in more difficult examination and treatment.

Food animals (cattle, sheep, swine) should be unloaded with a minimum of shouting, arm waving or excitement. Lead or herd them calmly to a holding pen or enclosed alleyway. Most presentations of food animals at a hospital involve purebred or show animals that usually are accustomed to being handled and moved about. Move confidently, yet cautiously, as even the most apparently passive 4-H cow may turn cantankerous and cause serious injury if mishandled.

Unannounced arrivals at the hospital usually find the veterinarian on call in the field. It is best to politely inform those clients of the doctor's rigorous schedule and suggest an appointment another day. However, many clients travel a considerable distance with trailer in tow, making a return trip most unattractive. In these cases, and in emergency situations, it is best to refer the client to another practitioner in the area or contact the doctor by radio or telephone, if possible, for advice.

LARGE ANIMAL MEDICAL RECORDS

History and Presenting Complaint

Horses

Before the horse is examined, either at the hospital or in the field, initial patient information must be obtained. Information on the age, sex, breed, color, registration (if applicable), and geographic location of stabling or pasture should be obtained. Specific information regarding previous illness or injury, diet, vaccination history, parasite control, type of housing, and animal contacts should be recorded. The presenting complaint should be noted, along with clinical signs, any abnormal behavior or recent changes in diet or location, vital signs, and location of injury or wound, if applicable. Copies of herd health records, if available, should be included with the record.

Any description of past illness or injury should include the date of illness, clinical signs, extent and location of any wound, treatment and length of illness. Any bad habits arising from the illness or manifesting themselves at other times should be recorded. These may include cribbing, head shaking or eating unusual objects (pica).

The immunization history is of critical importance in any medical record. An equine vaccination history should include the date of and age at vaccination and the type of vaccine used. There are many conflicting opinions regarding strangles vaccination. Current recommendations are to immunize the herd if one individual should contract the disease by placing the exudative pus from the infection in the feed of other horses. Venezuelan equine encephalomyelitis (VEE) has been largely eradicated, but vaccination may still be necessary in areas of outbreak.

Information on previous parasitic infections and results of treatment should be entered into the patient's file. Horses are affected by more than 75 internal parasites, with strongyles, ascarids, pinworms and bots being the most injurious. Prevention of internal parasites consists primarily of sanitary measures. An emaciated, unthrifty appearance generally indicates parasitism, but the diagnosis can only be confirmed by fecal examination.

External parasitisms include those by blowflies, mosquitos, lice, mites, screwworms, ticks and ringworm. Eradication programs involve sanitation, use of parasiticides and care of open wounds.

Information on the animal's housing or any history of confinement should be recorded. The mental state of the horse should be considered when dealing with a horse accustomed to confinement. Stables should be properly insulated and drained and ventilated. Horses may injure themselves if stalls and the stable have not been surveyed for sharp projections, broken rails or poorly insulated wiring. Be aware of these potential dangers when recording the medical history.

Pastured horses have the advantage of free grazing exercise but run the risk of poisonous plants, broken fences and poor pasture. Become informed of the poisonous plants in your geographic location. Some common poisonous plants and shrubs are hemlock, green bracken, laurel, ragwort and monkswood. Broken or poorly constructed fences may cause horses to become entangled in barbed wire, wounded on splintered boards or nails, or tangled in rope or baling wire. The time of entering information in the medical record is the ideal opportunity to alert both the veterinarian and client to potential hazards in housing by making an early note of it.

A notation in the medical record should be made regarding exposure to other animals. Respiratory infections are both very common and contagious among equidae. Joint pasturing also facilitates parasitism and spread of bacterial and viral diseases.

Food Animals

As with horses, specific information should be obtained regarding the individual, entire herd or flock when the initial complaint is discussed. When working with commercial operators, there are usually designated periods within the year when the entire herd is worked. Records should be updated at that time as to the current condition of the animals.

In commercial operations, herd records are updated when new calves are worked at 3-5 months of age. Separated calves are identified with ear tags, immunized, dehorned, castrated, weighed and branded. If older cows or bulls are worked at this time, the veterinarian may be involved in vaccinating, pregnancy and semen testing, deworming, recording weights and updating files.

Sheep are worked on a similar schedule, though that work is performed in shorter time due to the shorter gestation period and faster growth rate of sheep. Inquiry should be made into nutritional, reproductive and production programs for commercial flocks. The nutritional history should be compared with National Research Council nutrient and mineral requirements.

As for all patient records, questions should be asked regarding vaccination history, parasite control programs, parturition season and type of housing or shelter provided. Production records are critical tools for sheep and hog operations in monitoring drops in weaning percentages, birthing rates, and overall production levels. Such records are critical in commercial operations for superior returns and also enable the veterinarian to quickly and efficiently analyze the continuing needs of that operation.

Record systems for horses and food animals should include a treatment record and case summary. For entire herds this information may be incorporated into herd records. Records for purebred animals are handled somewhat differently, due to the commercial value of the animals involved. In purebred beef operations, each animal should be assigned its own record, allowing close assessment of its performance and tracking of the medical record. This assures a more individualized assessment of medical problems, subsequent treatment and production performance.

Case summary reports should be entered into each file after the animal is treated. Information regarding diagnosis, treatment procedures, dates of treatment and disposition of the animal should be included. When dealing with herd records, the number of swine farrowed, sheep docked or calves branded should be recorded. After creating each file, the summary report should be readily available for easy access of information.

PHYSICAL EXAMINATION OF LARGE ANIMALS

Horses

When a new patient is first examined, the vital signs and general appearance should be first evaluated. Table 9 summarizes the vital signs for horses and food animals. These values may be artificially elevated, depending on recent exercise, stress, general condition and stages of pregnancy or lactation. The technician should be adept at recording the vital signs to save time for the doctor.

When viewing a horse for the first time, stand back and inspect the animal from the side at 20-30 feet. Look for an alert attitude, with the horse standing squarely (resting one hind leg is normal, resting a foreleg indicates disease in that leg or elsewhere) and the ears erect and active. The eyes should be bright, the haircoat sleek and shiny in summer, but heavier in winter, and free of parasites or lesions. The hoof walls should be smooth and pliable, not misshapen or split. The frogs of the hoof should be well shaped and resilient, with no offensive odor or discharge from the cleft.

The animal in question should interact normally, if pastured with other horses. The appetite should be good, the droppings well formed and moist, with no parasites or mucus visible, and the urine thick and yellowish. Have the horse trotted and watch for soundness while observing the stride and gait. Watch for clumsy movement or a great deal of side movement. Make the visual appraisal while taking note of any abnormalities, and then begin a systematic examination of the organ systems.

Palpate and gently probe over the body of the horse. Take the extra time to calm the horse while searching for abnormalities or tender areas. The equine digestive system is unique because of its large cecum. Fluid contents forced from the cecum to the large intestine continues to be digested for several days, producing heat and gas.

Table 9. Normal Rectal Temperature, Heart Rate and Respiratory Rate for Horses, Cattle, Sheep and Swine

Species	Rectal Temp. (F)	Heart Rate (/min)	Resp. Rate (/min)
Horse	99.5-101.3	28-50	8-16
Cattle	100.5-103.0	40-70	10-30
Sheep	102.0-104.0	60-90	12-19
Swine	100.5-104.0	58-100	8-18

This process normally is accompanied by intestinal noises, or borborygmi, which are healthy, churning noises of the colon.

After the digestive tract, a horse's feet and legs create more medical problems than any other body system. The foot must be capable of absorbing tremendous shock during locomotion. The foot consists of a horny, somewhat elastic box enclosing the distal bones of the limb, which are cushioned by fibro-fatty pads. The most distal bone of the leg, the third phalanx, has elastic wings extending above the coronet, toward the heel. The more proximal second phalanx articulates with the third, forming the coffin joint. At the caudal aspect of this joint is the navicular bone, over which the flexor tendon courses. The sensitive sole covers the ventral aspect of the third phalanx, producing the overlying horny sole. The frog is formed on the ventral aspect of the plantar cushion.

A routine hoof-care program includes regular trimming and shoeing, daily use of a hoof pick, and painting with some type of hoof dressing to keep the hoof soft and free of cracks. Some hoof injuries can result in severe discomfort and lameness, sole bruises, corns, punctures, thrush, cracked hooves and heels, quittor, founder and laminitis.

Food Animals

As with horses, it is best to begin the physical examination by checking the vital signs and then moving to a visual appraisal for estimating general condition (Table 9). Food animals should be evaluated on the basis of their economically important anatomic systems.

Dairy cows should be evaluated on the basis of their milk production and udder health. The udder should be structurally sound in all quarters, with no ligament breakdown, signified by an asymmetric shape. Each teat should be examined for wounds, strictures, abnormal discharge or hardness, which may indicate mastitis. The feet and legs should also be observed for signs of lameness.

Dairy Herd Improvement Association (DHIA) records should be reviewed, noting any drops in milk production or butter fat content and increase in somatic cell counts. Be aware of the reproductive performance of each cow, noting abnormally long open (nonpregnant) periods and problems with dystocia. Keep in mind that production levels are critical in commercial herds. Good herd health programs ensure continued production at high levels. The AHT should be able to review these records and find areas of poor performance for the veterinarian to explore. As with dairy and beef records, sheep and swine production records should be closely scrutinized for problem areas in conception rates, weaning weights, feed conversion levels, mortality losses and areas of declining production levels.

Attention should be directed to proper conditioning of both sheep and swine. Both these species produce valuable meat cuts from the rear legs and loin. Examine their legs and palpate over the lumbar area for excessive fat or leanness. Avoid rough handling and excitement before shipping, if possible. Swine are very susceptible to stress and can develop the porcine stress syndrome, producing a soft, exudative cut of meat. Sheep should be closely examined for external parasites, such as mites, ticks and lice, that may destroy the quality of the fleece. Special note should be made of the condition of the fleece, with reference to fiber quality and density. Poor fleece condition may indicate improper nutrition.

Restraint of Horses

by J. T. Vaughan and R. Allen, Jr.

Despite the introduction of tranquilizers, sedatives, muscle relaxants and new anesthetic agents, restraint of horses remains an ability acquired through experience. More than any other large domestic animal, horses must be handled as individuals. They must be protected from abusive restraint and from accidental injury when restraint is applied.

There are basically 4 psychological categories of horses: the well-mannered horse that has had good training and proper handling; the unbroken horse that has had little or no training or handling and is easily frightened; the ill-mannered horse that has had unfavorable exposure to people and has been poorly trained; and the rogue horse that may have had good training and proper handling but still ferociously resists restraint for even the simplest procedures. Each of these types requires individual assessment as to the method and degree of restraint required. The ability to recognize individual differences and to take into account an animal's idiosyncrasies as reported by the owner or stable manager is necessary if minimal restraint is to be applied.

The method of restraint depends on many factors, including the animal's temperament, age, size, physical condition, procedure to be performed, and the equipment, help and drugs available. The duration of the procedure and the amount of pain or anxiety likely to be produced should be considered. The use of humane technics is imperative. A professional responsibility is acquired when a patient is accepted for treatment. It is assumed that the practitioner and technician will protect the patient's well-being and prevent injury, especially that resulting from unwise application of restraint.

Because individual horses may react differently in a given situation, the method and degree of restraint required are often a matter of experimentation. In general, one should apply the least restraint possible initially while judging the animal's reaction as a procedure progresses. The general methods of physical restraint, in increasing order of severity, include halter and lead, skin twitch, ear hold, and nose or lip twitch. Other methods, such as raising a limb, the tail hold, and use of stocks and breeding hobbles, are useful in certain situations.

Halters and Leads

The most important assistant is the one restraining the horse's head. Use the halter and lead to exert control just as a rider uses reins and bits. Never try to restrain a horse by the halter alone because a lead attached to it provides much more control. Always be alert to divert the horse's attention from work being done by the operator, who may be at the opposite end of the animal. The assistant should usually stand on the same side of the horse as the operator as this is the best position to prevent the animal from wheeling into or kicking the operator.

A horse should be led from the left or near side, the same side on which it is usually caught, bridled, saddled and mounted. When leading a horse during an examination, the assistant should walk or jog alongside the horse's head, facing the direction of travel and never looking back. If the horse does not follow willingly, it should be urged from behind by another person and not pulled by the halter. If there is only one assistant, a loop or rope can be dropped over the

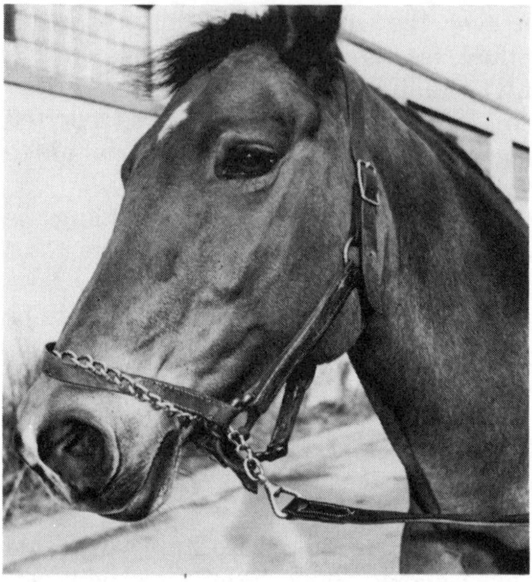

Fig 25. Use of a chain shank over the muzzle.

horse's hindquarters, crossed over the back and the ends passed up through the halter, to be pulled along with the lead to encourage the horse to advance. If this fails, the horse can be blindfolded and led or backed for short distances.

Halters are typically constructed of leather or braided rope (nylon or cotton). The latter are cheaper and stronger, and can be tied. They are used commonly with farm and western horses. Leather halters can be used with a chain shank for special restraint of spirited horses. The chain can be used over the muzzle, under the jaw, through the mouth, and over the gingiva (Figs 25-28). The last method has somewhat the effect of a war bridle and can be very effective in restraining horses that cannot be twitched or do not respond to a twitch. Chain shanks (leads) should not be used abusively, nor should they be used to tie a horse. When not used in the ways described, a chain shank is simply snapped in the halter ring at the bottom of the caveson (nose band) or doubled through the ring and snapped back on itself.

Special halters include heavy reinforced table halters for confining the animal to an operating table and the dental halter, with a rigid loop of steel incorporated into the nose band. Both have D-rings at the 4 quadrants of the nose band as well as the crown piece behind the poll, which make it possible to secure the head from any direction. The rigid nose band in the dental halter provides space to open the mouth for dental surgery without encroaching on the cheeks. The list

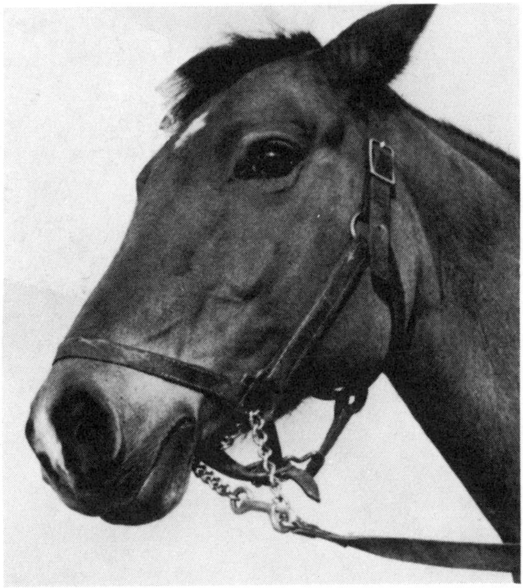

Fig 26. Use of a chain shank below the mandible.

of halter types also includes the stallion bridle, lunging caveson, Tennessee grass halters, and stable and track halters.

A word of caution is important at this point, however, concerning the use of cattle halters and temporary rope halters on horses. Both are "draw" halters, *ie,* they constrict around the head or muzzle when tightened. This can cause serious injury, especially if the horse is tied and attempts to escape. Trauma to the nasal bones and passages,

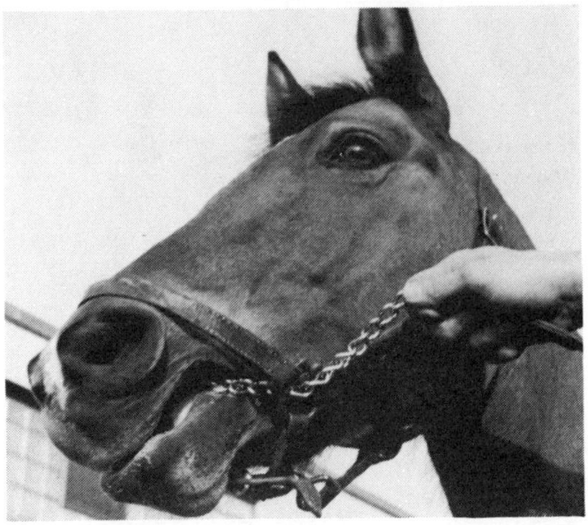

Fig 27. Use of a chain shank through the mouth.

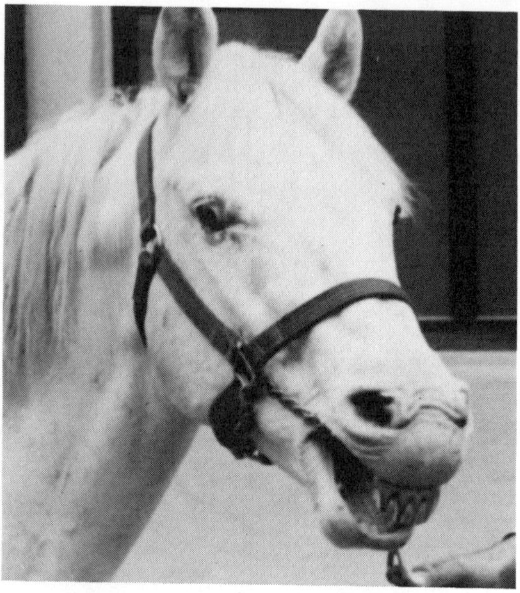

Fig 28. Use of a chain shank over the upper gingivae.

hemorrhage and asphyxia have resulted from use of such halters. If it is necessary to improvise, one should make a knot in the lead rope to prevent halter constriction.

A horse of unknown temperament should never be left unattended when tied because it may become excited and struggle to free itself. This is hazardous as the horse is likely to be injured or to injure persons nearby. One should never attempt to do anything to a tied horse,

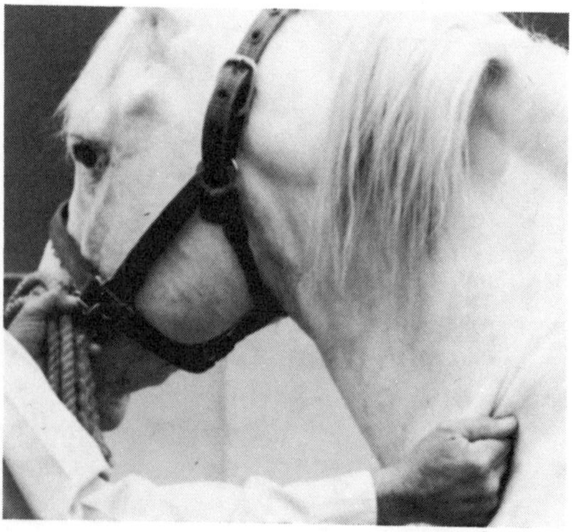

Fig 29. Application of the skin twitch to discourage a horse from striking.

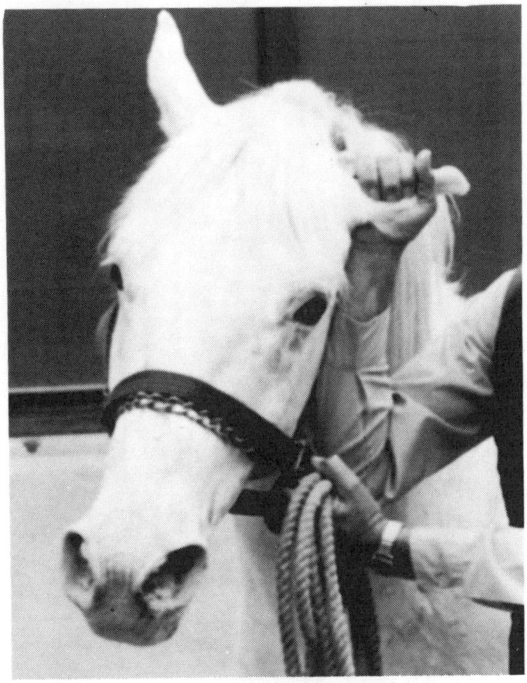

Fig 30. Grasping an ear to restrain the head.

even such seemingly minor operations as examining the incisor teeth, inspecting an eye or taking the pulse. Many horses use the slightest excuse to sit back on their halters, invariably breaking a piece of tack. These "halter breakers" frequently cannot be tied at all.

Skin Twitch

Another method of restraint, especially useful on horses prone to strike with the front feet, is the skin twitch. The skin twitch is applied by grasping a roll of skin over the shoulders with both hands (Fig 29). As with any other method of restraint, the skin twitch works well on some animals but not on others.

Ear Hold

Horses that do not respond to halter or skin twitch restraint may respond to the ear hold. The left ear is firmly grasped with the right hand, with the heel of the hand against the animal's scalp (Fig 30). The ear is squeezed and slight pressure is applied ventrad. The right forearm and elbow should be held firmly against the vertical ramus of the animal's left mandible, so the assistant is pushed away rather than hit in the face if the animal rears.

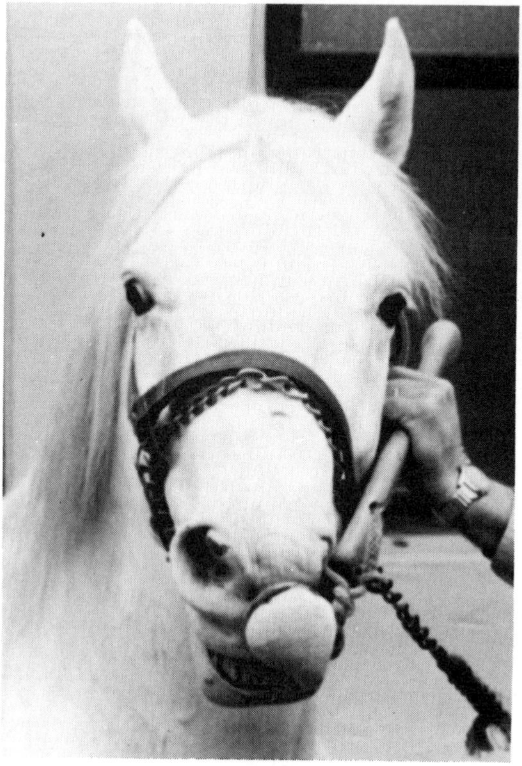

Fig 31. A rope twitch applied to the upper lip.

The ear hold can be very effective if correctly applied. However, it can result in a fallen ear or head-shy horse if applied abusively. The application of a rope or chain twitch to the ear is inhumane and usually results in permanent ear injury.

The ear hold should not be applied to show horses, such as the American Saddlebred, Tennessee Walking Horse, Hackney, Arabian, Morgan and others.

Lip Twitch

The twitch is one of the oldest and most widely used (and misused) restraint devices. Its exact effect on a horse has been argued, but nevertheless it effectively distracts the animal's attention and provides restraint. Twitching is most simply accomplished by firmly grasping the lip (usually upper) between the tips of the thumb and fingers. This often is necessary to hold the horse's head still long enough to apply the twitch to the lip. The conventional twitch consists of a loop of small chain or rope fixed to the end of a wooden handle about 36 inches long. The loop is applied over the lip, which is folded so that the mucosal surface is not exposed, and the loop is tightened by twisting the handle (Fig 31).

At this point some horses may strike or paw with one or both front feet. Therefore, the person holding the horse should be standing beside the left shoulder and the one twitching the horse should be beside or just in front of the first, so both are in a safe position. As the twitch handle is turned the last time, it should be held at its end so the handler will not lose control of the twitch if the horse pulls back or strikes. This is important because if the twitch is pulled from an assistant's grasp, the horse may use it as a flail and seriously injure anyone in the area. After the twitch has been applied an assistant can hold the halter lead and twitch. This is the customary restraint for routine procedures, such as passing a stomach tube.

Some horses should never be twitched. Because of past abuse, they greatly resent the twitch and fight it, even after it is applied. These animals should be restrained in some other way. A twitch is most effective when used as needed. Its effect is greatest when first applied and is lost if the lip becomes numb. Therefore, one should alternate the pressure of the loop around the lip so that maximum pressure is applied when needed. The pressure is then reduced enough to allow sensitivity and circulation to return. When the upper lip becomes numb or if there is some reason not to use it, the lower lip can be twitched with almost as good effect (Fig 32).

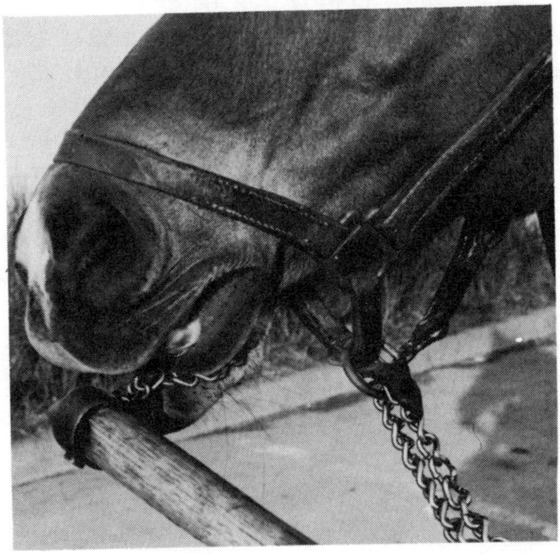

Fig 32. A chain twitch applied to the lower lip.

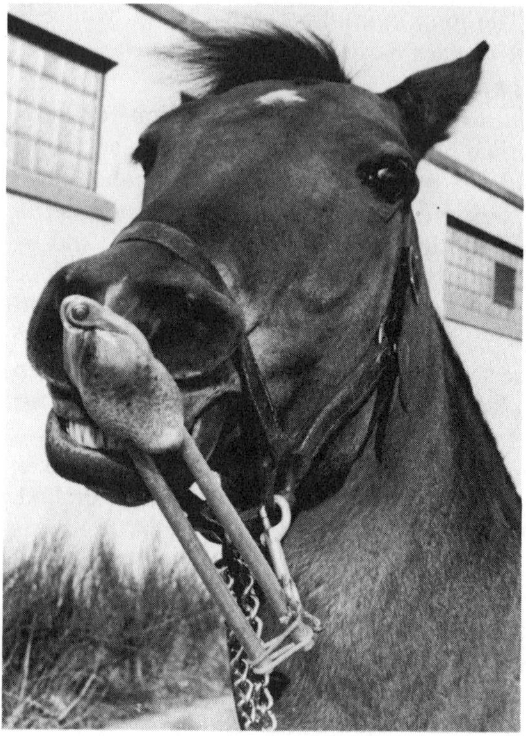

Fig 33. A clamp twitch applied to the upper lip is snapped on the halter.

The nose clamp has been used for many years (Fig 33). The modern version has a nylon cord and snap so it can be fixed to the halter, freeing one hand of the assistant.

War Bridle

This is a rope gag used to restrain a horse that tends to rear or resist a twitch. There are several variations, including Magner's modified war bridle (Fig 34). It should always be used in conjunction with a halter and lead, and never used to tie a horse. A war bridle can injure the horse if not used properly.

Another method of restraining the head involves holding the muzzle with the left hand and the nape of the neck with the right. The left thumb can be inserted under the noseband to prevent the horse from ducking its head. The right hand can grasp the mane or an ear for added restraint. This method is very useful for such procedures as floating teeth (Fig 35). Do not compress the nostrils and restrict breathing.

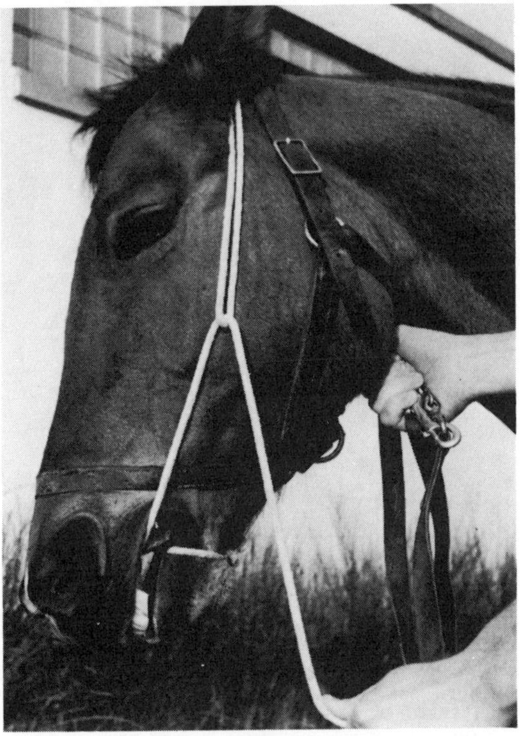

Fig 34. The war bridle.

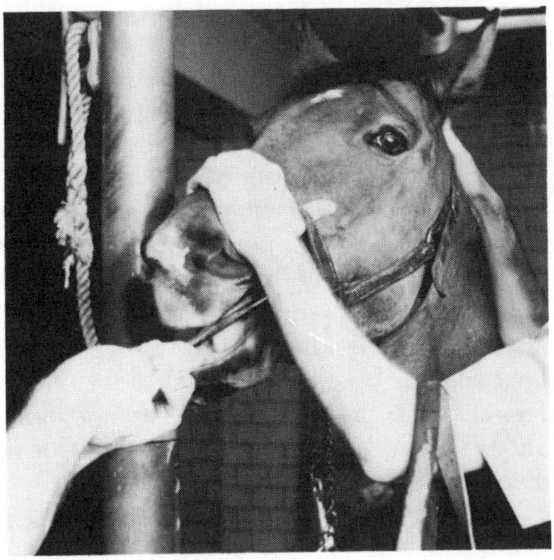

Fig 35. A method of head restraint for floating teeth.

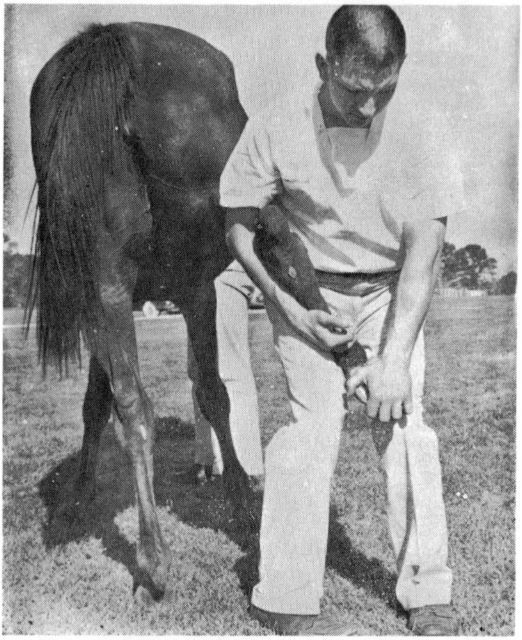

Fig 36. Position for examination or treatment of a hindfoot.

Restraint of the Feet

The manner in which the feet are restrained depends on how the horse has been handled. An animal that has been groomed daily and is accustomed to having its feet handled cooperates by picking up its feet. When the horse's feet have never been handled, some training may be required. Sedatives or tranquilizers are helpful. Regardless of the horse, the approach is the same. The assistant stands at the animal's head and the horse is encouraged to stand with its weight on all 4 legs so its weight can easily be shifted to 3 legs. The operator should make his presence and intentions known to the horse. If a front leg is to be raised, a hand is moved down the leg to the fetlock and the volar digital nerves are pinched or the hair below the fetlock is pulled. This usually prompts the horse to pick up the foot. Some horses require more force, such as pushing the animal onto the opposite leg while flexing the one being raised. If the horse's foot is held between the operator's knees to free his hands, the operator should crouch with his knees together and his toes pointed mediad. One should avoid pulling the horse's foot or leg laterad because it is uncomfortable for the animal.

Raising and holding a hindfoot can be more difficult. A horse that cannot be approached safely from behind usually gives warning by

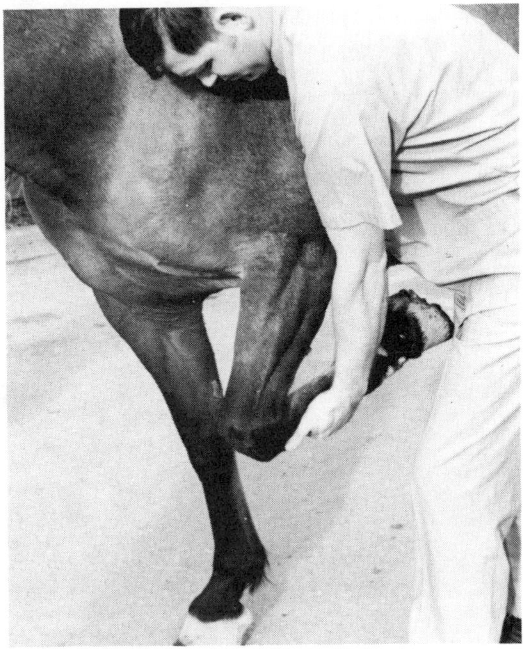

Fig 37. Manual restraint of a foreleg.

moving away, feinting with the hindleg that is being grasped, or merely taking weight off the leg so it can kick at any time. The operator's hand nearest the horse is kept on the animal's tuber coxae, while the other is moved down to the cannon bone to draw the leg craniad. The hock and toe are held in a flexed position when the leg is raised, partially restricting voluntary movement of that leg. As the leg is cradled between the operator's arm and leg nearer the horse, the cannon is propped on the inside of the thigh. The operator can then use his hands to clean the foot and perform the required procedure (Fig 36). The operator should position himself firmly so that he is not thrown off balance by the horse's struggling. When releasing the leg, the procedure is reversed: the operator's near hand is placed on the horse's tuber coxae and used to push himself to the front of the animal.

Many horses are accustomed to having all 4 feet examined and cleaned daily from the left side, with the operator reaching under and across when raising the feet on the right side. A front foot can be raised and held to prevent a horse from kicking with a hindfoot (Fig 37). The front foot on the same side as the operator should be lifted because the horse is then unable to kick with the rear leg on that side. When holding a front leg, one should avoid supporting the horse. A

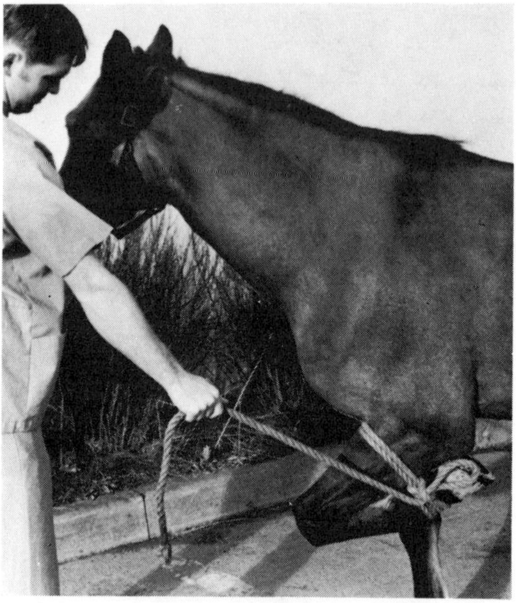

Fig 38. Restraint of a foreleg by tying.

front leg is occasionally tied for restraint of a mare during breeding or for rectal examination (Fig 38). The rope or strap should be tied in such a manner that it can be released quickly to prevent the animal from casting itself. Tying a hindleg involves the use of a single rope sideline. This does not permit a careful examination of the foot but may discourage kicking. For animals that resist these restraint methods, the use of tranquilizers or sedatives is indicated. Rope burns can be avoided by using hobbles or bandages (Fig 39).

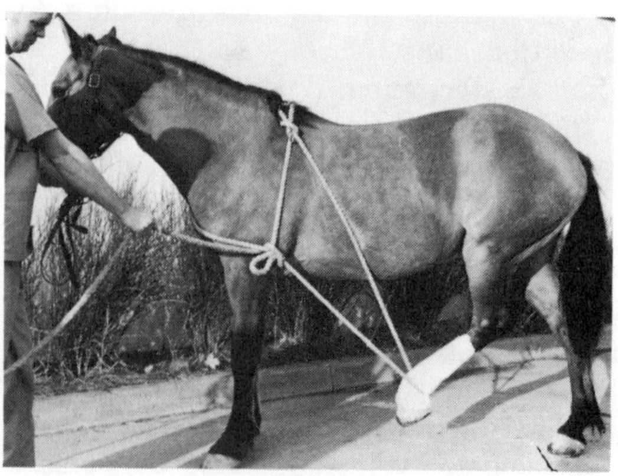

Fig 39. Use of a sideline to immobilize a hindlimb. The bandage on the immobilized leg prevents rope burns.

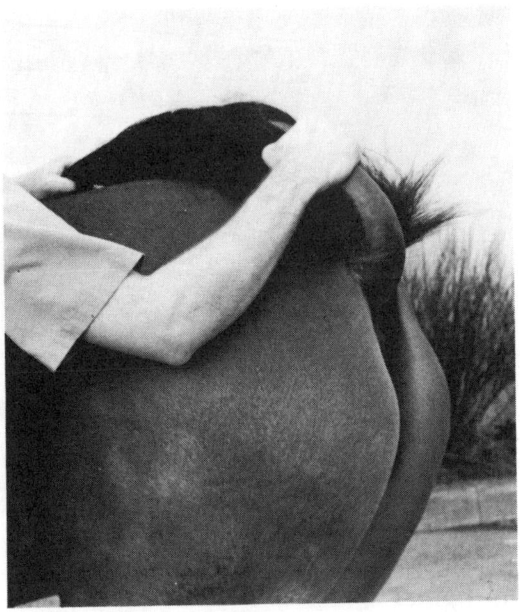

Fig 40. Manual displacement of the tail.

Tail Displacement

The tail is displaced for rectal or urogenital examinations, to discourage kicking, and to provide some support of the hindquarters during certain procedures, such as a standing castration and putting a horse on a surgery table. This can be done manually or with a rope tied in the end of the tail (Figs 40, 41). A tail rope is held and never tied to a stationary object if the horse is standing. When the animal is lying on a surgery table and secured by a halter and body belts, the

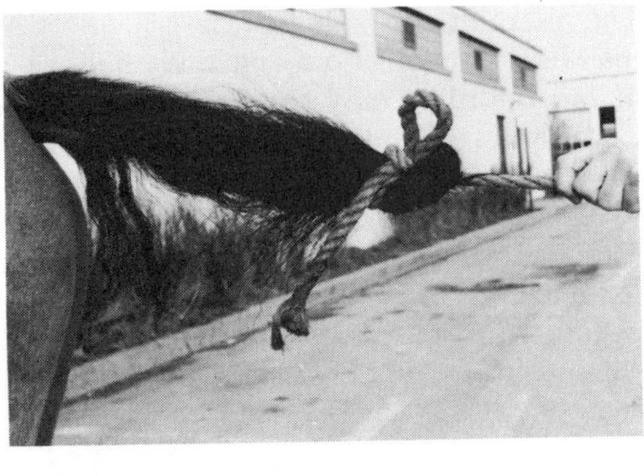

Fig 41. Use of a tail rope for restraint.

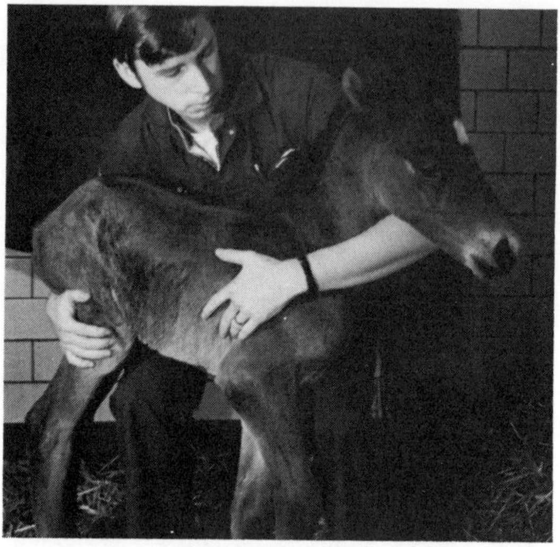

Fig 42. Restraint of a foal.

tail can be tied. As a horse is getting on its feet, it can be assisted by lifting the tail.

The tail can be used to subdue unmanageable ponies and weanlings. One person can often restrain such an animal by grasping the halter with one hand and the tail with the other. The tail is held firmly over the animal's back by grasping it near the base and pulling it craniad. If the horse is not haltered and is small enough, the base of the neck is cradled in the other arm. To restrain a larger weanling, it is helpful to push the animal beside a smooth wall and lean into it while holding its head and tail. It is even better to back the animal into a corner of a stall. This provides safe restraint for stomach intubation, injections and other short procedures.

Young horses often react to head restraint by rearing and may fall over backward, strike the head, and suffer concussions and fractures. The restraint methods just described are safer for young horses that may be unbroken or only partially halter-broken. Abusive application of tail restraint may cause fractures, especially in young animals. Coccygeal fractures can result in abnormal tail carriage due to pain, paralysis or bone distortion.

Restraint of Foals

Suckling foals require special handling and foals should never be separated from the dam unless kept in a safe place, preferably with a "baby-sitter." Foals can become very excited when left alone and may hurt themselves.

When restraining young foals or weanlings that have not been halter-broken (even though they may be wearing one), one should not grasp the halter or apply one and attempt to hold the animal with it. The foal's reaction usually is to rear back and fall. Instead, the foal should be cornered in a smooth-walled box stall free of buckets, tubs, sharp edges or other hazards, with the mare nearby, restrained by an assistant. The foal can then be cradled in the arms, one around the neck and the other around the rump (Fig 42).

Restraint in Stalls

Certain procedures are often more easily accomplished if performed in surroundings familiar to the animal. Passing a stomach tube, treating teeth, examining the eyes and medicating a wound are usually more easily accomplished in the animal's stall. Usually the best position for both the assistant and operator is the center of the stall, with the horse led beside a wall. A fractious horse is restrained more easily this way. The operator keeps to the inside (normally the left) shoulder of the horse. By taking a short hold on the lead shank and placing the elbow of the same arm squarely against the side of the horse's neck, it is possible to keep the horse's head turned toward the handler and its hindquarters away.

Slings

As a rule, the use of slings is indicated when the animal, once raised to a standing position, can and will support or partially support its own weight at least part of the time. If a horse will not support its weight at least partially, it is better off lying in a deep bed of clean, dry straw and turned or lifted at regular intervals. A sling may be used temporarily to raise a weakened animal to its feet. Horses have tolerated a sling well for many weeks (fracture cases), but in such cases the animal was able to bear its own weight and stand for long periods without the sling's support. When an animal hangs in a sling constantly, its death is certain.

There are many poor slings and a few good ones. The former are poorly constructed with inferior materials. A good sturdy, easily adjusted sling is a valuable possession. Although there are relatively few occasions for its use, nothing else will suffice when a sling is needed. The components of a sling are a wide belly band (the wider the better), a breast collar, breeching, a crupper, a single-tree, and a chain hoist (Fig 43). The breeching keeps the horse from falling out of the sling backward and must have the necessary straps to keep it from slipping up or down. The breast collar prevents the horse from slip-

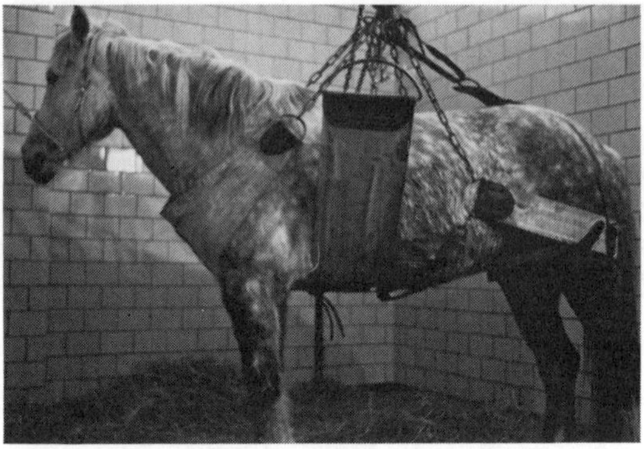

Fig 43. A satisfactory sling.

ping forward. All bands and straps should be buckled together in one unit and adjusted to fit the individual horse. The single-tree is the point of suspension above the horse and keeps the straps separated over the animal's back. The chain hoist is firmly anchored in the ceiling of the stall. It should be raised until the horse is lifted to a standing position and then lowered just enough to allow a hand to be slipped between the belly band and the horse when it is standing. This amount of clearance is necessary to remove constant pressure on the chest and abdomen. Otherwise, respiration and circulation are impaired.

The patient usually is tied loosely to one wall by the halter to prevent its turning in circles in the sling. This may not be necessary if the hoist has a swivel. Feed and water must be placed in easy access, and a hay net hung nearby is an added convenience. When first placed in a sling, the horse should be fully conscious. It is very difficult to put a partially anesthetized animal in a sling, especially if it is unable to use one or more legs. Tranquilization may help horses that rear and otherwise resist being placed in the sling. Time and patience are necessary until the patient adjusts to confinement.

Stocks

Stocks are very useful to simplify examination and treatment, and are especially suitable for dental procedures and surgery on standing horses (Fig 44). Animals unfamiliar with restraint in stocks should be introduced gradually before the need for such restraint arises.

The use of a kickboard in conjunction with stocks enables one to work with relative safety around the rear of a standing horse. This is a heavy half-door constructed of either oak boards or heavy marine

Fig 44. A well-constructed set of outdoor stocks. The hinged rear door is at the left and a padded neck cradle on the hinged front door is on the right.

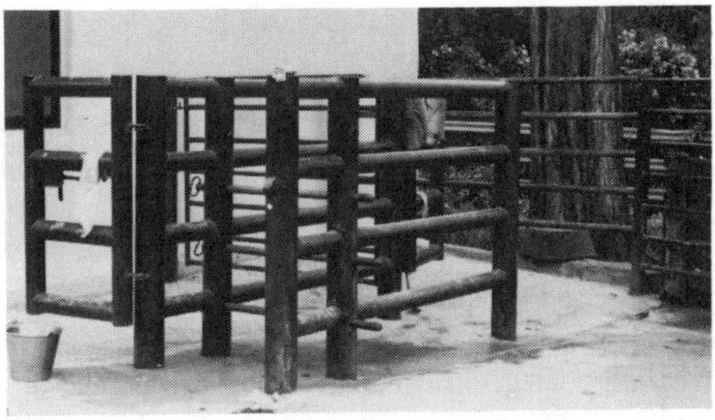

plywood with a reinforced backing. It can be hinged to swing open like half a Dutch door or can be slipped into the stocks behind the horse. It should be 40 inches high and wide enough to be braced against the uprights of the stocks. The side facing the horse should be smooth or padded, especially the top edge. The door should be fixed to the stocks with ropes or latches to keep it from falling forward against the horse. After the door is fixed in place, the horse should be backed against it. If allowed to move forward, the animal might be able to kick over the top of the door.

Casting Harnesses

Although casting harnesses are still used, such equipment is no longer required to restrain horses, and risks their injury. If casting harnesses are used, they should be employed in conjunction with tranquilizers, sedatives, general anesthetics and/or muscle relaxants to minimize the risk of injury. Many, if not most, horses are cast with the use of drugs alone. They can be held by a halter or snubbed to a ring in the wall or some other stationary object to prevent falling backward and possibly striking the head on the wall or floor. Once

Fig 45. Breeding hobbles applied to a mare.

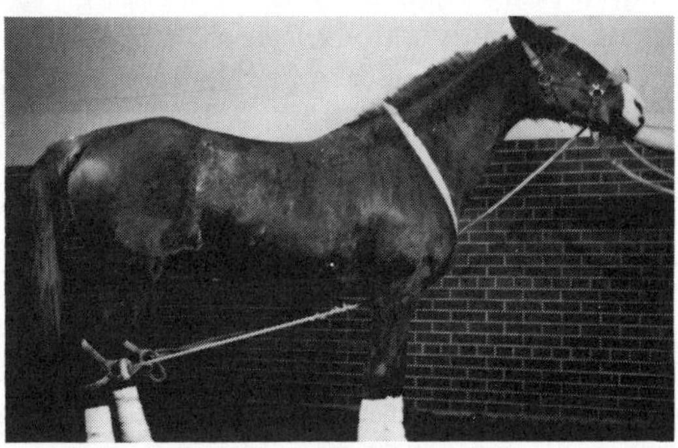

anesthesia has been induced, the analgesia and muscle relaxation achieved render restraining ropes and harness unnecessary except to maintain the position of the limbs. Tight ropes and strained positions are contraindicated because they often result in peripheral nerve injuries, especially of the hindlegs.

Breeding Hobbles

Breeding hobbles are used to prevent the mare from kicking during breeding. The restraining ropes extend from a breast collar, between the forelegs, and to the hocks or pasterns of the hindlegs (Fig 45). They also can be used for restraint during rectal examination or any operation around the hindquarters. One should adjust the hobbles properly to prevent any slack and also provide for quick release in case of such emergencies as the stallion's catching a leg in one of the ropes or casting of the mare.

Restraint of Cattle

by W. A. Aanes

Cattle may be restrained by many methods. The choice of a single method or combination of restraint methods depends on many factors. Careful consideration of these factors in selection of restraint should result in minimal stress to the animal and handler.

The response of most cattle to handling depends mostly on previous experiences. Beef cattle usually require more restraint than dairy cattle because they are handled less frequently and are commonly subjected to pain or discomfort when restrained. Dairy cows usually do not associate handling with pain, and their restraint should be minimal to avoid loss of milk production.

Bulls should never be trusted! Even a bull that appears to be gentle may suddenly change, especially during or after a painful procedure associated with restraint. The beef bull is usually less dangerous than a dairy bull, but there are enough exceptions to heed the statement "the only safe bull is a dead bull."

Factors that determine the methods of restraint to be applied include size, age, strength and disposition of the animal, and the availability of mechanical restraint equipment. The examination or treatment procedure(s), their duration, and the amount of pain to be inflicted also influence the extent of restraint. Because cattle have very sensitive skin, few procedures can be accomplished without causing some pain. Judicious use of tranquilizers, local anesthetics and general anesthetics is indicated, in conjunction with physical restraint, to handle cattle effectively. The general principle of "the least restraint necessary to satisfactorily accomplish the task at hand" should be followed at all times.

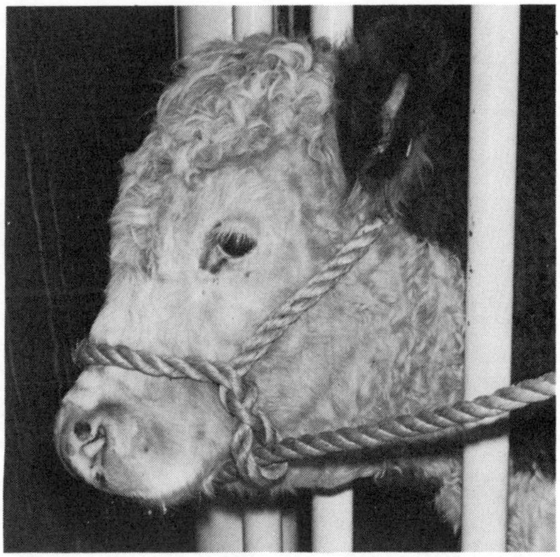

Fig 46. Properly applied rope halter.

Restraining the Head

Ordinary adjustable rope halters may be used to catch cattle in small pens. The halter should be adjusted so the crown of the halter can be dropped over the animal's head and the halter shank tightened under the jaw (Fig 46). The nose piece of the halter should be sufficiently long to keep the halter from damaging an eye or interfering

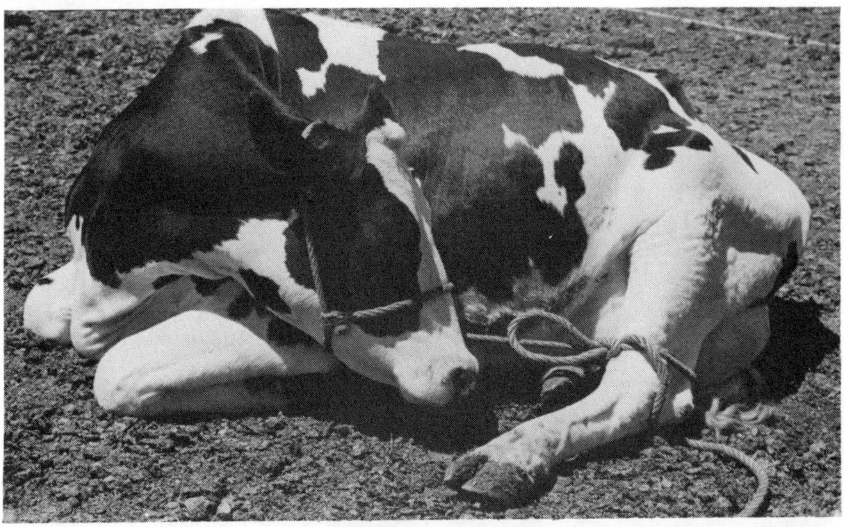

Fig 47. "Downer cow" restrained by the halter's shank tied back to the leg proximal to the hock.

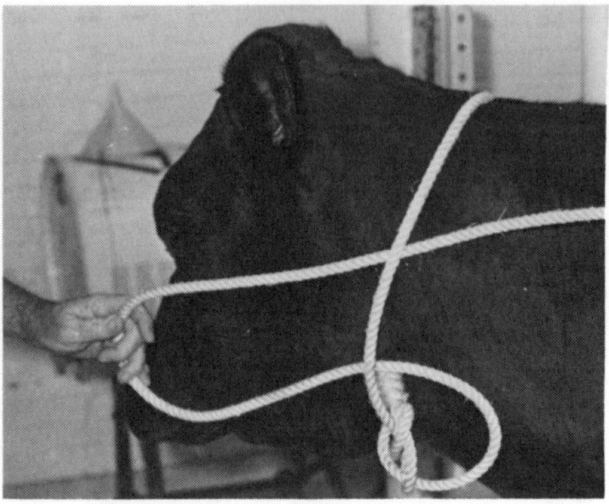

Fig 48. A temporary halter can be made by looping a lariat around the neck and pulling a bight through the loop toward the muzzle.

with respiration. A common error in applying the rope halter is reversing the crown position so the pull on the halter shank is across the poll of the animal; this reduces the effectiveness of the restraint. In larger pens a lariat may be used to catch the animal and then a halter applied to prevent choking. A halter can be used to effectively restrain the head of a "downer" cow during medication by tying the halter shank above the cow's hock (Fig 47).

If an ordinary rope halter is not available, an effective temporary halter can be made by putting the loop of a lariat around the animal's neck. A bight (loop) is formed in the standing part of the rope distal to the honda (eye at end of lariat). This bight is passed back to front through the lariat loop and adjusted over the nose. When properly ad-

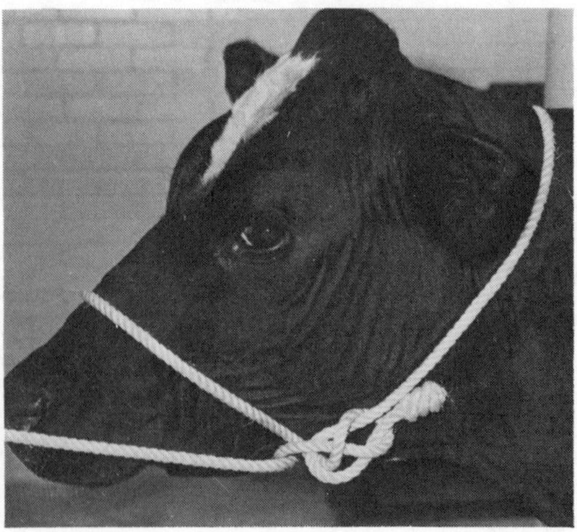

Fig 49. The bight is pulled over the bridge of the nose and adjusted.

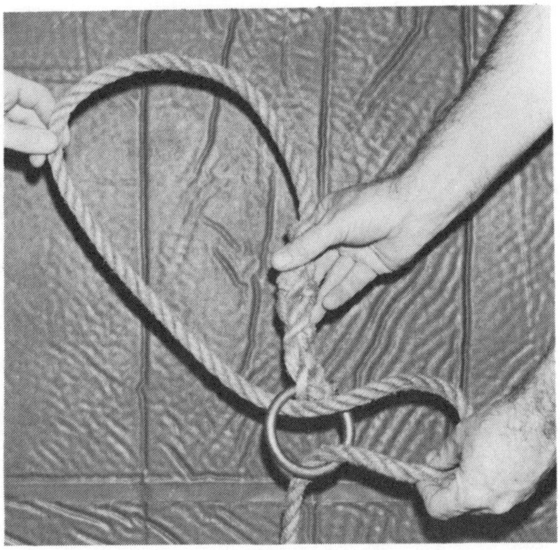

Fig 50. A Wyoming slip halter is made from a rope with an attached metal ring in one end.

justed, this temporary halter does not choke the animal. Any danger of choking can be avoided by tying the initial loop around the neck with a bowline (Figs 48, 49).

Another type of halter, called a "Wyoming slip halter," may be formed by splicing a metal ring into one end of a rope. A bight is formed in the standing part of the rope and is passed through the metal ring, forming 2 loops (Fig 50). The loop from the spliced end of the rope forms the crown of the halter and the bight through the ring

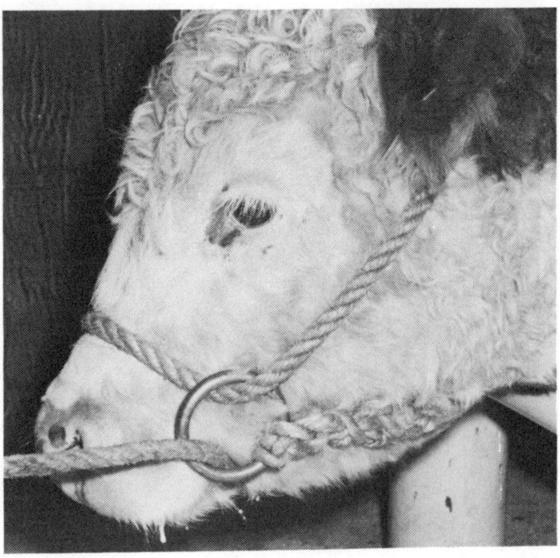

Fig 51. A bight is formed and pulled through the ring and over the bridge of the nose.

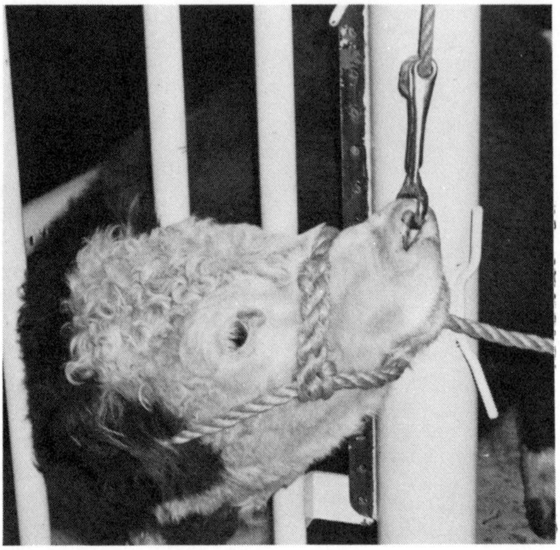

Fig 52. A nose lead should only be used with a halter.

forms the loop for the nose (Fig 51). Pressure on the standing part of the rope shank tightens the loop around the nose. This halter is easily released by pulling the loop from the nose.

A nose lead (bull leader) used in conjunction with a halter is an excellent device for restraining cattle (Fig 52). The nose lead causes temporary pain and thus diverts the animal's attention. Pressure on the lead should be in a dorsal direction, against the alar cartilages, to avoid tearing the nose. There should be sufficient tension on the

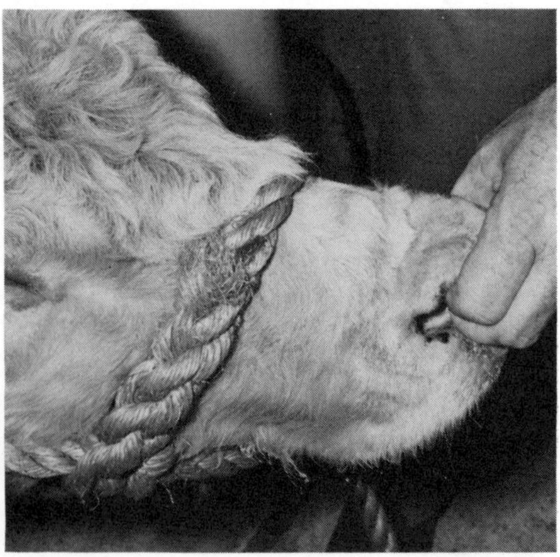

Fig 53. Cattle can be temporarily restrained by grasping the nasal septum with the thumb and forefinger.

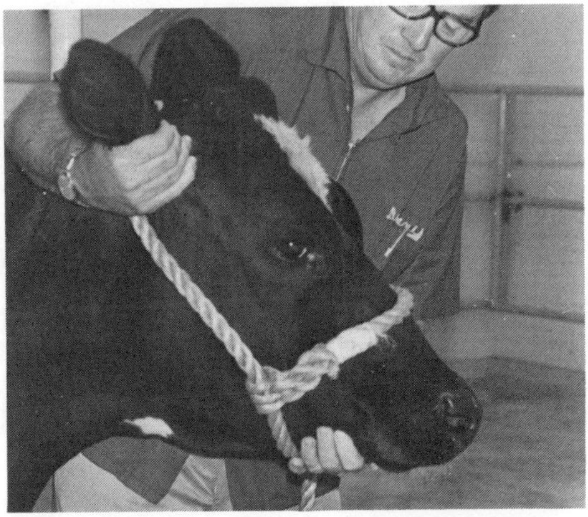

Fig 54. A cow in a stanchion can be restrained by holding the head against your hip.

halter shank to prevent the entire weight of the animal from pulling on the nose lead. If a nose lead is not available, the same type of restraint can be applied by grasping the nasal septum with the thumb and forefinger of one hand and supporting the animal's head with the other hand (Fig 53). The effectiveness of this restraint is limited by the strength of the individual applying it; it is a poor substitute for a nose lead.

The head of a gentle young animal may be held for simple examination and minor treatments by grasping the base of an ear with one hand, applying pressure against the head, and stabilizing the head with the other hand placed beneath the jaw. The head of an animal confined in a chute or stanchion may be examined by facing in the

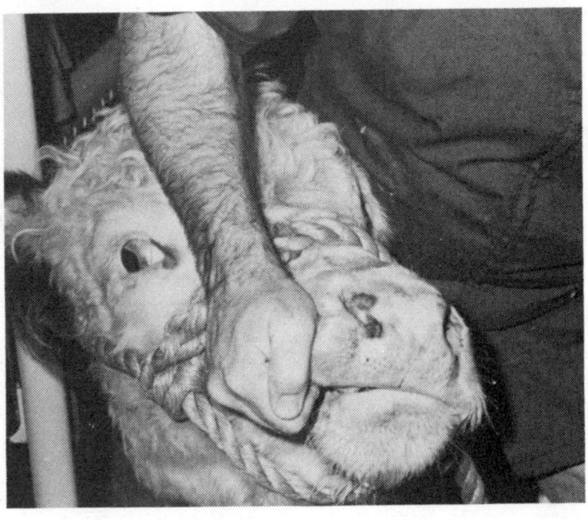

Fig 55. Grasping the upper lip facilitates oral examination and administration of medication.

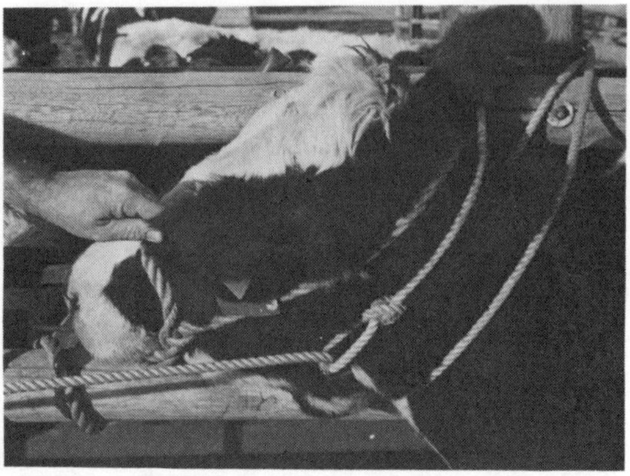

Fig 56. The head is secured to a fence in preparation for dehorning.

same direction as the animal, grasping its head, and holding it securely against the hip (Fig 54). Additional restraint can be applied by firmly grasping the animal's upper lip between the thumb and fingers of a hand passed across the nose of the animal (Fig 55). This restraint is effective for oral examination and medication.

To restrain the neck of the animal during dehorning when a chute or head stanchion is unavailable, a bight can be formed in the loop of a lariat. This bight is then placed over a fence post and the collapsed loop is passed under and around the animal's neck. A second bight is formed in the loop and placed over the first bight on the post. The honda is drawn tightly to secure the animal's neck to the post (Fig 56). A nose lead can then be used to control the position of the animal's head for examination or dehorning.

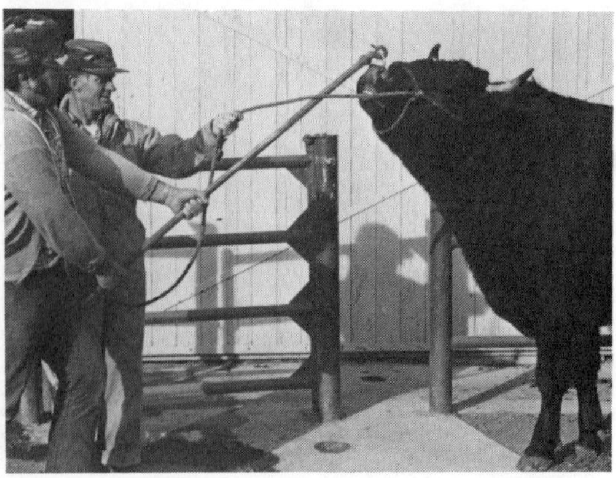

Fig 57. A bull staff is inserted through a bull's nose ring to control the animal.

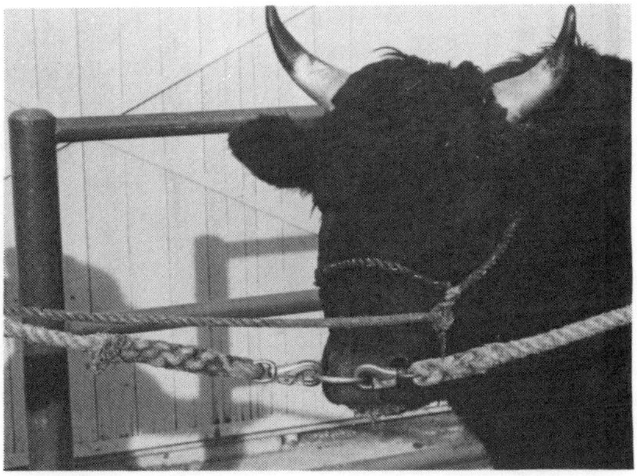

Fig 58. Control of a bull with 2 long lead shanks through the nose ring.

Restraint of a Bull's Head

Use of a hood that completely blindfolds or allows the bull to see only in a ventral direction may aid in handling and moving bad-tempered individuals. A hood can also be used to protect the animal's eyes when it is being cast.

A nose ring is one of the most effective devices for restraint of a bull's head. Nose rings are commonly used on diary bulls and should also be used on beef bulls that have bad temperaments or are handled frequently. The nose ring restrains by causing pain, thus diverting the animal's attention from the handler. A nose ring should not be used as the primary method of head restraint because the nose may be torn, resulting in loss of this important method of restraint. A bull lead and halter should be used for primary restraint of the head for examination and treatment.

When moving bulls, a commercial bull staff may be snapped into the ring to aid control of the head (Fig 57). It is safer to use 2 long lead shanks snapped into the ring; each shank is held by a separate handler on each side of the bull (Fig 58).

When moving "unbroken" cattle where adequate corrals or chute systems are not available, the animal should be "double haltered" with a shank held to each side of the animal for control. An alternate method is to apply a single halter and lariat to a foreleg to reduce forward speed, thus throwing the animal off balance should it attempt to escape.

Restraint of the Body and Limbs

If a chute or stock is not available, uncooperative animals may be examined by securing the head to a strong fence post and applying a

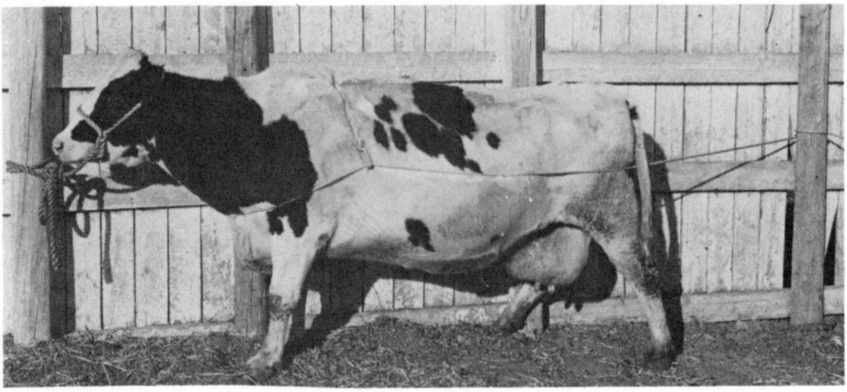

Fig 59. A halter secures the cow's head and a side line keeps the animal against the wall.

nonslip loop around the animal's neck. The standing part of the rope is then brought along the animal's side and tied to another fence post behind the rear legs. After pulling the animal snugly against the fence, the handlers can approach and examine it (Fig 59).

Several methods of restraint may be employed to reduce or prevent kicking:

Tail restraint is applied by grasping the base of the tail firmly with both hands and bending it sharply in a dorsal direction (Fig 60). This causes pain and diverts the animal's attention when its legs, udder or external genitalia are examined and when performing minor operations. Care must be taken to bend the tail at the base because lateral movement may cause pain and fractures of the vertebrae without pro-

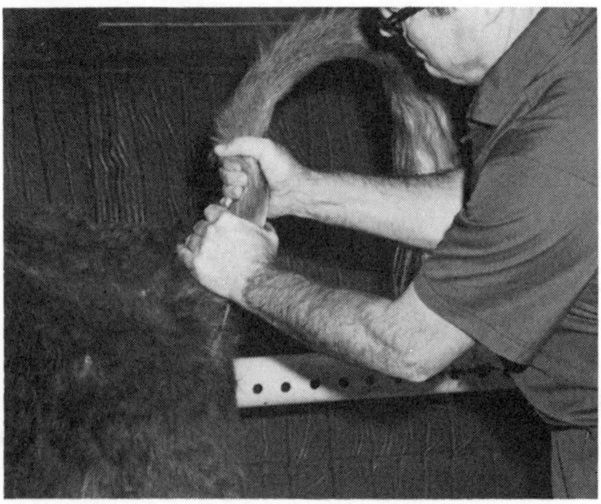

Fig 60. Restraining a beef cow by bending the tail dorsad.

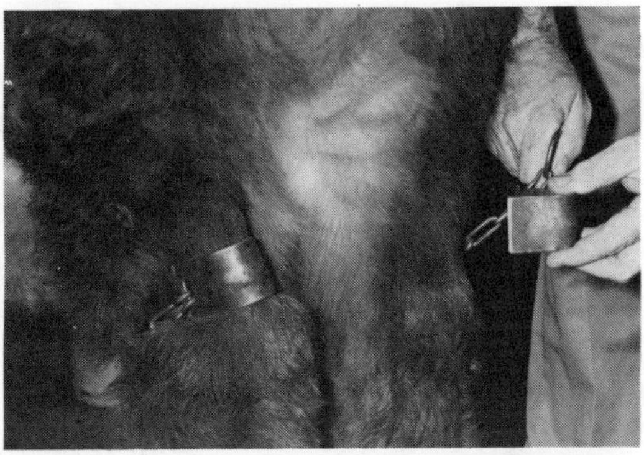

Fig 61. Milking hobbles applied to the rear legs to prevent kicking.

ducing the desired restraint. Tail restraint is often used in conjunction with a bull leader for minor procedures.

Milking hobbles may be applied to the hindlimbs to prevent kicking (Fig 61). This restraint device is used most commonly on dairy cattle to prevent kicking. It is applied over the Achilles tendons, proximal to the hocks, and pulled sufficiently tight to prevent kicking. The device works well when cows are accustomed to its use. The hobbles should be applied cautiously because the hindlegs may easily be injured when animals are not accustomed to this restraint.

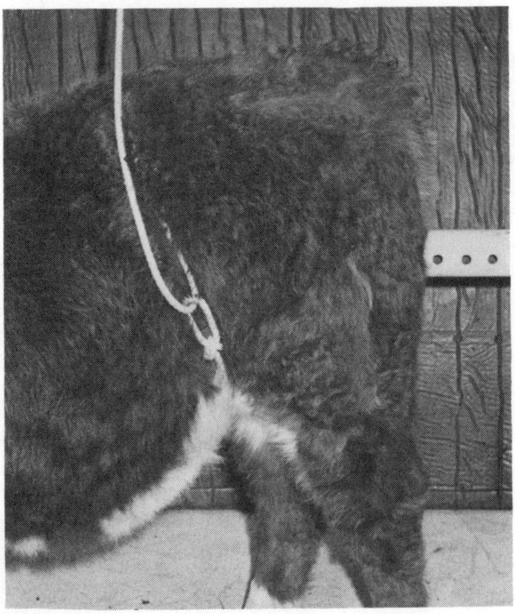

Fig 62. Flank rope used to prevent kicking.

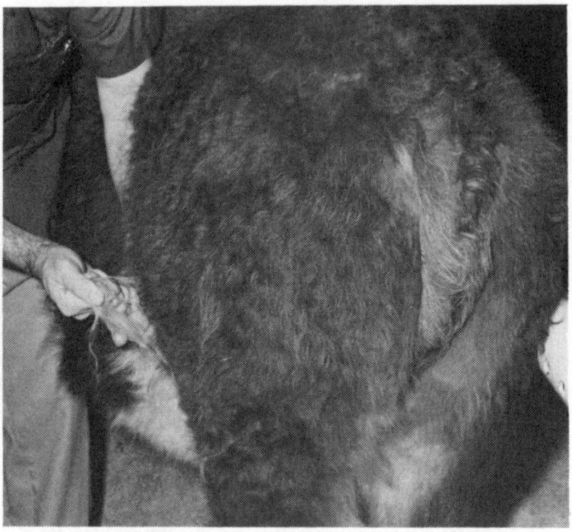

Fig 63. The tail is pulled between the rear legs to restrain the legs.

A *flank rope* is effective for reducing kicking (Fig 62). This involves placing a lariat around the flank area, just cranial to the tuber coxae. The rope is tightened to reduce kicking. Excessive pressure may cause the animal to fall.

For minor examinations of the hindquarters of smaller animals, the *tail* can be *pulled* between the hindquarters and flank (Fig 63).

A *hock twitch* may be applied to a hindlimb just proximal to the point of the hock (Figs 64-66). This restraint device consists of a piece of cotton rope about 20 inches long, with a loop braided in each end. A stick about 12 inches long is threaded through the loops of the rope and twisted until the rope binds the limb tightly. Pressure on the Achilles tendon tends to prevent flexion of the limb and aids in examination of the hindleg.

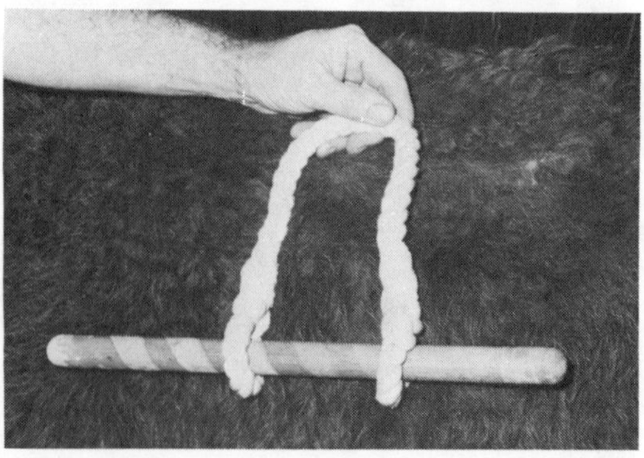

Fig 64. A hock twitch consists of 20 inches of rope with a foot-long stick inserted through the end loops.

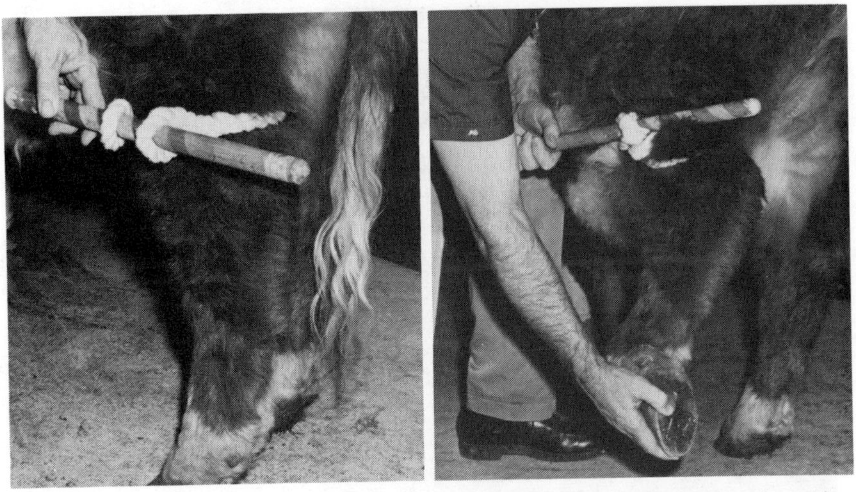

Figs 65, 66. The hock twitch is applied by looping the rope around the hock and inserting the stick through the rope's end loops. The stick is twisted until the rope constricts the hock, allowing examination of the foot.

A *tail rope* effectively controls tail movements and is essential for reduction of contamination during surgical procedures (Fig 67). The switch of the tail is tied to a small (¼-inch diameter) cotton rope with a quick release knot (Weaver's). The opposite end of the rope is then secured to the neck, horns or opposite foreleg of the animal. The rope should *never* be tied to a fixed object because the tail may be lost if the animal escapes the restraint when the tail is still secured.

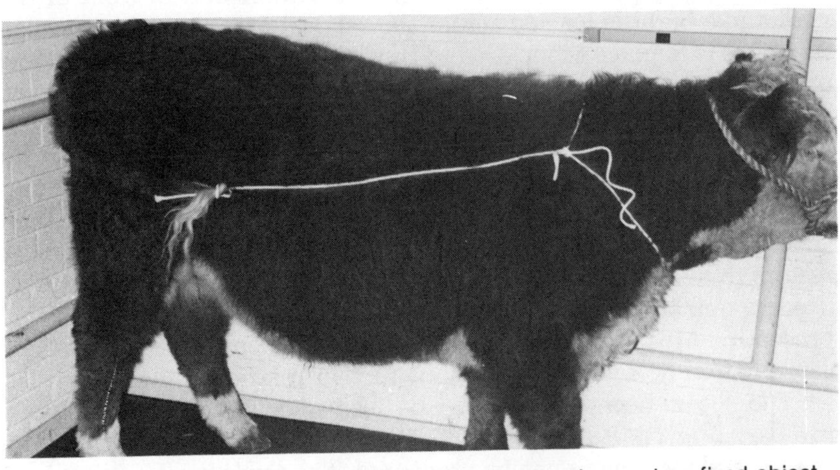

Fig 67. A tail rope should only be tied to the animal and never to a fixed object.

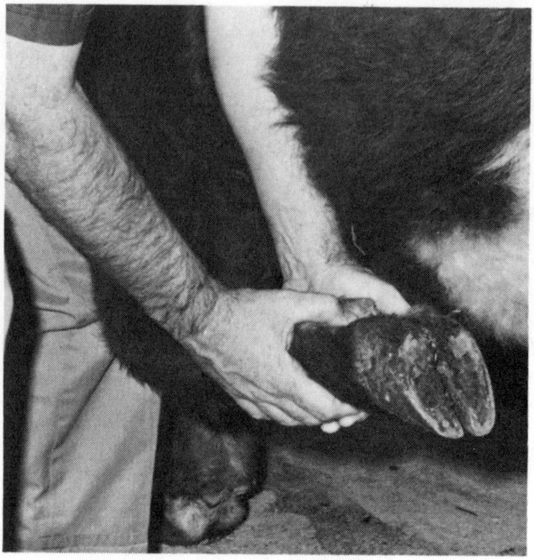

Fig 68. Raising a front foot for examination.

An *electroejaculator* can be used effectively to restrain the hindquarters for minor procedures. Excessive stimulation may cause the animal to "go down" or damage the muscles of the hindquarters.

A front foot is properly picked up by manually flexing the carpus and pulling the limb into a flexed position (Fig 68). Most cattle have a tendency to lie down when a front foot is flexed, however, making this manipulation difficult. A rope can be used to assist examination of a front foot by placing a loop around the pastern (Fig 69). The standing part of the rope is then passed over the withers and in front of the neck and a bight is formed across the vertical part of the rope. An alternative is to place a loop around the forelimb, proximal to the elbow and secure the loop to a beam above the animal. This supports the animal's weight while the operator examines the foot.

The hindfoot of a gentle cow can be raised for examination by grasping the limb at the fetlock, slightly flexing the limb, and supporting the animal's weight with a hand or knee (Fig 70). The limb should be retained in a slightly flexed position because extending it results in kicking and loss of control of the limb. A nose lead can be used to pull the animal's head to the opposite side to facilitate this procedure. Most cattle do not cooperate sufficiently for satisfactory examination of a hindlimb without further restraint.

The "beam hook method" can be used when cows are stanchioned in a barn (Fig 71). For such restraint the animal must be positioned so that lateral movement can be prevented. The cow's head is restrained

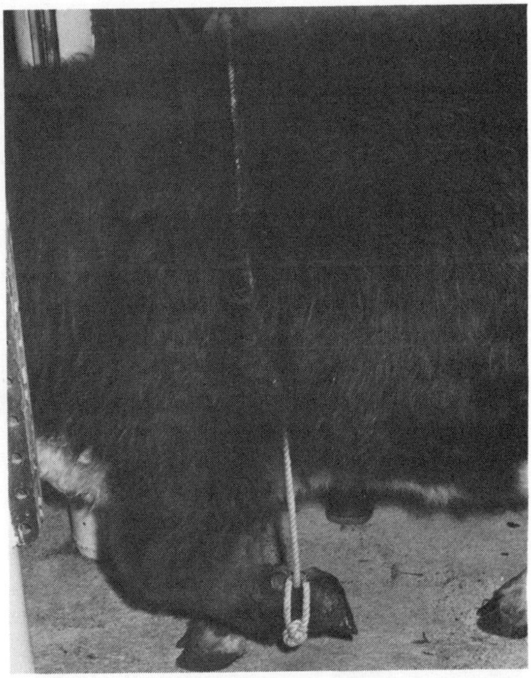

Fig 69. Rope looped over the pastern and led up over the back aids examination of a front foot.

with a nose lead, pulled to the side opposite the leg to be examined, and a beam hook is fastened above and behind the cow. A loop of rope is then placed around the pastern of the hindleg to be lifted. The opposite end is passed through the ring of the beam hook so that the free end goes toward the head of the cow. The standing part of the rope is

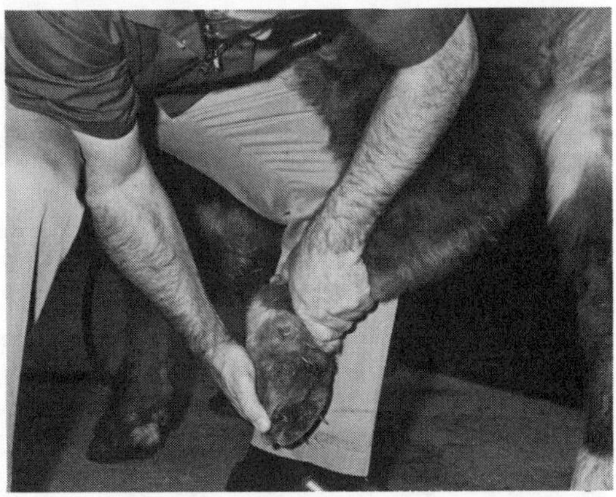

Fig 70. Examining a rear foot by flexing the limb and supporting the animal's weight with the knee.

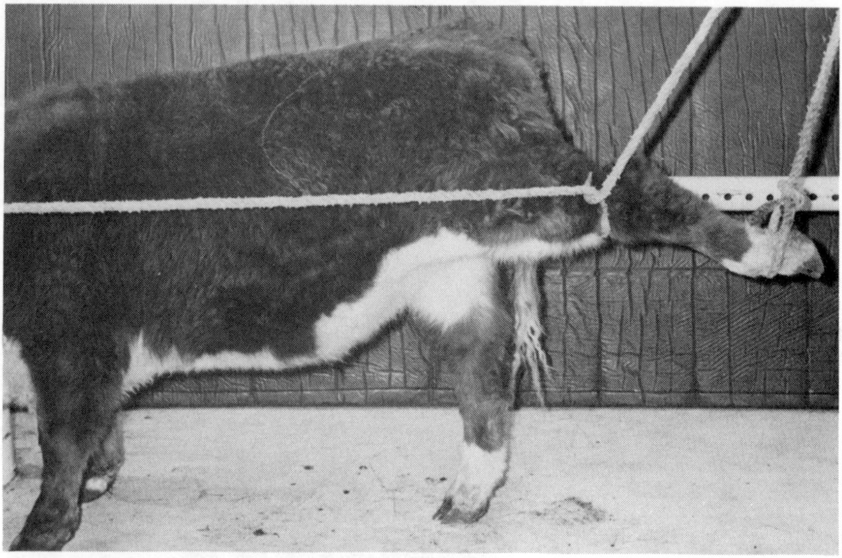

Fig 71. Rope is looped around the pastern and led up over a beam hook and back down to the hock for examination of a rear foot.

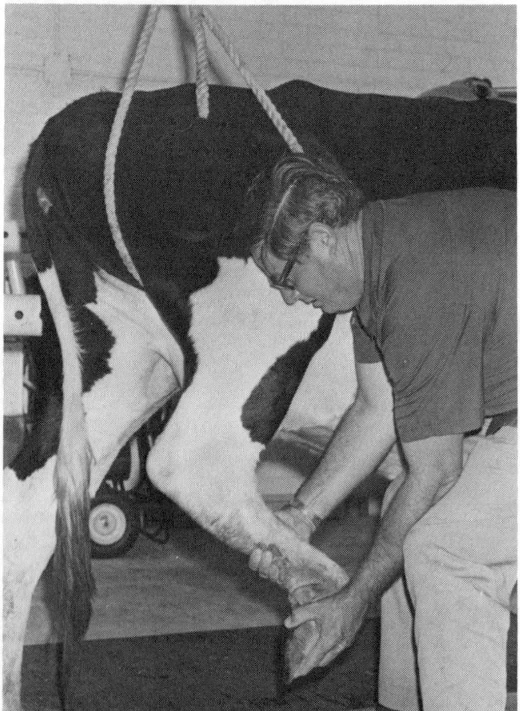

Fig 72. Placing a fixed loop around the proximal rear leg helps support the animal's weight during examination of the foot.

passed medial to the limb to be raised, brought around the limb craniodorsal to the hock, and a bight is formed around the standing part of the rope. The end of the rope is then carried forward and wrapped around a fixed object (stanchion). The foot to be examined is lifted off the ground and the slack in the rope is removed. The animal will struggle when the foot is lifted and care must be taken to prevent its being injured.

Another method of examining a hindfoot of a standing animal involves placing a fixed loop of rope around the limb (Fig 72). The loop is attached to a beam above the animal with a block and tackle to support the animal's weight so that the fetlock can be flexed to examine the foot.

The methods described so far are adequate for examination and treatment of many animals. Others, because of their temperament or the procedure, do not allow adequate examination and/or treatment. Other types of restraint are thus necessary.

There are several methods of casting cattle, each with its advantages and disadvantages. The animal's rumen should be empty when casting to avoid discomfort and possibly death from bloating. Though cattle are relatively easy to cast, care should be taken to select a place on which bruising will be minimal.

The "double half-hitch" method of casting is used commonly to restrain cattle (Figs 73, 74). It involves tying the animal's head in a fixed position with a halter. A loop of cotton rope is placed around the neck and secured with a nonslip knot, such as a bowline. The loop is made large enough to prevent excessive pressure on the trachea during casting. The standing part of the rope is then used to form a half-

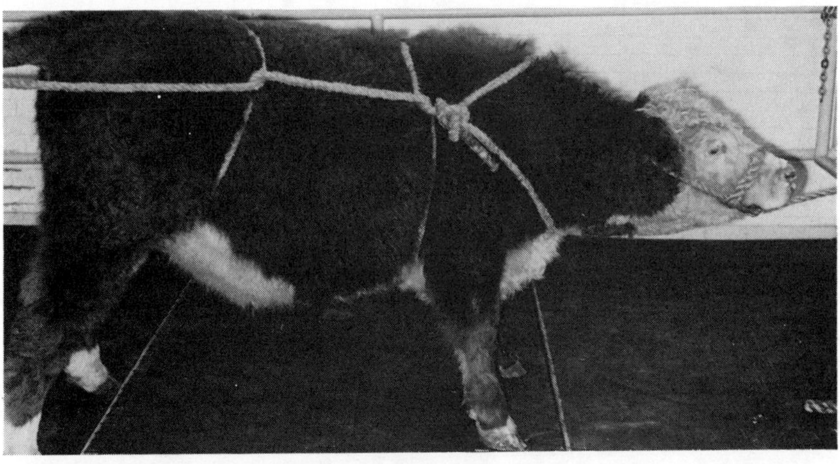

Fig 73. A double half-hitch is used to cast an animal.

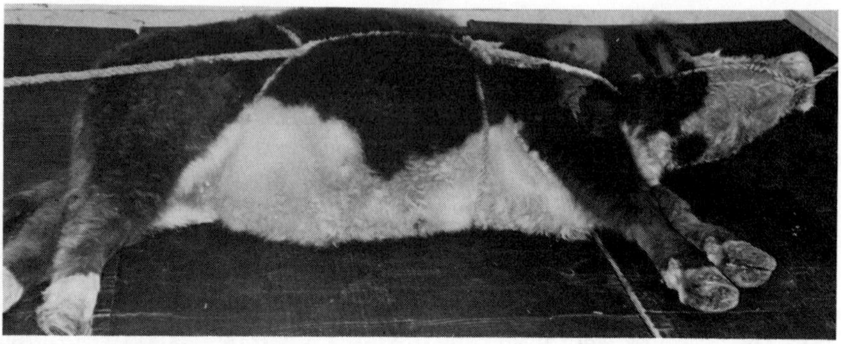

Fig 74. Tightening the half-hitches by pulling caudad causes the animal to lie down.

hitch around the thorax, just caudal to the forelegs. A second half-hitch is made in the flank area, cranial to the tuber coxae. The half-hitches are tightened; pressure exerted on the standing part of the rope causes the animal to lie down. Most cattle are cast relatively easily in this manner. Constant pressure must be kept on the casting rope to keep the animal down; otherwise ropes are applied to the fore- and hindlimbs and secured to fixed objects. This method of casting places pressure on the thorax and mammary vessels of a cow or external genitalia of a bull.

The "Burley method" of casting cattle involves using a 40-foot cotton rope (Figs 75-77). The cow's head is secured by a halter rope to a fixed object. The middle of the rope is placed over the neck of the cow cranial to the withers. The ends of the rope are carried between the front legs and crossed at the sternum. One end is carried up each

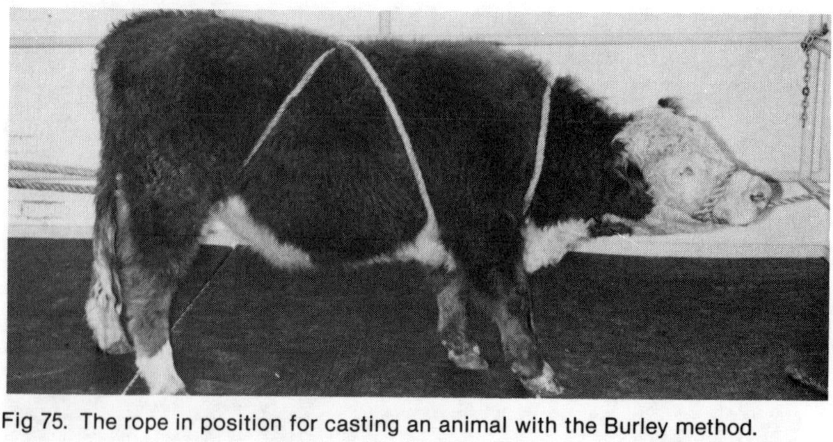

Fig 75. The rope in position for casting an animal with the Burley method.

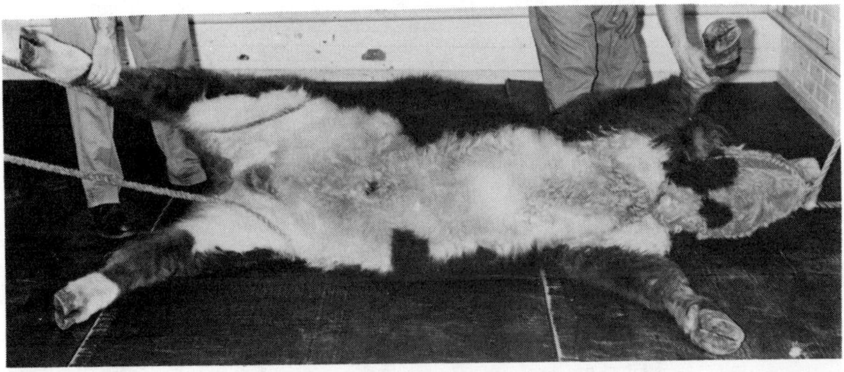

Fig 76. Pulling the ropes caudad causes the animal to fall.

side of the animal's thorax and the 2 ends are crossed again over the back. Each end is then passed down to the flank and caudad on the medial aspect of the hindlimb. When the ends of the ropes are pulled backward simultaneously, the animal falls. The direction of the fall may be controlled by applying pressure to one side with both ends of the casting rope. The upper hindlimb can be tied while flexed by sliding the upper rope along the medial surface of the leg to the pastern, where a loop is formed. The limb is then flexed and tied with one or more "figure 8's" and secured with a half-hitch. The upper forelimb can then be secured to the casting rope by flexing the limb and wrapping a cord around it several times. The cord is attached to the casting rope cranial to the sternum. The animal is turned and the opposite limbs are tied similarly.

The Burley casting method requires application of more pressure on the ropes to cast most animals than the double half-hitch. It has the advantages, however, of exerting less pressure on the thorax and

Fig 77. A loop is tied around the pastern of the flexed rear limb, followed by a figure 8 and a half-hitch.

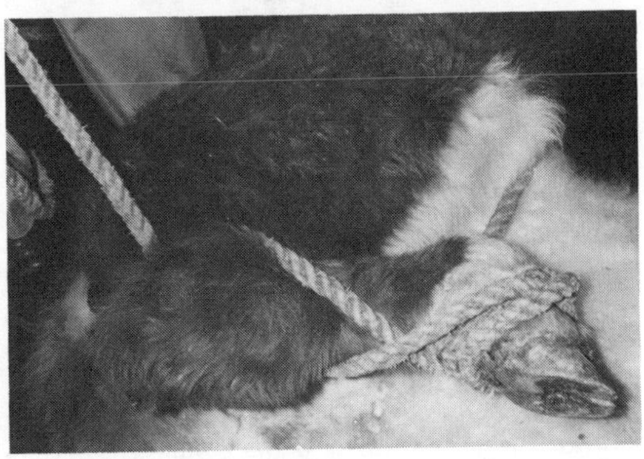

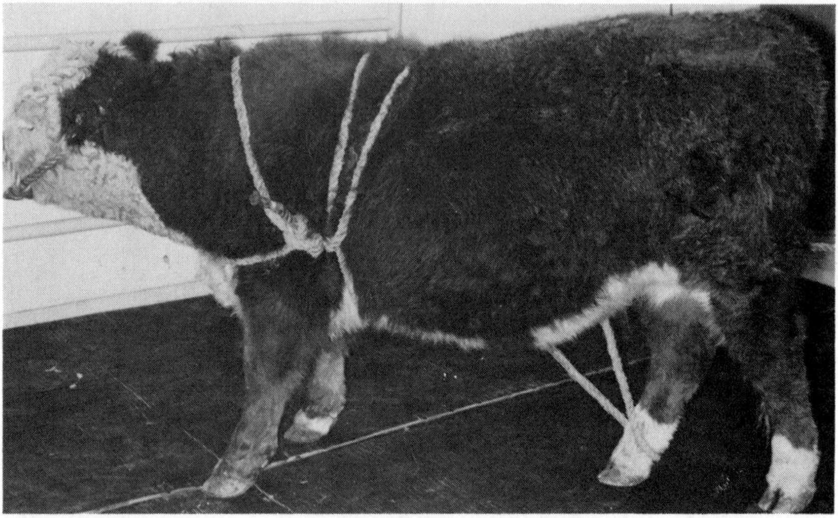

Fig 78. Rope in position for the modified half-hitch method of casting.

avoiding any pressure on the mammary vessels of cows or the external genitalia of bulls.

A modified half-hitch method of casting and completely restraining cattle is especially effective in an open area where only one fixed object is available to restrain the animal (Figs 78-80). It involves tying the animal to a fixed object with a halter shank. A loop of cotton rope is placed around the animal's neck and secured with a nonslip knot (bowline). A half-hitch is then formed around the thorax

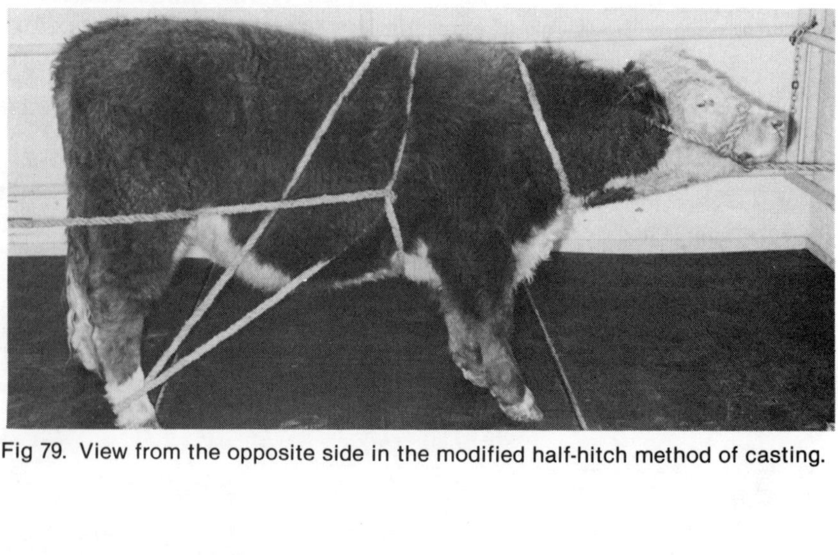

Fig 79. View from the opposite side in the modified half-hitch method of casting.

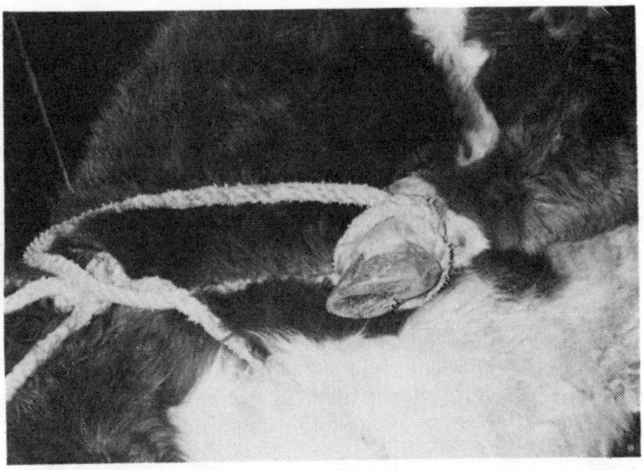

Fig 80. After the ropes are pulled and the animal falls, the rear leg is tied forward.

caudal to the forelegs. The half-hitch is positioned at the level of the left elbow if the animal is to be cast on its right side. The standing part of the rope is passed over the back and mediad to the right hindlimb. The end of the rope is brought forward on the lateral side of the right hindlimb and passed beneath the rope around the thorax. The bight formed by the rope around the hindlimb is then dropped to the pastern distal to the dewclaws. At this point all slack is removed from the entire rope and the right hindfoot is pulled craniad to the thorax. The standing part of the rope is pulled caudad and the animal is cast on its right side. After readjusting the rope to remove all slack,

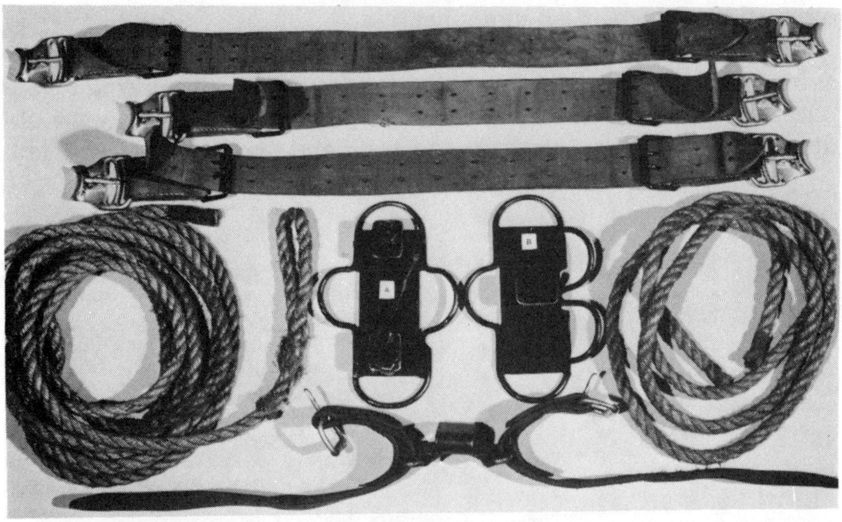

Fig 81. Bovine casting harness consisting of 2 metal plates (A,B), 3 adjustable leather straps, 2 ropes (1 with a loop braided in), and adjustable hobbles for the front legs.

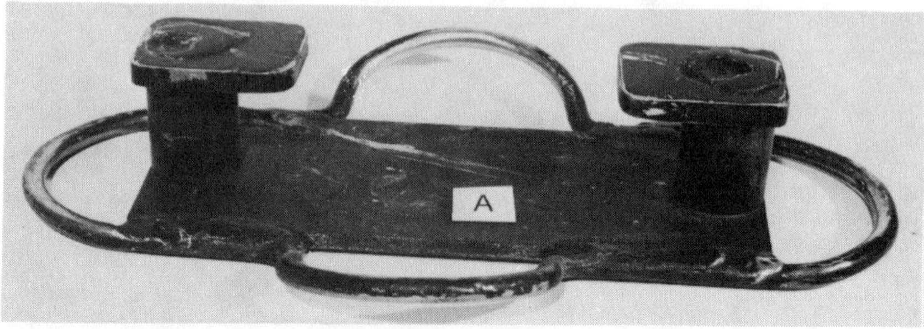

Fig 82. Closeup view of metal plate A.

the standing part of the rope is brought to the left (upper side of the animal) and an overhand knot is placed around the rope on the thorax. The standing part of the rope is then passed around the left hind pastern (from medial to lateral). The left hindlimb is pulled craniad to the thorax and secured with 2 half-hitches on the left hind pastern. The forelimbs are restrained by tying a Tom Fool's knot near the honda of a lariat, placing the knot over the pasterns of both forefeet, and pulling the feet up to the sternum with the standing part of the rope over the withers secured to the honda with a halter tie. When the animal attempts to extend the hindlimbs, the pressure of the standing part of the rope tightens the half-hitch around the thorax, tending to recast the animal. The animal can be cast on the left side by reversing the method of application.

If properly applied, this restraint affords complete control of the animal. It is essential that no slack develop in the rope during its application. If the half-hitch around the thorax slips back to the abdomen, there will be slack in the rope and the restraint will fail.

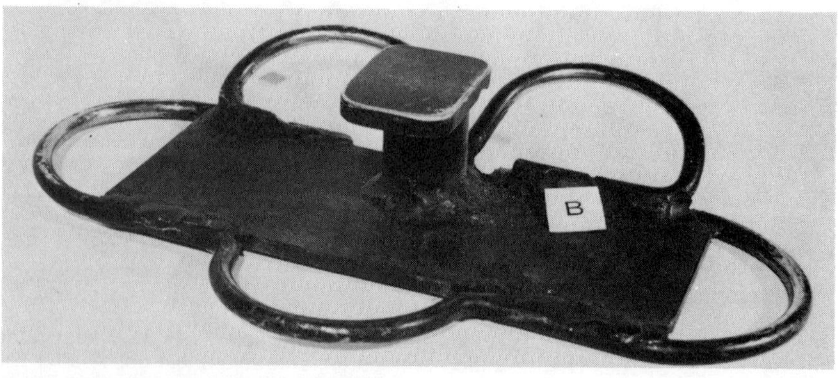

Fig 83. Closeup view of metal plate B.

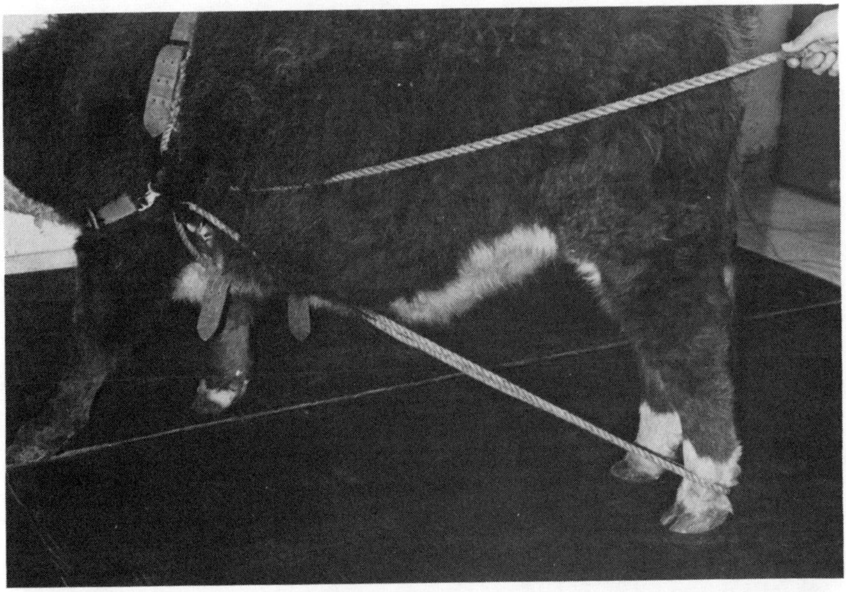

Fig 84. Casting harness in position, with metal plate A on the animal's left side.

Veterinarians and handlers have been reluctant to use this excellent method of restraint because of failures resulting from inadequate attention to keeping the rope taut at all times. I have developed a modification of this method that involves using the principle of the modified half-hitch method, together with a casting harness that eliminates this problem (Figs 81-88). This harness (Lane Manufacturing Co, Denver) includes 2 metal plates; plate A has 4 metal loops and 2 metal pegs and plate B has 5 metal loops and a metal hook. The plates are joined with 3 adjustable leather straps designed so that animals of different sizes can be cast on the right or left side. The leather straps attach to the plates with tackleberry buckles; the length of the straps can be adjusted by "D" buckles. Adjustable hobbles are used to restrain the forelegs after the animal is cast and the hindlegs are tied in the restrained position. Two ropes, one with a loop braided in one end, complete the harness.

The harness is placed on the animal and adjusted so that the plates (A and B) are located over the opposite sides of the thorax at the level of the shoulders. The adjustable leather straps are used to join the metal plates, one over the back caudal to the withers (back strap), one cranial to the forelegs (breast strap), and a third caudal to the forelegs under the sternum (belly strap).

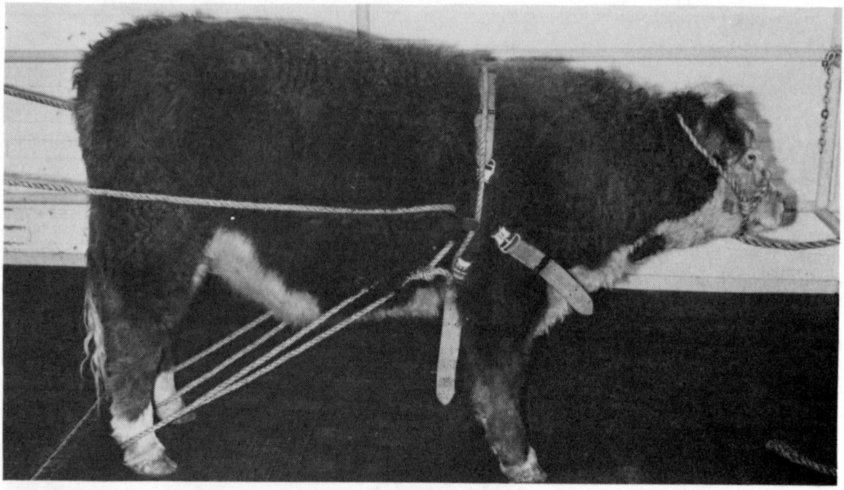

Fig 85. Casting harness in position, with metal plate B on the animal's right side.

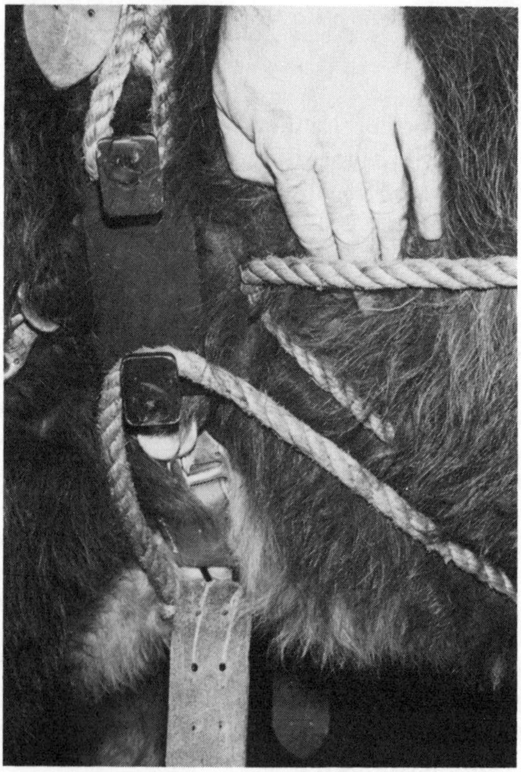

Fig 86. Closeup view of ropes coursing around metal plate A.

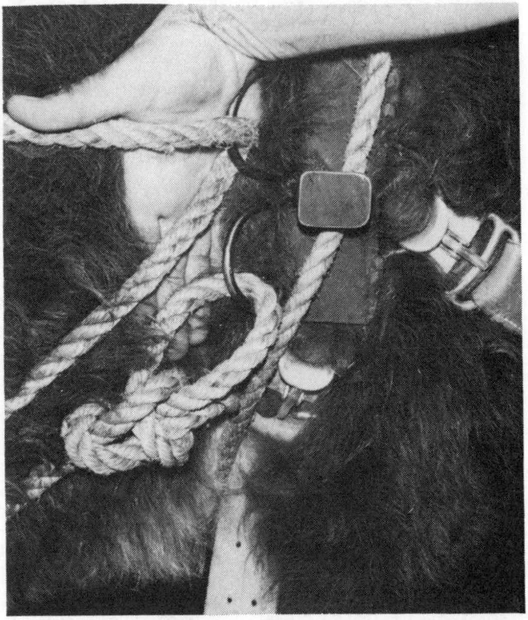

Fig 87. Closeup view of ropes coursing around metal plate B.

The braided loop of rope is secured over the upper peg of plate A and passed over the withers, cranial to the hook in plate B. The rope is then guided under the sternum, behind the forelegs and over the lower peg on plate A, passing from the front toward the back. It is then passed around the pastern of the hindleg on the side of plate A from the inside (medial) out (lateral). The end of the rope is passed through a single metal loop on the back (caudal) side of plate A. The rope is now in position to cast the animal. A second rope is tied (bowline) to 1 of 2 loops on the caudal edge of plate B. This rope is passed from the inside outward, around the pastern of the hindleg on the same side as plate B and through the second loop on the caudal edge of plate B.

After the animal's head is secured to a fixed object, the rope on the side of plate A is pulled caudad to cast the animal (a sleeve is provided on each peg of plate A to facilitate proper tightening of the rope around the thorax). The hindleg is pulled craniad, toward the casting harness, and the animal usually goes down on this side (plate A). Tension is maintained on the rope while it is secured to itself by a halter tie behind plate A. An alternative and usually simpler procedure is to maintain tension on the rope at plate A after the animal is cast and tie the upper hindlimb to plate B after pulling the hindlimb close to the plate and securing the rope with a hitch. The animal is then rolled

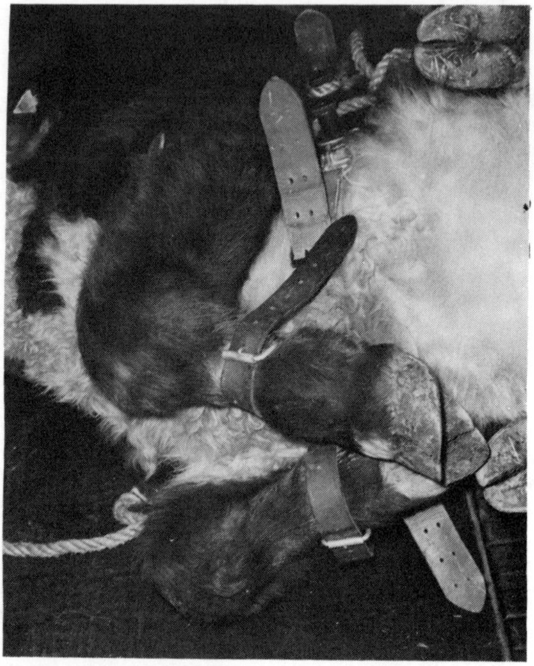

Fig 88. Forelegs restrained with hobbles.

to the opposite side and the rope is tied at plate A as described previously. The forelegs are secured to leather hobbles attached to the belly strap after the animal is cast and the hindlegs are secured. At this time the animal is completely restrained and can be positioned as the handler desires.

This harness can be used to cast animals of all sizes. In mature cattle a sedative or tranquilizer should be given before applying it. With this harness, cattle can be cast on either the left or right side or placed on their back. After the animal is cast and properly tied, the harness keeps the animal in the cast position until it is released.

Restraint of Calves

Small calves can be efficiently restrained by hand by adequately trained handlers. The method is rapid and effective for such procedures as branding, vaccinating and castrating. In "flanking" a calf to lateral recumbency, the handler grasps the animal and stands at its side while facing the calf, reaches over its back, and holds the loose skin at the flank with one hand and places the other one under the forelimb (Figs 89-91). With a knee pressed against the calf's side, the calf is lifted off its feet so it falls to the ground in lateral recumbency.

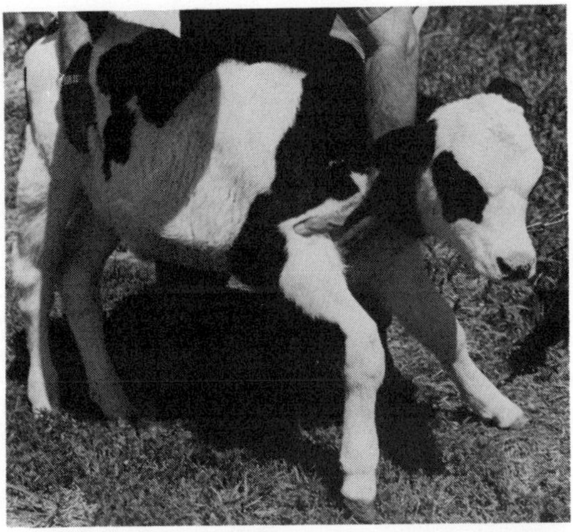

Fig 89. To "flank" a calf to lateral recumbency, the foreleg and skin of the flank are grasped.

The upper foreleg is held in complete flexion and a knee is placed across the calf's neck to keep it restrained. If another assistant is available, this person can aid in restraining the calf by sitting on the ground behind the animal and holding the upper hindleg and extending the lower hindleg forward by placing a foot on the Achilles tendon above the hock and applying enough pressure to prevent kicking (Fig 92).

Another method of casting a calf is to grasp its flank and foreleg nearest to the handler. By a rapid, coordinated movement, the calf is lifted so it falls on the opposite side. The operator then steps across

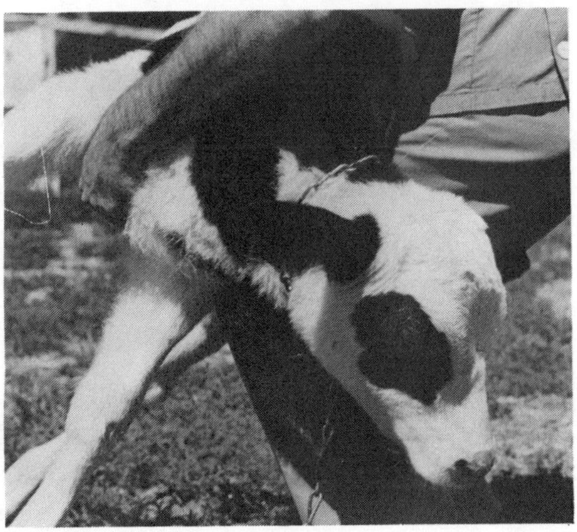

Fig 90. The operator's knees are used to raise the animal as it is flopped onto its side.

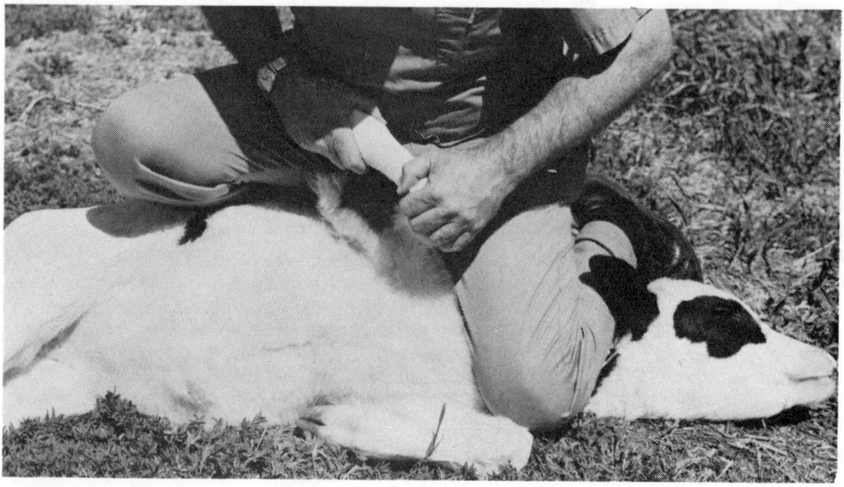

Fig 91. The operator's knee is placed on the calf's neck as the foreleg is held.

the calf, placing his knee over the calf's neck, and maintains the upper forelimb in a flexed position (Figs 93-96).

In a third method of laying a calf on its side, the halter shank is passed around the hindlimb from inside out, proximal to the hock. The end of the shank is then passed around the standing part of the rope and the hindlimb is pulled craniad. This pulls the head to the same side, causing the calf to lose its balance (Figs 97, 98). After a calf is cast, it can be "hog tied" by placing a loop of rope around a forelimb above the fetlock and pulling the hindlimbs craniad to the

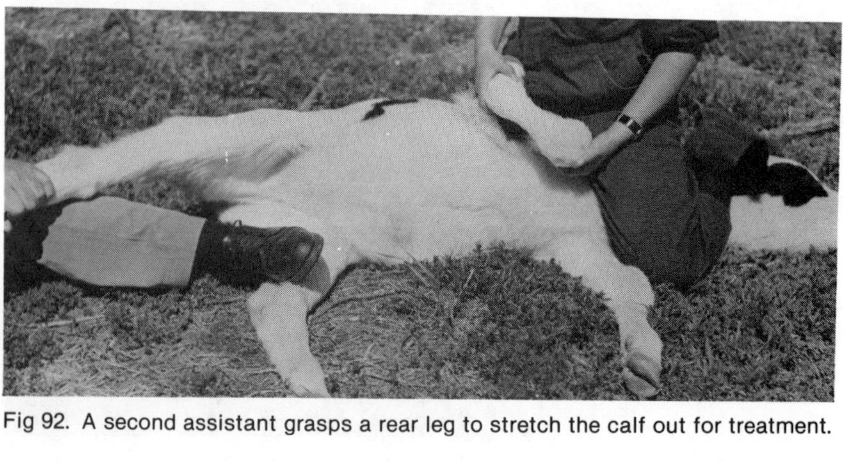

Fig 92. A second assistant grasps a rear leg to stretch the calf out for treatment.

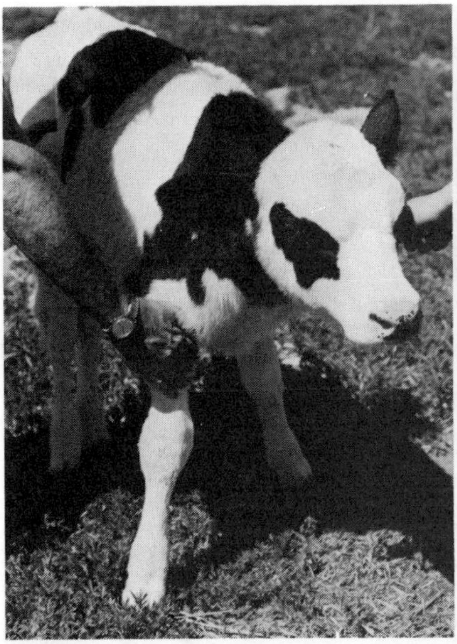
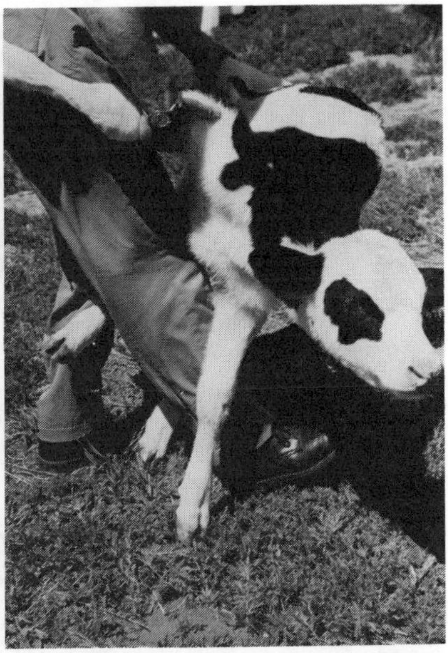

Figs 93, 94. Position to "flank" a calf from the near side is similar to that for flanking on the far side. The operator steps forward as the calf is lifted.

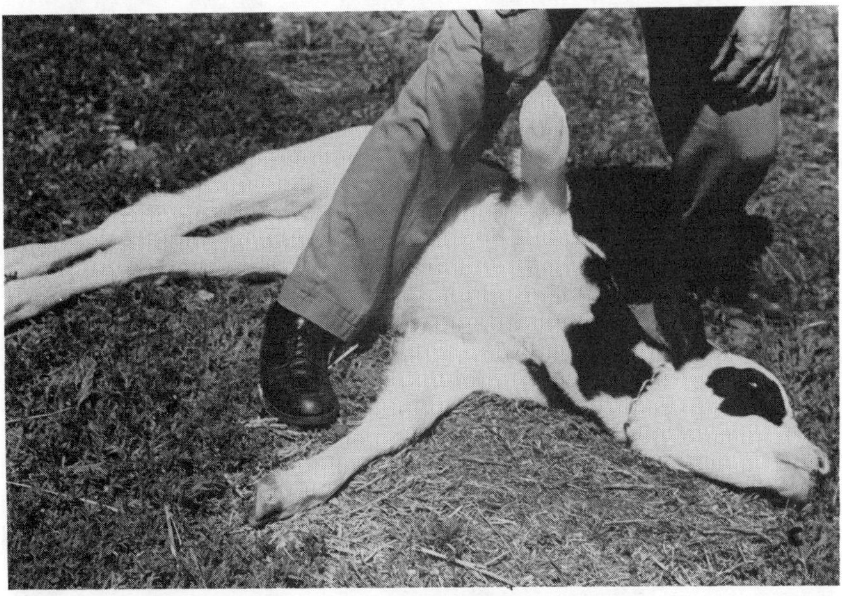

Fig 95. The operator's left leg is thrown over the calf as it falls and the foreleg is held.

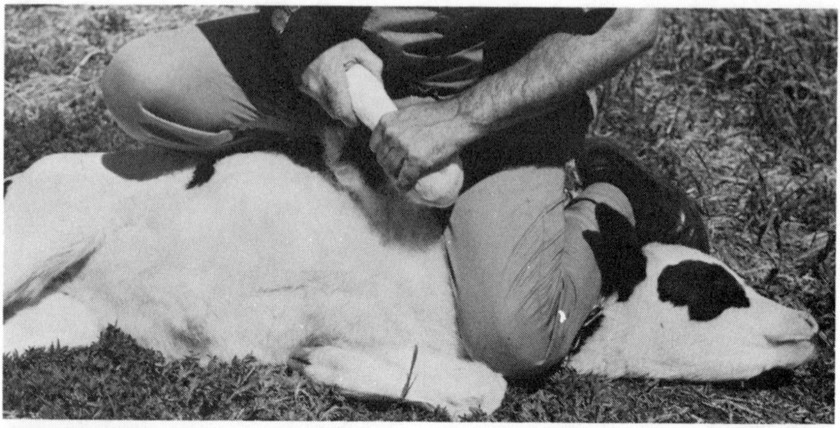

Fig 96. The knee is placed on the calf's neck while the foreleg is held.

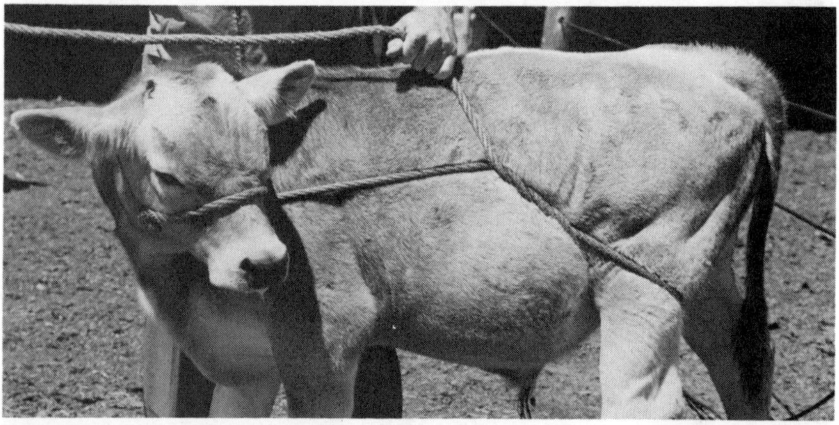

Fig 97. A halter shank is looped around the hindlimb to pull it forward.

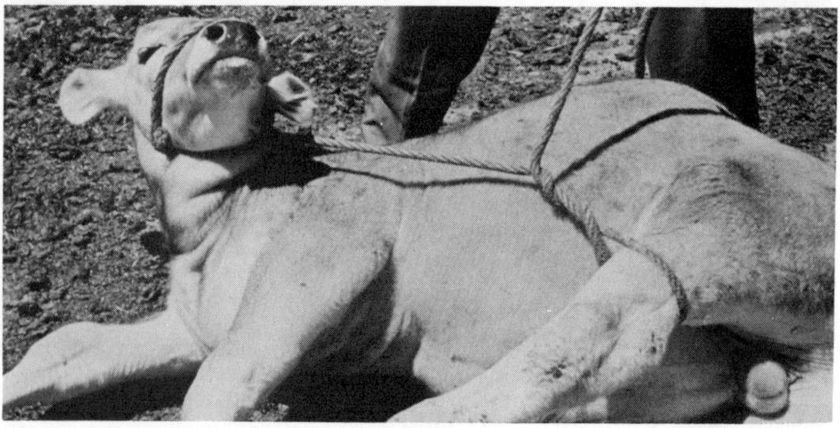

Fig 98. Tightening the rope pulls the head toward the rear, causing the calf to fall.

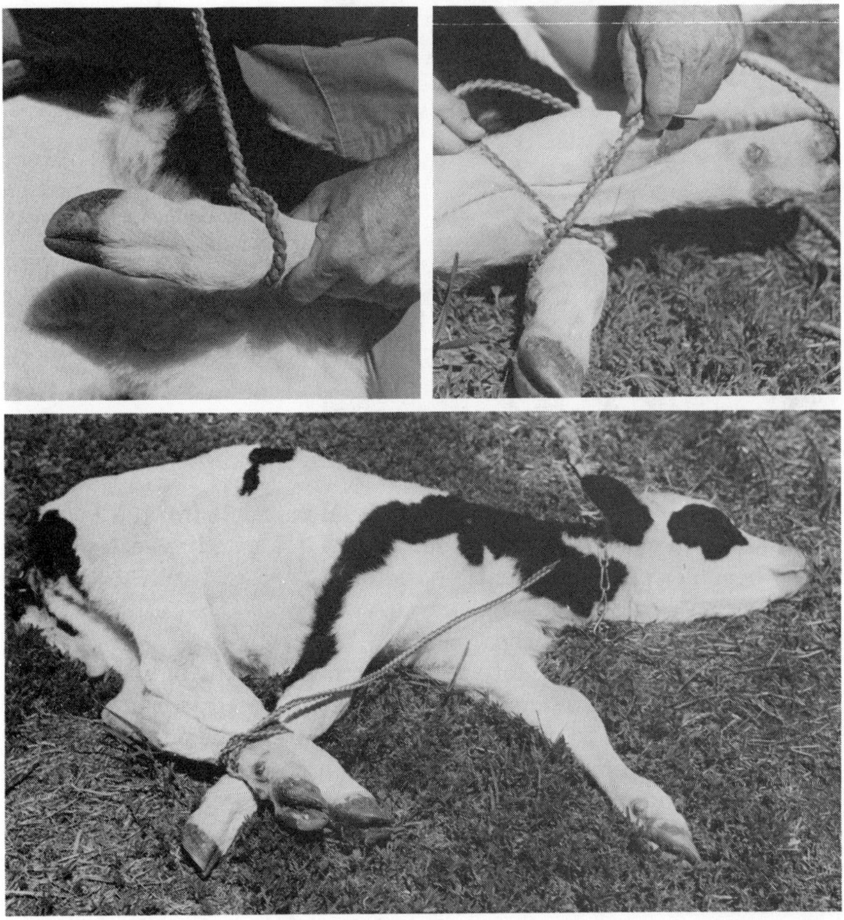

Figs 99-101. Hog tying. First, a loop is made proximal to the front fetlock. The front leg is then brought back to the rear legs and all are secured with loops around them. A half-hitch secures the hog-tied calf.

forelimb. One or 2 loops are then passed around the forelimb and both hindlimbs proximal to the fetlocks, followed by 1 or 2 half-hitches (Figs 99-101). "Hog tying" adult animals may cause injuries.

Restraint of Sheep
by K. Faler and K. Faler

Sheep do not bite, strike or kick. Their only method of defense is running away or butting. Handlers must be steady, calm and patient, as excited sheep may exhaust themselves running, suffer from hyperthermia (especially if they are heavily wooled and it is a hot day), or

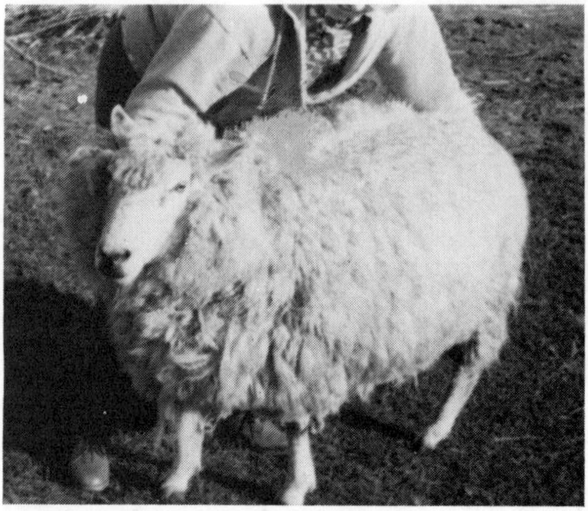

Fig 102. Sheep can be restrained with one arm placed under the chin and the other behind the animal's rump.

injure themselves. They have strong social instincts (form a flock); a single sheep in a pen is harder to catch than if left with several others. Sheep become tame with gentle handling.

Catching and Moving Sheep

Drive a group of sheep into a pen, narrow alleyway or chute before attempting to single one out. Most domestic sheep will not jump a barrier over 1.2 m (4 ft) high. Once the sheep are in the pen, an individual can be singled out by guiding it into a corner with a wooden or wire panel, or by calmly entering the group and catching the selected one as it flees past, with an arm under the chin or around the breast (Fig 102). A shepherd's crook can be used to pull an individual from a group by snaring it above the hock. Never grab a sheep by its wool or

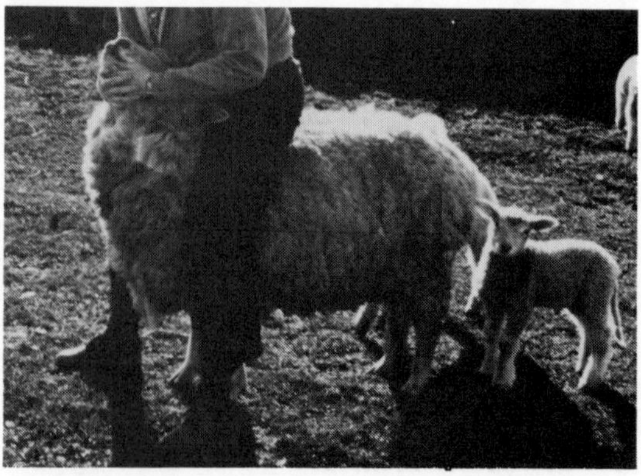

Fig 103. Sheep restrained for administration of oral medication.

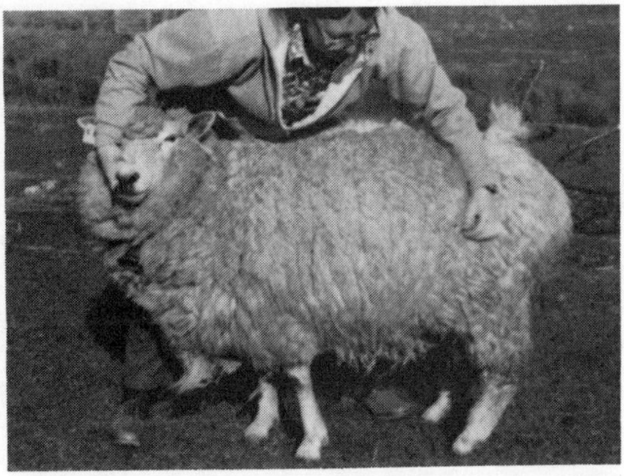

Fig 104. In the first step in setting up a sheep, the animal is pulled toward the operator by its muzzle and flank.

skin as the wool may pull out, the skin may tear, or the underlying tissue may be bruised.

Sheep may be led by grasping under the chin and around the tail and guiding the animal in the desired direction. Sheep can be taught to lead, using a halter or collar.

Restraint of Adult Sheep

Only 2 basic methods of restraint are used for adult sheep. The animal can be straddled at the shoulder, between the handler's legs, and the chin restrained in one hand for medication with a balling gun or drench (Fig 103). The mouth can be opened by pressing a thumb in the interdental space (behind the incisors, where the bit would rest in a horse's mouth). To limit motion, as a tall sheep may give the operator an unexpected ride, back the sheep into a corner before straddling it.

For examination of the oral cavity, udder, prepuce and testes or to trim the hooves, the sheep is set up on its rump, with all 4 feet in the air, by unbalancing it and rolling it over the handler's knee. It is not lifted off the ground, as the object is to unbalance the animal rather than "muscling" it into position. To set up the sheep, stand at the animal's side, grasping the web of the flank in one hand and the muzzle with the other (Fig 104). Bend the sheep's head backward, beside the neck, while pulling up and toward yourself with the flank. A bent knee can be used as a lever to help roll the sheep over (Fig 105). The most important thing is to bend the head back as far as you can, rather than lifting it up and over the back. Improper technic results in the struggling sheep pivoting around the handler. Rather than bending its neck, small sheep can be set up by reaching over the back and under the animal's chest to grasp the front leg nearest the

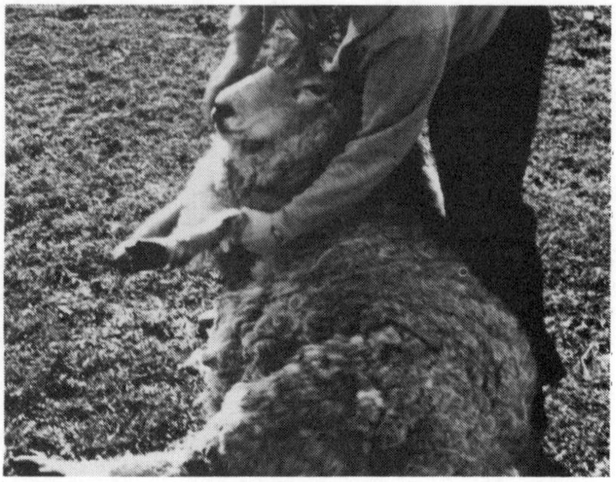

Fig 105. The sheep is rolled onto its side and set up, using the knee as a lever.

handler. The leg is used as a handle (holding it above the knee) to rotate the sheep up onto its rump.

Once the sheep is set up, it is held between the handler's slightly spread knees (sheep's withers) and feet (sheep's rump) and slumped to one side (60° off vertical). The front legs are held to stabilize the position and prevent flailing. The sheep's head may be tucked under one of the handler's arms for jugular venipuncture (Fig 106). Most sheep are extremely docile and quiet once they are set up.

Tying 3 feet together with a thong or string after the sheep is set up allows immobilization in recumbency for most short procedures.

Head-locking systems, ranging from a pole set in the ground with a strap around the top to table-top stanchions, are useful when help is limited.

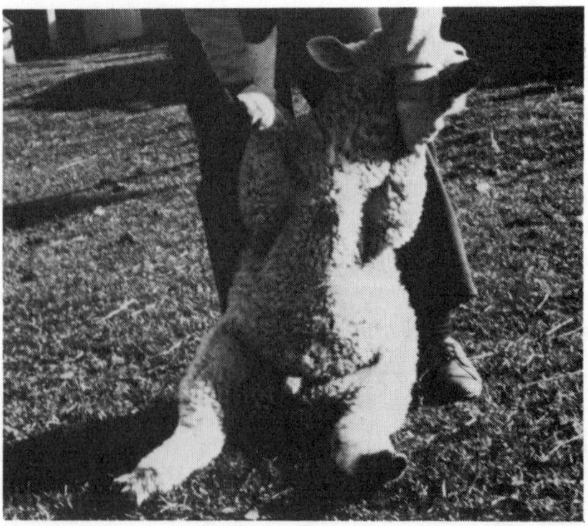

Fig 106. The sheep's head can be tucked under an arm for jugular venipuncture.

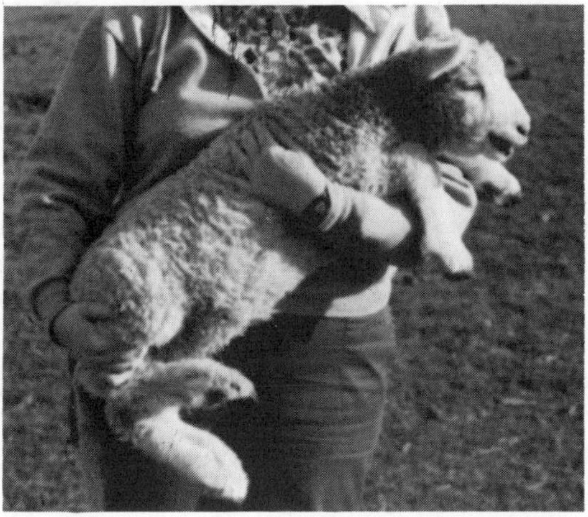

Fig 107. A lamb is supported by an arm under the rump and another under the chest.

Restraint of Lambs

Lambs are carried cradled next to the handler's chest, with one arm around the animal's breast and another around its tail (Fig 107). Lambs are presented for tail docking and/or castration by placing them on their back and grasping one front leg and one rear leg in each hand (Fig 108). This can be done over the handler's extended knee or while sitting.

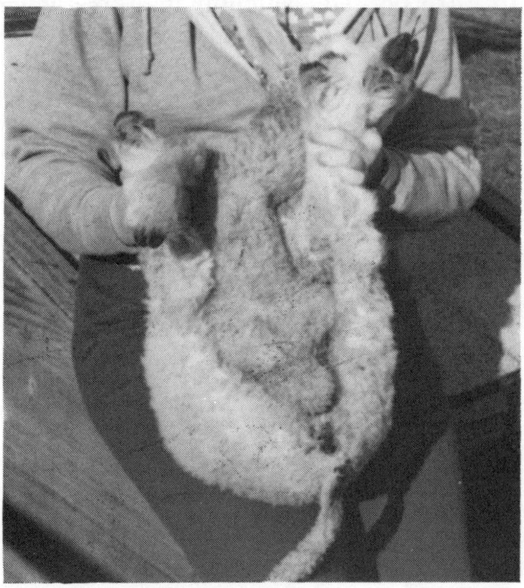

Fig 108. Lamb properly restrained for castration or tail docking.

Restraint of Swine
by K. Faler and K. Faler

The main danger of swine is their bite. Even baby pigs have sharp, pointed teeth that can inflict damage. Adult boars have tusks formed from elongated canine teeth. Due to their poor vision, pigs try to force their way through any small opening, even if it is between the handler's legs. Some tame pigs can be handled with a minimum of restraint, soft talk and gentle scratching of the skin. However, swine can move swiftly and the animal's head should always be watched as they can turn and bite suddenly.

Individual behavior varies, but swine generally are unpredictable. It is best not to enter a pen without a readily accessible escape route. Sows with baby pigs and boars are especially aggressive. The streamlined body and tightly adhered skin of swine offer no handholds for grasping, except the legs. They are especially slippery when wet.

Swine can become stressed or hyperthermic (especially on a hot day) if chased or excited or if they struggle excessively when restrained. A calm, purposeful approach should be used during capture and the rectal temperature monitored on a restrained animal for signs of hyperthermia.

A hog that is rushing toward a handler may be discouraged by slapping it on the nose with a board or cane (pain can, however, cause further aggression); do not use a hand or foot, as the pig may bite it.

Most pigs squeal loudly in protest when they are restrained, even when they are not in discomfort. Squealing may excite other pigs, especially sows, but there is no physical way to stop it.

Never mix pigs of various sizes or add anesthetized or bleeding pigs to pens with normal animals, as they may be attacked by their penmates.

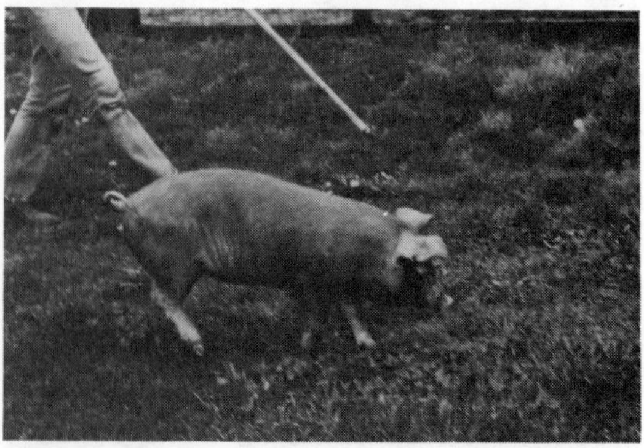

Fig 109. Pig being driven with a cane.

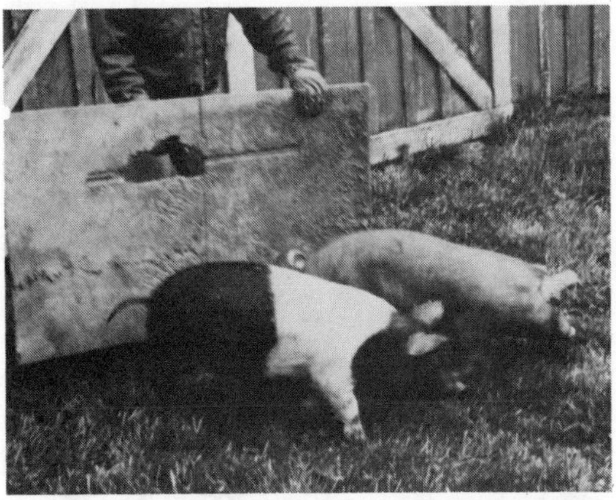

Fig 110. Wooden panel being used to drive swine.

Moving Pigs

Pigs are very stubborn and cannot be led, as they usually move in the direction opposite from that desired by the handler. Swine should be handled in small pens or chutes. Trained pigs can be moved by using a wooden cane to tap them on the side of the head, turning them away from the cane (Fig 109).

A wood or wire panel is a good way to guide pigs or to pin them in a corner for closer examination. Keep the shield close to the floor or ground and tilt the bottom toward the pig so it cannot get its snout under the bottom and toss the barrier aside (Fig 110).

A pig will back away from a bucket or blindfold placed over its head. This behavior can be used to guide the pig backwards in the desired direction. One hand or a second person pulling on the tail is an additional help while backing the animal (Fig 111).

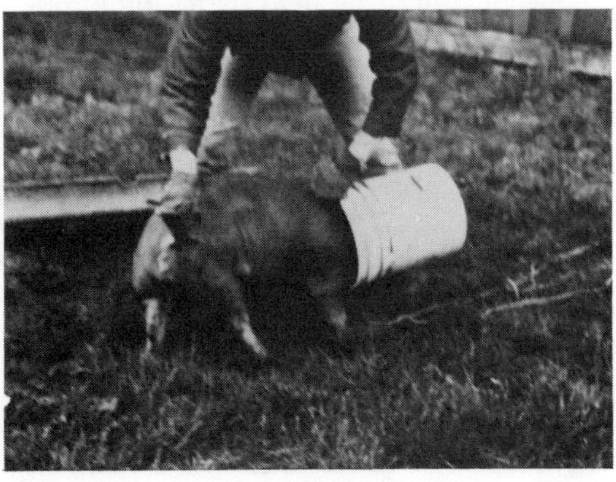

Fig 111. Pig restrained with a bucket over the head and hand on the tail.

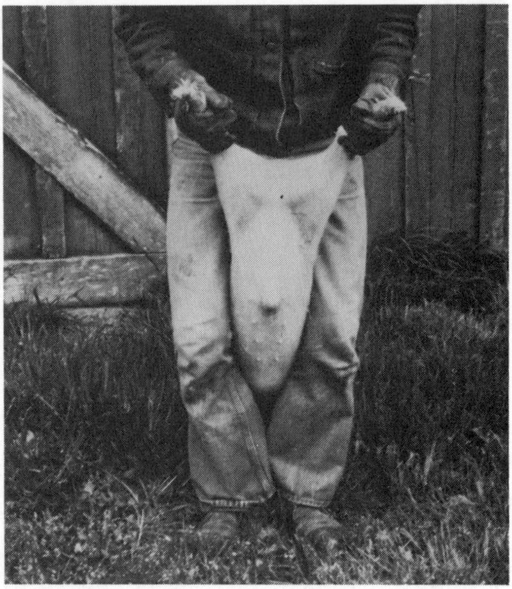

Fig 112. Pig held upside down and between the operator's knees.

Stationary Restraint

Small to medium-sized pigs (under 100 lb) are often restrained by holding them up by their front or rear legs by the standing handler. The pig's back or head can be held between the handler's knees, depending on the amount of struggling, for additional control (Fig 112). The pig can be held facing either direction but keep in mind that it may be able to bite. If the pig is held so that its feet touch the ground, it will struggle less and it is not so tiring for the handler, as the pig's legs support some of its weight. The rear legs should be held above the hocks and care taken not to twist the pig's legs.

Swine cannot be held by a single rope around their necks, as their response to such restraint is to back up and evade the noose. How-

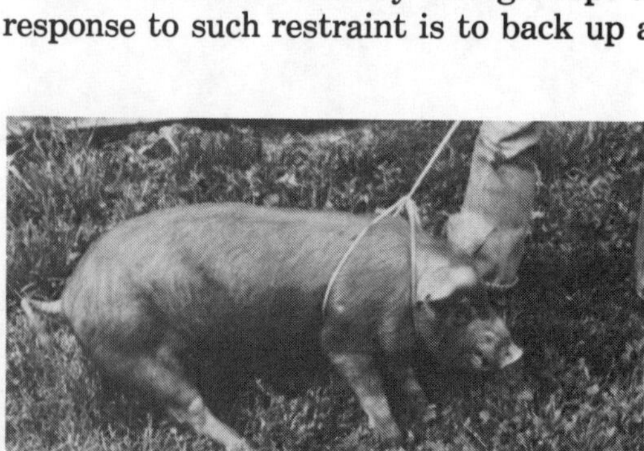

Fig 113. A half-hitch is combined with a loop around the pig's neck to form a harness.

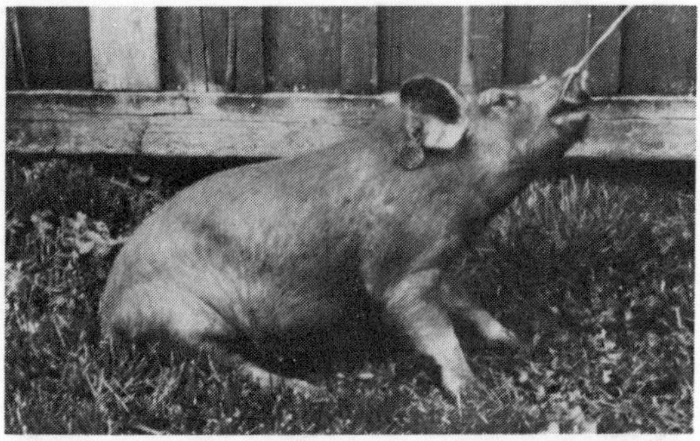

Fig 114. Pigs reflexively back up when a rope is thrown over their snout.

ever, a loop over the head can be combined with a half-hitch behind the front legs to form a harness that can be used to tie up or hold a pig (Fig 113). The first loop is applied over the neck without tightening it (or the pig will back up). The half-hitch is threaded around the pig or it is preformed and the pig encouraged to step through it. The handler should stand behind and to the side of the pig to cause it to move forward.

The snout rope or snare is used for pigs as the halter is for horses. It consists of a loop of 1/8- to 1/2-inch rope or cable placed behind the canine teeth and around the maxilla (snout). The pig automatically pulls back as the rope tightens and can be held or tied up for examination or treatment (Fig 114). Once the noose is tightened around the snout, constant pressure must be maintained on the end of the rope to prevent it from slipping out from behind the canine teeth. The handler stands directly in front of the pig. This technic does not usually work for baby pigs. Snout ropes should not be left on for longer than 15 minutes, as they act as a tourniquet, cutting off the blood supply to the snout. Watch carefully that the animal does not chew through the rope while it is being restrained or that the rope does not slacken.

To place the snare around the snout, form a loop (through a honda or permanent eye on the end of the rope) and hold it in both hands. Approach from the side and rear of a quiet or confined animal. In many cases, the pig will open its mouth to chew on the rope, which is then tightened over the snout. However, pigs that have previously been restrained by this method may need to have the snare forced into the mouth by holding each side of the loop and "sawing" it back and forth while pulling toward the tail. If the pig moves during this process, the handler must move with it.

"Hog tongs," a large, blunted, pincer-like instrument, can be used behind the ears to temporarily immobilize the head and snare the snout of a resisting pig by causing it to squeal and open its mouth.

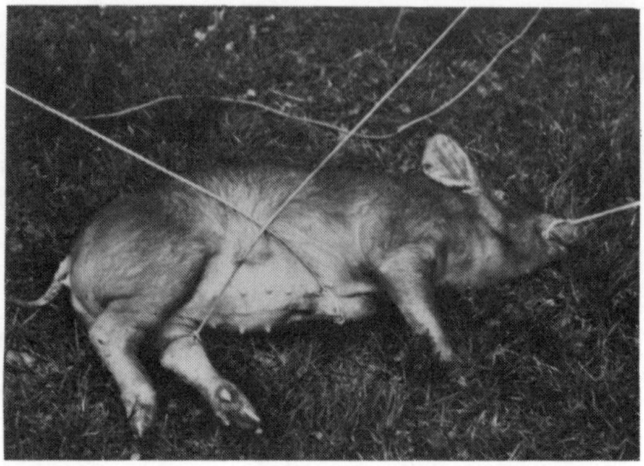

Fig 115. Pig restrained in lateral recumbency with a rope on the snout and ropes on the front and rear legs next to the ground.

The tongs are removed once the snare is in place. Tongs cannot be used effectively on pigs over 100 lb due to their thick neck.

A variety of snares with handles are available to make catching pigs easier and to lessen the danger by allowing distance between the handler and the pig. These snares consist of a loop, with the tail of the rope threaded through a tube. Once the loop is around the snout, it is tightened against the end of the tube (some types have a locking mechanism).

Casting Swine

A small pig may be laid on its side by reaching under its abdomen and pulling the legs farthest from the handler out from under the animal. This can also be done with ropes around one rear and one front leg; the free ends are passed across the abdomen and over the back (Fig 115). The legs should be tied together once the pig is on its side.

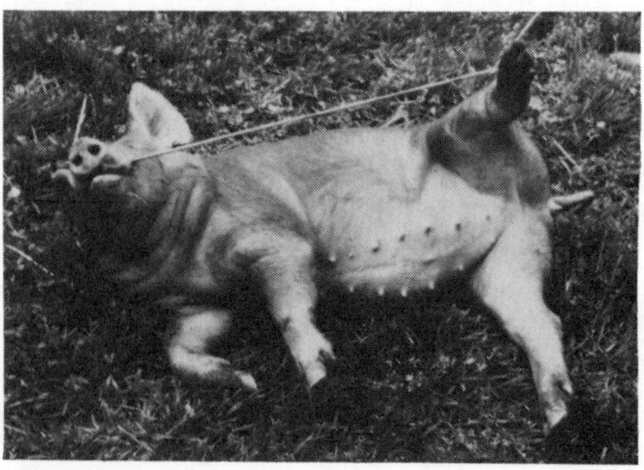

Fig 116. Pig restrained for castration with a snout rope led back to a half-hitch around the rear leg.

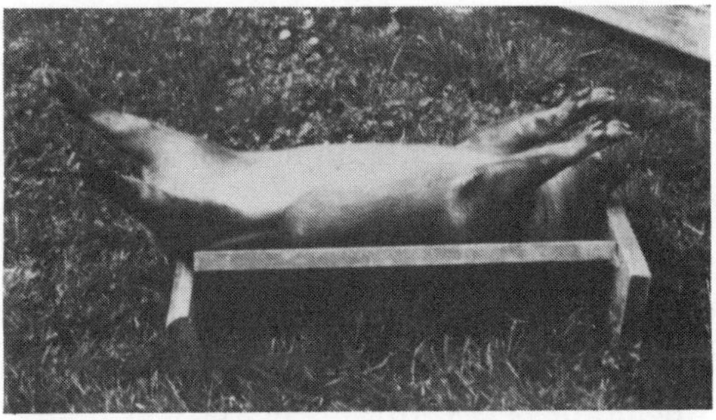

Fig 117. Pig restrained in dorsal recumbency in a trough.

A pig restrained with a snout snare may be stretched out by tying another rope above both the hocks and pulling the rear feet back, fixing the pig between the 2 ropes on its side or back. A "bar hobble" or "hog shackle" works well for this and spreads the rear legs for castration or other procedures. It consists of 2 loops of chain on each end of a bar. Each loop is placed above a hock and tightened with a common rope. Most pigs do not object to having their feet lifted to apply the chains.

A common method of casting pigs is to take the snout rope back along the animal's side, keeping constant tension on it, and make a half-hitch above a hock. Pulling on the end of the rope causes the pig to lie down on its side, with the half-hitch up (Fig 116). This is a good position for castration.

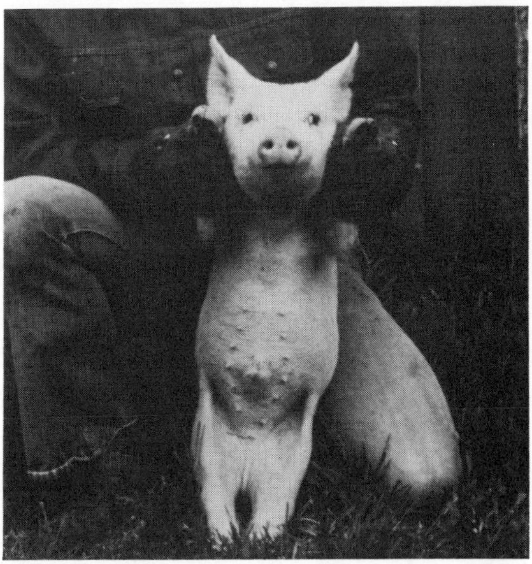

Fig 118. Baby pig restrained between operator's knees.

For further restraint once the pig is cast, the legs may be trussed together or a person may kneel on the pig's neck or back.

Various types of troughs or cradles are used to hold pigs on their backs for surgery, examination and venipuncture (Fig 117). A bar or rope over the snout is used to hold the head down and the legs are tied or strapped down. Squeeze chutes or cages are used for bigger swine.

Restraint of Baby Pigs

Baby pigs should be captured with a minimum of chasing. They should be seized from behind by gripping them over the shoulder or by one or both rear legs. They are lifted up by both hind legs or scooped up with a hand under the animal's chest and over its back. Never lift them by a tail or ear only. They can be restrained between the knees of a sitting handler (Fig 118). Always restrain the sow before handling its babies because their squeals can make the sow very aggressive. Holding baby pigs with their heads down often quiets them.

Recommended Reading for Restraint of Animals

1. Leahy and Burrow: *Restraint of Animals.* Cornell Campus Store, Ithaca, NY, 1953.
2. Fowler: *Restraint and Handling of Wild and Domestic Animals.* Iowa State Univ Press, Ames, 1978.

3

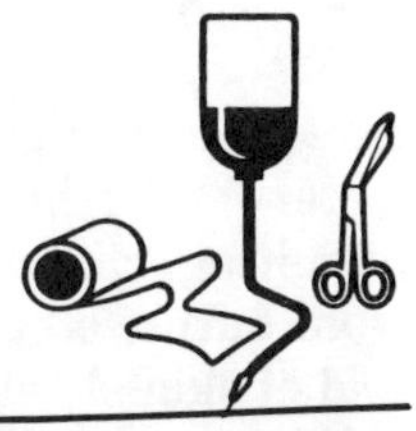

supportive care

K. FALER & K. FALER

FLUID THERAPY

Animals are 55-67% water by weight. The water is held within cells, between cells and in body cavities, and circulates in the blood, lymph and cerebrospinal fluid. Water is a solvent for chemicals, enters into chemical reactions, is involved in temperature regulation, acts as a lubricant and is a transport medium for nutrients and waste products. When more water is lost from the body than is taken in, the animal becomes dehydrated and many necessary functions are interrupted. If enough water is lost, the animal dies. Therefore, replacing lost fluid, maintaining hydration and monitoring fluid balance are all important aspects of health care.

Determining Degree of Dehydration

There are several methods to estimate how much fluid an animal has lost, and often more than one is used in the final assessment.

History

When the patient's history is taken, the frequency of urination, vomiting and/or diarrhea should be noted and the amount estimated. Fever, heat, stress, severe sneezing or coughing, neglect of stall-fed livestock or drought conditions can all contribute to dehydration and should be noted on the medical record.

Skin Fold Pinch

During physical examination, the percent dehydration can be estimated by the "4-6-8" rule. Loss of 4% of the body water is not evident clinically but is assumed if the animal has not taken in food or water for 24 hours, or if there has been water loss by any means (vomiting, diarrhea, excessive urination, blood loss, serum leakage from burns, etc). A 6% loss (moderate) is indicated when a pinched fold of skin slowly returns to its normal position, rather than quickly springing back. In addition, the eyes may be dull due to dryness and the animal may be depressed. At 8% dehydration (severe), the animal's skin stays in a tented position when pinched and feels coarse and leathery. The eyes are sunken into their sockets and the animal only sluggishly responds to any stimulus. When an animal is 12-15% dehydrated, death is imminent and the animal may be in shock and may twitch due to muscle tremors.

Packed Cell Volume

A third way to determine dehydration, one that is used to monitor the patient's condition, uses the packed cell volume (PCV) and the total plasma protein level. Loss of fluid elevates the PCV and proteins in the blood.

Evaluation of dehydration in large animals is more difficult to assess than in small animals. Loss of skin elasticity, sunken eyes, a rapid weak pulse, weight loss, dry mucous membranes, cold extremities and a low urine volume are all indications of a deficient fluid volume. The severity of signs varies with the degree of dehydration. An improvement in the patient's condition with fluid therapy may be the only sign dehydration was present.

Small animals dehydrate more rapidly than large animals due to their greater surface area in proportion to their smaller total fluid volume. Young animals, especially puppies, kittens, calves and foals, may quickly reach a critical level of dehydration with only mild vomiting or diarrhea when they are not consuming liquids.

Hydration

Volume

To hydrate an animal, lost fluids must be replaced, maintenance fluid needs met and any continuing losses offset. If the patient is consuming liquids, the amount can be subtracted from the volume given to hydrate the animal.

The required amount of maintenance fluids is estimated by multiplying the animal's body weight by 45 ml/kg (20 ml/lb). Percent dehydration is multiplied by the body weight to determine the percentage of body weight reduced due to fluid loss (*eg,* a 15-kg dog that is 6%

dehydrated has lost 0.06 x 15 = 0.9); as 1 L (1000 ml) = 1 kg, then the loss in body weight can be converted to volume (*eg,* 0.9 x 1000 ml = 900 ml lost). Continuing losses are estimated by observing the volume of vomit, diarrhea, etc. Adding maintenance needs to the amount of dehydration and any continuing fluid losses gives the approximate volume of fluids to be replaced.

If too large a volume of fluid is given IV, it passes out of the blood and into the air spaces in the lungs, "drowning" the animal. This occurs because the small blood vessels in the lungs are thinly separated from the air for effective exchange of O_2 and CO_2. When giving fluids IV, no more than one-quarter of the total volume needed should be given in the first hour and one-quarter the second hour. The remaining half should be distributed over the rest of the day. Following this guide when giving large volumes of fluids IV prevents additional stress on an already compromised animal.

The amount of fluid given to an animal varies with kidney function, lung status, cardiovascular integrity and other factors. Therefore, the technician should always consult with the veterinarian regarding the volume of fluid to be replaced before starting therapy.

Routes of Administration

Fluids can be introduced into the body in several ways. They can be added directly to the blood stream (IV), injected under the skin (SC), deposited in the abdominal cavity (IP), or given by mouth or tube directly into the stomach (oral, per os or PO). Each method has advantages and disadvantages. The type of fluid necessary may influence the route of administration.

Fluid should be administered at room temperature or warmed to body temperature (floating the container in a sink of warm water works well) for severely debilitated or very small animals.

IV Administration: Adding fluids directly to the blood stream is the quickest way to hydrate the animal. Because the solution is diluted by the blood, many substances that are irritating when given IM or SC can be safely administered by this route. However, fluids that contain excessive potassium (K), calcium (Ca) or glucose should not be given IV.

To give fluids IV, a needle or catheter is inserted into a large vein, usually the cephalic or jugular (see Chapter 4), a piece of tubing connected to it, and the tubing attached to a bottle or bag of fluids. The tubing allows the fluid container to be held above body level so the solution can flow in by gravity. The fluid bottle is attached to the IV unit by puncturing the bottle's rubber stopper with a large needle or prong on the end of the tubing opposite that which is connected to the needle or catheter in the animal's vein. This end also usually has a clear, bubble-like container so drip speed can be visualized. For large animals, the IV unit may simply consist of a rubber tube with a flared end, which is slipped over the neck of the fluid bottle.

An air vent allows pressures to equalize as fluid leaves the bottle. The air vent may be built into the IV unit or created by puncturing the tubing with a needle inserted into the air space near the neck of the fluid container. Fluid flow is regulated by compressing the tubing or by using needles with different diameters (gauge) in the animal's veins. The IV unit should be sterile, as the fluid moving through it is introduced into the blood and any microorganisms or chemical residues present may be harmful. Contaminated lines should be discarded, autoclaved if made from hard plastic or rubber, gas sterilized if made of thin plastic, or cold sterilized with a disinfectant and thoroughly washed with sterile water before reuse.

Most IV drip lines deliver 15 drops/ml but microdrip units deliver 60 drops/ml and are used for long-term, slow infusion.

The speed of fluid administration varies with the percent dehydration, condition of the animal and the vein used. Giving fluids rapidly stresses the cardiovascular system but may be necessary in an emergency. Due to the great fluid capacity of large animals, solutions are often administered as fast as they can flow and in emergencies a pump (pressure cuff around the container) or more than one line may be used. The optimal rate of fluid administration in drops/minute can be estimated based on the volume to be administered in an hour and the delivery rate of the line (*eg,* 15 drops/ml x 250 ml fluid = 3750 drops ÷ 60 minutes/hour = 60-65 drops/minute or about 1 drop/second). It is best to consult with the veterinarian regarding the speed of fluid administration for each patient, then take care not to exceed it.

Check the patient periodically while IV fluids are being administered. Lung sounds should be normal (no wheezing or "wet," fluid sounds) and the pulse regular. If the catheter or needle has been dislodged from the vein, fluid flow into the patient stops or a SC swelling forms around the vein due to fluid accumulating outside of the vessel. If either of these situations occurs, rethread the needle in the vein or replace the catheter. Before rethreading the needle, run a small amount of fluid through it to make sure it is free of blood clots. Do not try to unplug a needle or catheter while it is in the vein or the clot will enter the circulation and may occlude a small vessel (such as the coronary artery, which may cause a heart attack).

The drip may also stop if the air vent is obstructed, the line is kinked, the vein is blocked (*eg,* by flexing the limb or with a pressure bandage), or if the bottle is not held above the level of the vein.

Shut off the fluid flow before the bottle is completely empty to prevent air from entering the blood stream. Air emboli (circulating bubbles) are thought to be an infrequent cause of death but they should be avoided. If air enters the line, close the tubing below the bubble and inject enough additional fluid into the line with a syringe to push the air back into the bottle, withdraw the air bubble with a syringe, or detach the line from the vein and run fluid through the tubing to push the air out.

After the fluid flow is stopped, the bottle can be changed or the therapy ended. A needle is withdrawn from the vein but a cap can be applied to the end of a catheter and taped in place for later use. If the catheter is not removed, a small amount of heparin (about 0.1 ml of 1000 units/ml) is injected through the catheter to prevent blood from clotting in the tube. The IV line can be reused if only sterile fluids have contacted the inside surface.

SC Administration: In dogs and cats, the skin is loosely attached to the underlying tissue, creating a large potential space for fluid to be deposited. It is then slowly absorbed as the body needs it. Horses and cattle generally have skin too tightly attached for SC fluid therapy, though this route is sometimes used for small volumes of fluid.

Fluid for SC injection should be similar to plasma in composition (isotonic); 10-200 ml can be deposited in one area, depending on the size of the patient. More than one site can be used in an individual at the same time. In small animals, the back, from shoulders to tail, is used, but in swine the flank area is the best site (where the rear legs join the body at the abdomen) to use. The fluid is delivered from a syringe or IV line (see Chapter 4).

The more dehydrated the animal is, the faster fluid is absorbed. Periodically checking the fluid deposit under the skin indicates how often to repeat the therapy. Pinching the needle hole in the skin after the needle has been withdrawn helps prevent leakage from the site due to fluid pressure. Fluids given SC take less time to administer than those given IV but the return to normal hydration is slower.

IP Administration: The space around the abdominal organs (peritoneal cavity) offers a potential depot for fluids. They are absorbed more rapidly from this space than if given SC, but not as quickly as the IV route. Large volumes can be given, 100 ml to several liters, depending on the size of the animal, but the fluids should be of a plasma-like composition. The method has a potential hazard of puncturing an organ but is still relatively safe (see Chapter 4). It is used in both small and large animal medicine for fluid therapy.

Because the peritoneum (membrane lining the abdominal cavity) has a good blood supply and is semipermeable, fluids deposited in the abdominal cavity equilibrate with the blood stream. Thus, the blood can be gradually cleared of many toxins by adding fluids to the abdominal cavity, letting diffusion take place and removing the fluid and accumulated material. The technic is called peritoneal dialysis and is used in treating kidney failure and poisoning. Using a needle or dialysis catheter, 200 ml-2 L of fluid are injected into the abdomen and withdrawn after about an hour. In severe cases, dialysis is repeated 3-5 times a day. The volume of fluid collected after each treatment should be recorded and the whole procedure done as aseptically as possible because peritonitis (inflammation of the peritoneum) is a constant danger.

Oral Administration: Giving fluids by stomach tube, force feeding or pharyngostomy tube (see Chapter 4) is the ideal way to hydrate an animal (Fig 1). Fluid volume and composition are of lesser importance than for other routes, as the animal's body selectively absorbs what is needed. The method is less traumatic to tissues and more natural than other technics. In addition, it is the only way to administer adequate nutrients to an anorectic animal. Oral fluids need not be sterile and can be mixed in the veterinary clinic, so are less expensive than purchased fluids.

The route is not used when vomiting, diarrhea, enteritis (intestinal inflammation) or GI obstruction is present, to avoid additional stress to the digestive system.

Fluid Types

Fluids for therapy consist of water and various electrolytes, amino acids, carbohydrates and vitamins. Electrolytes are ionic particles that can conduct electricity when in solution. Ionic particles are atoms charged by losing or gaining electrons. Common ions are K^+, Ca^+, Na^+ (sodium), Mg^{++} (magnesium), Cl^- (chloride), and HCO_3^- (bicarbonate). Electrolytes are necessary for the many chemical reactions in the body's normal function.

Different diseases cause different ion imbalances, so the fluid type for therapy depends on the animal's condition. For example, vomiting causes loss of HCl (hydrochloric acid) from the stomach. The Cl in HCl is normally recycled by the body during digestion, so Cl lost by vomiting should be replaced by administering a fluid rich in Cl. If a solution low in Cl is given, the patient's condition would worsen rather than improve as a result of the therapy. For this reason, always consult with the veterinarian regarding the type of fluid to give each patient.

In addition to considering the type of electrolyte present, the overall balance of all electrolytes in a solution is important. If the

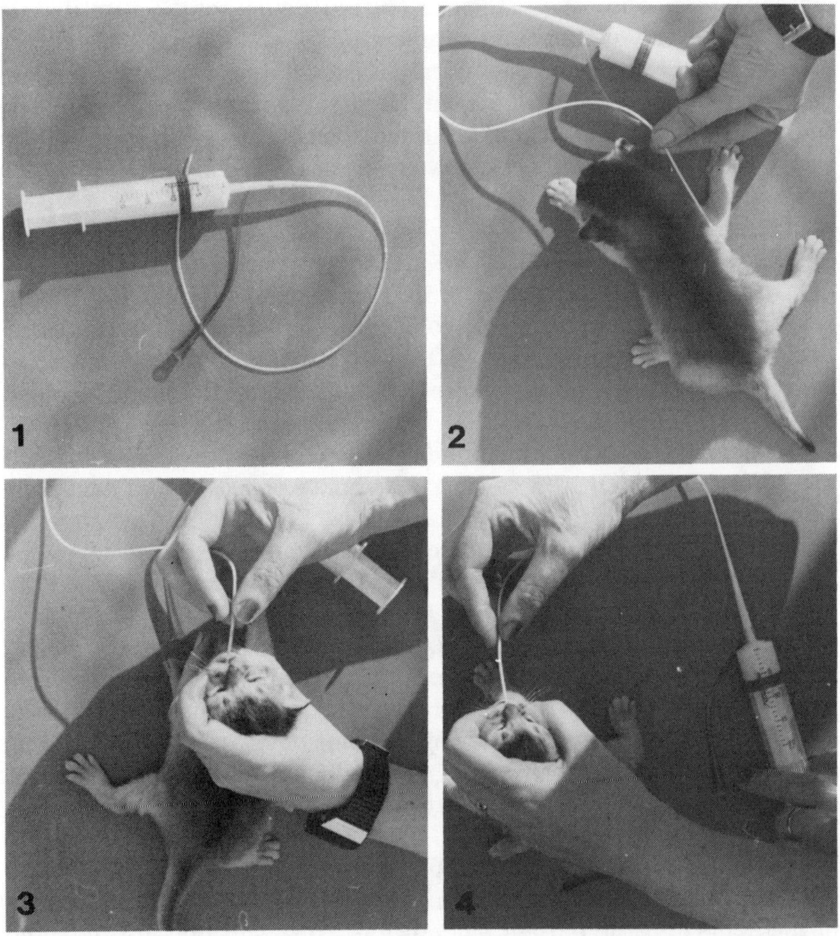

Fig 1. Tube feeding an orphan kitten. 1. The formula is placed in a large syringe attached to a plastic urinary catheter or rubber feeding tube. 2. The feeding tube is held next to the kitten to measure the distance from the tip of the nose to the last rib, to determine how far the feeding tube must be inserted. 3. The syringe plunger is depressed to fill the tube with formula and expel the air before the tube is inserted into the kitten's mouth. With the kitten held firmly, the mouth is pried open with the thumb and forefinger while the tube is inserted with the other hand. 4. The tube is inserted to the predetermined length and an assistant slowly dispenses the formula from the syringe. (Photos courtesy of TFH Publications)

balance is similar to that of plasma, the fluid is called isotonic. If there are more electrolytes than in plasma, it is called hypertonic and if less than plasma it is hypotonic.

Body fluids can move through tissues, so they stay in the same concentration throughout the animal (with only a few exceptions). If, for example, hypertonic solution is give SC, fluid moves out of the animal's body into the SC space to dilute the solution until it is isotonic and the overall fluid composition of the animal is balanced. The patient is now more dehydrated, except for the SC space, than before therapy. Isotonic fluids can be given by any route, but hypertonic or hypotonic solutions are only given IV or PO. Hypertonic or hypotonic fluids should be given IV slowly and with constant monitoring.

Isotonic solutions include whole blood, plasma, 0.9% sodium chloride (physiologic saline), 5% dextrose (glucose) in water, 2.5% dextrose in half-strength lactate, 1/6 M (a measure of mass in a liter of solution), or lactated Ringer's solution (a balanced electrolyte solution, with lactate for energy). A plasma substitute (Dextran) is also isotonic and contains large molecules to help hold fluids in the blood stream.

Hypertonic solutions include 50% dextrose, 3% saline (table salt or sodium chloride), 10% calcium gluconate or 5% amino acid solution. Lactated Ringer's with 2% glucose, Peridial 1.5% or Inpersol 1.5% are hypertonic solutions used for peritoneal dialysis.

Hypotonic solutions are plain water or 2% dextrose.

Storage and Handling of Fluids

Fluids should be stored at room temperature and protected from excessive heat or cold. Expiration dates should be observed and supplies rotated to prevent outdating of solutions. Inspect the seals on any new container before using it to make sure it is sterile. Discard any solution that appears cloudy or contains a precipitate (visible solid material).

Determining the amount, route, rate and type of fluid therapy should be left to the veterinarian as it requires a detailed knowledge of medicine and the patient's condition. However, giving fluids and monitoring hydration are valuable services the technician can contribute to patient care.

Fluid therapy has saved the lives of many patients but it is a supportive or symptomatic treatment. The underlying cause of the fluid loss must be corrected and the animal must maintain its own fluid balance before the prognosis (predicted outcome of the case) becomes more favorable.

OXYGEN THERAPY

Oxygen (O_2) therapy is indicated when respiration is impaired. Oxygen deprivation (hypoxia) requires immediate attention, as it may be rapidly fatal. Administration of O_2 is a temporary measure until the condition that caused the poor oxygenation can be corrected. Typical uses of O_2 include supporting the newborn animal that is weak from a difficult or prolonged delivery (dystocia), aiding the patient with a blocked trachea (windpipe), or assisting a patient in respiratory distress due to heatstroke, etc. If the hypoxia is due to airway obstruction, removal of the blockage may be adequate to restore normal breathing without O_2 therapy. When hypoxia is due to decreased numbers of circulating RBC, a transfusion may be necessary before O_2 therapy is effective. Shock, reduced cardiac output, circulatory failure or anesthetic overdoses all cause hypoxia because blood is not adequately circulated to the tissues to deliver O_2.

A significant stimulus for respiration is high blood carbon dioxide (CO_2) levels. When the brain's respiratory center is depressed by drugs, trauma, chronic respiratory disease or anesthetic overdose, the body's sensitivity to CO_2 may be reduced and the animal depends on low blood levels of O_2 to trigger respiration. If O_2 is given to such an animal, the elevation in O_2 lowers the "hypoxic drive," resulting in a depressed respiratory rate and an increased O_2 deficit. For this reason, animals with chronic O_2 deprivation should be watched carefully for respiratory depression when pure O_2 is administered (the patient must breathe for O_2 to enter the lungs).

The nervous system is very sensitive to hypoxia and is the tissue damaged first when blood O_2 levels fall below normal. The interval between O_2 deprivation and tissue damage depends on a number of factors, including the animal's age, condition, activity and temperature. As a rule of thumb, 4 minutes of hypoxia causes irreversible brain damage in a normal animal, but neonates (newborn animals) may tolerate up to 10 minutes without harm. Resuscitative efforts may continue for longer than 10 minutes when O_2 therapy has been given or when the animal is colder than normal (hypothermia due to immersion in cold water or exposure to cold temperatures).

If O_2 therapy is necessary for more than 2-3 days on a continuous basis, it may be prohibitively expensive.

Equipment for O_2 Therapy

Pure O_2 gas is compressed to 1900-2500 lb/square inch (psi) of pressure (at 70 F) and stored in thick, green, metal cylinders. Large tanks (G tanks) hold about 6000-7000 L and small tanks (E tanks) hold 500-600 L. Tanks are usually rented from and filled by commercial suppliers.

The cylinder is fitted with a gauge on the top (threaded onto the tank top) that indicates the amount of pressure in the tank, which is a direct reflection of the volume of O_2 in the tank, as gases expand to fill all space available. Tanks should be changed before they are completely empty to avoid running out of O_2 while treating a patient. Most tanks have a tag with perforations that is marked "Full," "In Use," "Empty," and sections of the tag are torn off as the tank is used so that its status is clear to everyone.

In addition to the gauge, a regulator is attached to the top of the tank. It reduces the pressure of the O_2 leaving the tank to $\leq$60 psi, as the immense, unregulated pressure in the cylinder would otherwise damage lung tissue. The gauge and regulator are often combined into one device. A handle on top of the cylinder opens or closes the tank.

Because the tank is under pressure, opening it without a regulator attached (or with a poor one) or puncturing the cylinder may cause it to be propelled like a rocket by escaping gas. This can be very dangerous, depending on the volume of O_2 in the tank. For this reason, tanks should be handled gently, opened gradually and fixed firmly in position by chaining them to a wall when not in use. Tanks in use should be well attached to the anesthetic machine or a solid surface to prevent knocking the regulator off if the cylinder falls.

Oxygen itself is not flammable, but it supports fire (like "fanning the flames"). It should be kept away from cigarettes, open flames and electrical connections, such as electrocautery equipment. It is explosive in combination with other substances, such as cyclopropane, grease and oil. Valves and fittings should not be lubricated with oil or grease if they are used with O_2. Only equipment designed for O_2 use at the pressure delivered should be used.

Administration of O_2

The tank can be hooked up to a variety of devices to deliver O_2 to the patient. A simple tube can be attached and held to the patient's

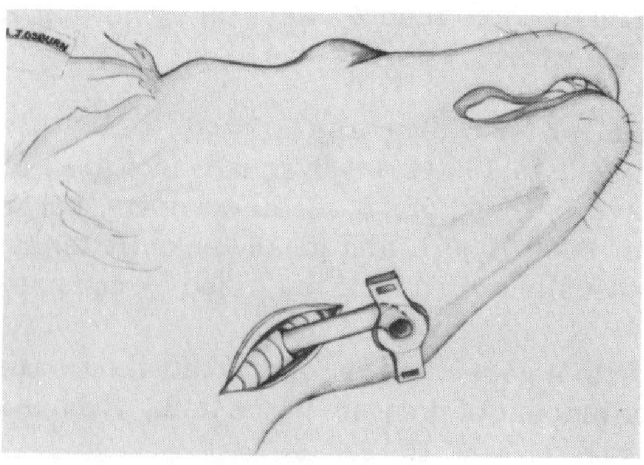

Fig 2. After incising the skin on the ventral midline of the neck and the ligament between 2 tracheal rings, a tracheostomy tube is inserted.

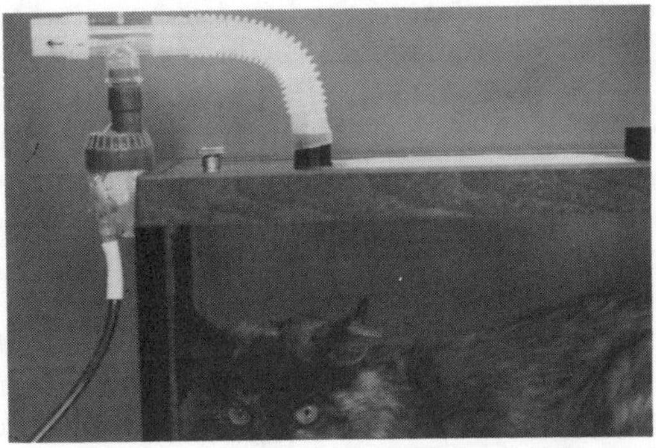

Fig 3. Anesthetic induction chamber used as a nebulization chamber for small animals.

nose, inserted through an incision in the trachea, passed into the pharynx (back of the throat) or run into an oxygen chamber (aquarium, closed cage, etc) (Figs 2, 3). Oxygen can be delivered through an endotracheal tube (tube in the windpipe) or nose cone. It can also be forced into the lungs using a rebreathing bag, Ambu bag or positive-pressure ventilation system (Fig 4). The rebreathing bag fills with O_2 due to flow from the tank. The Ambu bag automatically refills when the pressure applied to it is released. The positive-pressure system uses a machine that takes over or assists respiration (see Chapter 1).

To administer pure O_2, the delivery system must be sealed so that no air mixes with gas from the cylinder. The flow of O_2 from the tank is regulated by a flow meter (often attached to the anesthetic machine), which delivers gas at 5 ml-15 L/minute at room temperature under normal atmospheric conditions. The flow meter serves as

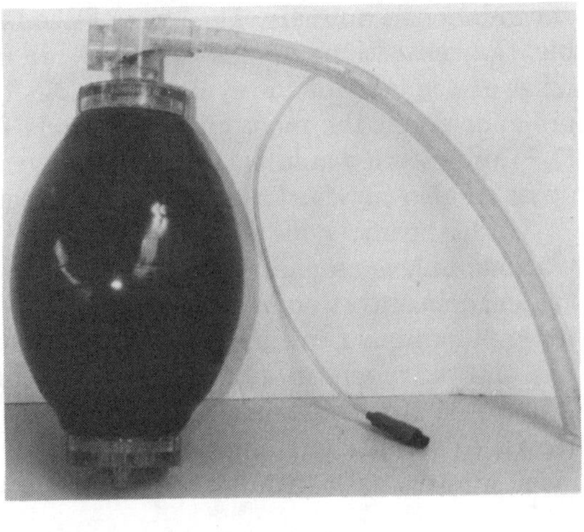

Fig 4. Ambu bag attached to an endotracheal tube, used for positive-pressure ventilation.

another regulator to reduce the pressure of the gas leaving the tank, preventing damage to the lungs.

The correct level of O_2 flow for the patient is determined by the minute volume of the animal's breathing and gas leakage of the delivery system. Minute volume is the amount of air breathed per minute and is calculated by multiplying the tidal volume (amount of air exchanged in a resting breath) by the number of breaths per minute. Tidal volume can be estimated by assuming that 10 ml of air/kg of body weight are exchanged in one breath (5 ml/lb). (This figure is not valid for very large or very small animals). For example, a 10-kg animal taking 10 breaths per minute would require an O_2 flow of 1 L per minute (10 kg x 10 ml/kg = 100 ml x 10 breaths/minute = 1000 ml/minute).

The greater the number of leaks in the delivery system (*eg*, semi-open anesthetic machine), the higher the flow must be to deliver the necessary amount of O_2. A loose-fitting mask or vented O_2 cage may require 10-20 times the O_2 flow as that given by endotracheal tube.

The percentage of O_2 (50-100%) given to a patient varies with the cause of the respiratory distress and the length of therapy needed. Most of the O_2 is carried by hemoglobin in RBC and only a small fraction is dissolved in the plasma. Once RBC are saturated by O_2, increasing the percentage of O_2 administered has little effect on the animal. On the other hand, if the hemoglobin is not saturated, increasing the percentage of O_2 above that in normal room air (about 16%) aids hypoxic patients. Poor oxgenation of RBC occurs when the respiratory rate is depressed, cardiac function is poor, alveolar (air sacs in the lungs) walls are too thick for good gas exchange, etc.

Pure (100%) O_2 can be administered in emergencies, but severe toxicity occurs within 10 hours (at 2 atmospheres of pressure) in warm-blooded animals. The eyes of neonates are especially susceptible. Concentrations of less than 35% do not affect the retina (visual layer at the back of the eye) and in dogs the first 21 days after birth are considered the most critical periods for eye damage from 100% O_2.[1] Cold-blooded animals are not damaged by long-term pure O_2 therapy and also survive O_2 deprivation better than mammals and birds.

Under normal conditions, it is difficult to obtain 100% O_2 concentrations unless an endotracheal tube is used for administration. The typical concentration in an O_2 cage is 30-50%. When using an O_2 cage for small animals, initial flows of 10 L/minute are needed to wash out residual nitrogen in the cage; levels are then decreased to 5-8 L/minute for maintenance. Oxygen cages are the best way to administer O_2 to a conscious animal without constant supervision. Using a mask may cause the animal to struggle, compounding the respiratory distress by using up more O_2 in muscular activity. In sealed O_2 cages, CO_2 levels should be maintained at less than 1.5% using an absorber containing soda lime.

The most efficient temperature for giving O_2 is 65-70 F, as the concentration of gas particles varies with temperature changes.

Pure O_2 decreases blood flow through the lungs. This reduces the volume of secretions by the respiratory tract and increases the thickness of mucus. The respiratory system is constantly exposed to foreign material and microorganisms from inhaled air. Mucus and other secretions trap inhaled particles and are swept out of the lungs and up the airways, clearing them of potentially harmful materials. Interference with this process increases an animal's susceptibility to respiratory tract disease. Clearance of respiratory secretions is greatly delayed in dogs given 100% O_2 because of thickened mucus. In addition, pure O_2 further narrows airways in patients with severe pulmonary (lung) disease. Evidence of inflammation of the airways occurs in dogs after breathing pure O_2 for 6 hours or 75% for 12 hours.

As there is no treatment for oxygen toxicity, do not administer 100% O_2 for more than 5 hours without consulting the veterinarian.

In most instances, 30-60% O_2 is adequate for hypoxic patients and there is no risk of toxicity. Increasing the humidity of the O_2 (40-60% humidity is ideal) by bubbling it through ice water before it enters the O_2 cage helps prevent respiratory irritation due to high concentrations of O_2.

For cattle, an adaption of the "Venti-Mask," designed for people, successfully delivers an O_2 flow of 12 L/minute at 28% (due to the air vents). Oxygen is usually administered to large animals by face mask, endotracheal tube or nasal catheter (through the nose by tube).

In summary, to administer O_2 to a conscious patient, use an O_2 cage for small animals or a nasal catheter for large animals. If the patient is unconscious, use an endotracheal tube or face mask. Animals that are not breathing spontaneously must be assisted with an Ambu bag, rebreathing bag, positive-pressure ventilation machine (respirator), closed-chest massage, etc. The oxygen flow is turned on by twisting the handle on top of the tank and the flow is regulated by setting the meter. Pure O_2 can be safely given for up to 5 hours. Closely monitor the patient's pulse rate, mucous membrane color, and respiratory rate and depth.

ARTIFICIAL ALIMENTATION

The best diet is useless unless it is eaten, and many hospitalized animals refuse to eat. This is especially a problem with cats, young horses and small dogs. Often the animal can be supported with forced feedings until its appetite returns with its health and it adjusts to the clinic environment.

The process of supplying nutrients to animals that cannot (due to face, mouth or throat injury or surgery) or will not eat is called artificial alimentation. Nutrients can be supplied by IV injection or orally.

Oral Alimentation

Forcing nutrients into an animal orally is less time consuming, expensive and risky than IV feedings. It allows the body to digest the food naturally and is the best way to supply a complete diet artificially. A functional digestive system (not inflamed or blocked) is necessary and the animal should not have vomiting or diarrhea.

Solid chunks of food, gruel and liquids can be administered as if they were medication, by "pilling" or "drenching" the animal (see Chapter 4). This method requires a docile patient with a pain-free, uninjured mouth, tongue, throat and esophagus (tube leading from the throat to the stomach). Due to the large volume of food required, it is not a practical method of feeding horses and cattle.

Slurries of food can be deposited directly into the stomach with a tube passed through the mouth for small animals or nose for large animals (see Chapter 4). For small animals, a nutritionally balanced, canned food mixed with water (using a blender) is ideal. Mix one-quarter of a 1-lb can with 175 ml of water and divide it into 3-4 feedings/day for a 5-lb animal. Giving some of the fluid by SC injection and using concentrated food sources (*eg,* egg yolk, baby food) reduce the volume and number of feedings/day.

For horses, a mixture of electrolytes, dextrose, dehydrated cottage cheese and 6-7 L of water can be used.[3] In cattle, use of a blend of vitamins, minerals, dextrose, dried skim milk, soybean meal and water is recommended.[4] Exact recipes, volumes and number of feedings should be left up to the veterinarian. Make sure all food particles are small enough to pass easily through the tube.

For long-term artificial alimentation, a pharyngostomy tube may be surgically implanted by the veterinarian (Fig 5). One end of the tube extends out of the esophagus, through the skin of the neck, near the jaw, and the other rests in the stomach. Food is given through the tube, which eliminates the need for repeated oral passage of a stomach tube. Pharyngostomy tubes are well tolerated by most animals and may remain in place for weeks. The skin around the tube and the incision (tube is sutured in place) should be washed daily with a mild antiseptic (*eg,* povidone-iodine) and water. The tube should be capped when not in use to prevent air from entering the stomach.

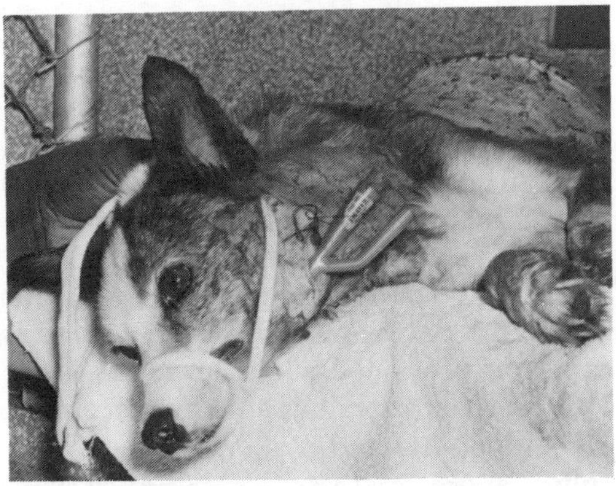

Fig 5. Pharyngostomy tube implanted in the esophagus of a dog, for artificial alimentation.

Concentrated nutrients are available in liquid or gel form (*eg,* Pet Kalorie, Sustagen) and can supplement the patient temporarily, but they are expensive and may cause diarrhea if given in large amounts or over an extended period.

Force feedings should not be continued longer than necessary. The patient should be encouraged to eat on its own by offering highly palatable food frequently.

Parenteral Hyperalimentation

An animal that is severely malnourished may not have adequate energy to digest its food. In addition, patients with serious digestive tract disease, chronic vomiting and/or diarrhea, acute kidney failure, inflammation of the pancreas, or GI surgery may (before or after) benefit from nutrients given IV. As with all artificial alimentation, the goal is to assist the animal while the condition preventing normal eating is resolved.

Parenteral hyperalimentation involves continuous IV administration of a hypertonic solution containing calories, proteins, vitamins, electrolytes and water. Calories are provided by fat (lipids) and sugars. Solutions typically contain 10% dextrose, crystalline amino acids, K, phosphate, Na, Mg, Cl, and vitamins B and C. Copper, zinc and multiple vitamins are added if therapy continues for more than a week. Some B vitamins and vitamin K must be given IM, as they are destroyed (oxidized) if placed in a high-glucose solution. Adding HCO_3 (bicarbonate) to the solution causes precipitation of Ca and Mg. The veterinarian may rotate the solutions to be used.

If a solution with more than 10% glucose is used, it should be administered through a large central vein, such as the jugular. Lipids are added (10-20%) by allowing a second, high-fat solution to mix with other infused fluids just before they flow into the vein. This method prevents the lipid from separating out from the rest of the solution (as happens with oil and water in salad dressings). If a high-fat solution is used to provide calories, the fluids may be given in a smaller vein in a limb, such as the cephalic.

The solution is best administered with an infusion pump, but any conventional unit (including microdrip) may be used. When administration of hyperalimentation solution is stopped, IV administration of 5% dextrose should be continued for a short time to gradually taper off the blood sugar level. As the patient begins to eat food, hyperalimentation is gradually discontinued.

Patients treated by hyperalimentation should be monitored carefully. Laboratory tests to determine the patient's response to therapy should be done regularly on blood, plasma and urine. Hydration status, body temperature, weight, and pulse and respiratory rates should be checked frequently. The IV catheter should be kept clean and dressings to hold it in place changed frequently. Any sign of localized or generalized infection should be reported to the veterinarian immediately.

CRITICAL CARE MONITORING

Ideally, every patient in critical condition should be observed 24 hours a day by a veterinarian. However, this is also physically and financially impractical, so the technician must aid the veterinarian by reporting anything important to the doctor.

A significant part of any technician's job is observation. Consider clients who did not know their animal was sick until the signs were so advanced it seemed impossible anyone could be unaware of the problem. These clients were not good observers and their animals may have suffered because of it.

Careful observation is a learned skill that develops with practice. It involves comparing normal behavior or appearance against abnormal signs, and drawing conclusions. The more time spent observing normal and sick animals, both as individuals and as members of a species, the better judgement a technician has when monitoring critically ill patients. Time spent observing, touching, hearing or smelling hospitalized animals is never wasted, as it is gathering data for decision making. Part of the reason animals are hospitalized is so they can be observed frequently by someone capable of recognizing minute changes that could herald a problem.

Pulse, respiratory and heart rates all vary significantly in normal animals, due to exercise, excitement, environmental temperature, etc.

However, an increase or decrease can also indicate a metabolic problem or other disease.

Consult with the veterinarian regarding how often to check vital signs and monitor the patient. As a rule of thumb for non-life-threatening cases, check the patient every 15 minutes for the first hour after hospitalization, every 30 minutes until the animal is stabilized, and every hour thereafter. Animals near death may have to be watched almost continuously. It is difficult to over-monitor a patient and usually the animal's condition indicates how often observation is necessary. Experience adds confidence in making this judgement.

Temperature

Most mammals and birds can regulate their body temperature within a very narrow range. The range varies with the species and allows for internal conditions optimal for chemical reactions (homeostasis).

Monitoring body temperature is not useful in cold-blooded animals, such as snakes, lizards and other reptiles, because they equilibrate with the environmental temperature. However, they also have an optimal temperature for body functions and when ill should be kept in that range by using an artificial heat source.

Warm-blooded patients sometimes lose control of their ability to regulate temperature. Elevated temperatures occur with heatstroke (see Chapter 1), infections, tight bandages, some poisonings, etc. Heatstroke causes the temperature to rise high and fast, and due to loss of temperature-regulating ability, the animal may easily be over-cooled during treatment. Infection with bacteria or viruses elevates normal temperatures, similar to turning up a thermostat. The way the temperature fluctuates varies with the disease. Some infections cause chronic low-grade fevers, others a sharp fever spike, and sometimes the temperature oscillates up and down. Close monitoring may provide clues to the source of the fever. Temperatures that rise rapidly usually indicate a worse prognosis than slowly rising fevers.

Temperatures may be measured rectally (see Chapter 2). However, the animal's behavior may also indicate that internal temperatures are not optimal. Animals with a fever may be depressed, have a dry nose, huddle in a corner or with other animals, feel warm to the touch, and/or drink excessive amounts of water. Animals with a subnormal temperature may also seek a source of warmth, be depressed, and/or have cold extremities. In both cases, the patient often is anorectic (inappetent) and unusually quiet and withdrawn.

A rectal temperature elevated 3 F (2 C) above normal is considered a fever. Excitement or extremely hot weather may increase a temperature 2 F (1 C), but only in unusual circumstances will it go higher. Allowing the animal time to adjust, then retaking the temperature, and considering other clinical signs, usually eliminates excitement as a cause of a fever.

The higher the rectal temperature goes, the more concerned a technician should be. Most thermometers do not measure beyond 106 F (42 C) and at 105 F (41 C), except for birds, the fever becomes harmful. The nervous system is especially susceptible to damage by fever. Fevers of 103-105 F (39-41 C) should be closely monitored and brought to the veterinarian's attention. The animal should be kept warm and quiet, and encouraged to drink liquids, and any other clinical signs treated. Animals with a fever above 105 F (41 C) should be treated by applications of ice packs or immersion in cold water, and/or drug administration. Any fever this high should be treated as an emergency.

The rectal temperature may be low when an animal is in shock, severely debilitated, suffering from cold exposure (hypothermia) or recovering from anesthesia. Conserve body heat by covering the animal and insulating it from cold surfaces, especially stainless steel. If the temperature drops to about 98 F (37 C), warm the patient with hot-water bottles, a heat lamp or heating pad. Be very careful that the patient does not get overheated by checking the temperature of the skin nearest the heat source frequently. Severely depressed animals may suffer burns as they cannot move away from an overly hot heat source. If the temperature drops below about 94 F (34.4 C), the animal may be near death and emergency measures must be taken to warm it. Immersion in lukewarm water is a quick way to increase temperature. The water may be gradually warmed to normal body temperature. Be sure to thoroughly dry the coat afterward to prevent chilling. Animals have survived with a body temperature as low as 75 F (24 C) when cooled in cold water or during open-heart surgery, but these are exceptional circumstances.

Young or old animals are less able to regulate their body temperature and should be watched carefully for chilling or overheating.

Due to their greater body mass, horses and cattle typically have slower temperature changes in disease and therapy than small animals.

Cardiovascular Function

Pulse

A pulse is created in arteries by expansion and contraction of the vessel walls with each heart beat. It does not normally happen in veins, as their anatomic structure tends to moderate pressure changes in these vessels.

A change in pulse rate or character indicates a difference in heart function or blood flow volume. However, the rate varies widely in normal animals due to excitement, anxiety or even normal respiration. An intermittent pulse (occasional pause between regular pulses) may be present in normal animals. Thus, judgement must be exercised when evaluating the pulse.

The character of the pulse usually is firm and regular. However, its rate and character may vary as the heartbeat does, becoming harder or softer, larger or shorter, depending on the amount of blood flowing through the vessel.

If the pulse abnormality is due to a heart defect, the veterinarian has usually detected it and the technician's main concern is a change in pulse, especially if it is gradually deteriorating in strength and/or rate.

A slow, soft pulse (thready) that is barely perceptible can occur with shock, diminished heart contraction strength or constriction of the heart by fluid in the pericardial sac (membrane around the heart). A fast pulse may occur when the tissues are not getting enough oxygen and the heart compensates by increasing its speed and subsequent blood flow.

A pulse deficit occurs when there are more heart beats than pulses present in a given time span (both must be monitored at the same time). The heart pumps blood inefficiently on abnormal beats, so no pulse may be felt then.

Pulse frequency (rate in beats/minute) is easy to evaluate but character (soft, hard, long, short, etc) is much more difficult to assess. The strength of the pulse (amplitude) can be estimated by determining the amount of pressure needed to close off the vessel. Spending time feeling pulses gradually increases digital sensitivity and the value of this in critical care monitoring.

Mucous Membranes

Color: The protective, keratinized layer of the skin's surface is absent in areas of the body that are moist and protected from injury and invasion by other means. These areas are called mucous membranes (mucosae) and line the body orifices. Because mucous membranes are hairless and thin, the blood within small vessels colors the tissue (unless the skin is naturally pigmented). This color serves as an important indicator of body condition.

The best areas to examine for mucous membrane color are the inside surface of the lip, gums (gingivae), tongue, inner eyelid, surface of the eye (sclera), and inner vulva or sheath. Most people find the lips and gums easiest to examine but the surface should not have any dark pigment that obscures the normal pink color. Good lighting is necessary to evaluate the color. Studies have shown that viewers may disagree on the depth of color of the mucous membrane.

If the mucosa appears blue-purple (cyanosis), the blood is low in O_2 content or blood flow to the tissue is decreased, so more O_2 is being extracted from the blood. Unoxygenated blood is dark red, but combined with skin pigment appears blue. Cyanosis could be due to impairment in delivery of O_2 to the lungs or in circulating O_2. Either instance is cause for concern and usually must be attended to immediately, though some heart conditions cause chronic, low-grade cyanosis). The deeper the shade of blue-purple, the more severe the condition, as the proportion of unoxygenated to oxygenated blood is greater.

Anemic patients may be low in blood O_2 but not cyanotic, due to low levels of functioning hemoglobin. This must always be kept in mind when monitoring such animals. If the cyanosis is due to low blood O_2, then O_2 therapy is of benefit. On the other hand, if it is caused by poor blood flow to a tissue, O_2 therapy is not beneficial to the patient.

If an animal is cyanotic, check cardiac and respiratory function first. If neither is working, initiate cardiopulmonary resuscitation (CPR). If the heart is beating but the animal is not breathing, pass an endotracheal tube if possible and assist respiration with an Ambu bag, mouth-to-nose artificial respiration, manual compression of the lungs, etc (see Chapter 1). Oxygen therapy during this time may also be helpful. If the animal is breathing but the heart is not beating, electric shock, compression or injection of a stimulant may start it. If a cyanotic animal is breathing and the heart is beating, administer O_2. If O_2 does not improve the color, therapy to increase blood flow, volume or quality may be needed. In all situations, notify the veterinarian as soon as possible.

When the amount of blood flowing through the vessels in a mucous membrane is low, the tissue becomes pale or white (pallor). This could be due to shock (as the blood is pooled elsewhere), loss of blood, or anemia. Whole blood transfusions may be necessary if the number of circulating RBC is very low.

Mucous membranes may also be bright red, as in carbon monoxide poisoning, or muddy brown, as in nitrate toxicity.

Develop the habit of checking the mucous membrane color whenever an animal is examined.

Capillary Refill Time: The smallest blood vessels in the body are the capillaries. They join the arteries and veins to make a continuous vascular circuit. Not all capillaries are filled with blood at one time or there would not be enough blood left in the large vessels to circulate (this is an indication of the vast number of capillaries in the body). However, enough are normally filled in an area to color the mucosae pink.

A good measure of cardiovascular function is to determine how rapidly capillaries refill with blood after their supply has been shut off with pressure. To determine capillary refill time, gently press on the mucous membrane (usually the gum) with the tip of a finger (not the fingernail) until it blanches white. Then quickly remove the finger and note the time it takes for the color to return, which normally is in less than 1 second. Diseases that lower cardiac output (the amount of blood leaving the heart), impair circulation or delay capillary refill time include shock, heart valve abnormalities and fluid in the pericardial sac.

Heart Rate

Interpretation of the various heart sounds is complex and usually requires a veterinarian to recognize any heart defect. Thus, patient monitoring involves primarily checking the rate of the beats. This can be done by palpation (feeling), auscultation (listening with a stethoscope) or indirectly by counting the pulse rate (see Chapter 2).

Report any of the following to the veterinarian: a progressively decreasing or increasing rate, a highly irregular beat, long pauses between beats or a countinuously rapid rate.

Respiration

Interference with respiration can occur in the upper respiratory tract (nose, mouth, throat) or the lower respiratory tract (trachea, bronchi, lungs). It can involve a simple physical blockage of air conduction or a subtle thickening of alveoli walls preventing gas exchange. Structures associated with the respiratory tract can affect breathing, such as the pleura (membrane covering the lungs) or ribs. Even diseases not associated with the respiratory tract, such as heart disease, anemia or gastric (stomach) dilation, can influence breathing. However, regardless of the cause of respiratory difficulty, it should be viewed as an emergency as adequate O_2 intake and CO_2 removal are essential for life. When establishing priorities in an emergency, adequate respiration should be the first concern as apnea (no breathing) and subsequent asphyxia (O_2 starvation) are the quickest cause of death.

The respiratory and cardiovascular systems are closely linked, so a change in one is usually reflected in the other. Pulse rate and character, mucous membrane color and respiration all change as blood gas levels become abnormal.

Changes in respiratory rate, depth or pattern can be detected by observation, palpation, or auscultation (see Chapter 2). Certain individuals or breeds may have variations in breathing that are considered normal. Respiratory sounds are usually harsher in young and/or small dogs and cats than in older or larger animals.

Respiratory Rate

The respiratory rate may be elevated with exercise, excitement, obesity, environmental heat, pain, structural changes in the lungs, low O_2 availability or change in the body's pH balance (measure of acidity or alkalinity). Animals acclimated to cold may show a rate increase of 6-8 times normal when brought indoors. Hyperventilation (prolonged, rapid, deep breathing) can cause loss of consciousness unless the extra O_2 is used up (*eg*, by exercise). Panting is normal in most animals but it does not elevate the body's O_2 level because the breaths are too shallow to exchange much air. The cause of fast breathing must be determined before it can be corrected. Excited animals may be calmed by moving them to a quieter location, blocking their view of other animals or using tranquilizers. Fever, pain and abnormal pH may be treated with drugs or specific treatment (cold-water baths, etc). Oxygen can be given if rapid breathing is due to hypoxia, but do not administer O_2 if the animal is already hyperventilated.

Low respiratory rates can occur with poisoning, overly deep general anesthesia or alkalosis (high blood pH). As therapy for hypoventilation (reduced breathing), the effects of some anesthetics may be reversed with antagonists, respiration may be stimulated with drugs or the pH can be adjusted with certain IV fluids. Oxygen should be given if the animal is cyanotic.

Depth of Respiration

The lungs are inflated by expansion of the thorax (chest), contraction of the diaphragm (drum-like muscle that separates the thoracic and abdominal cavities) and outward rotation of the ribs. Normally both the chest (thoracic breathing) and the abdomen (abdominal breathing) move with each breath. Pressure on the diaphragm from an enlarged structure (*eg,* the liver) or fluid in the abdominal cavity (ascites), and paralysis of the diaphragm may result in thoracic breathing only. Thoracic pain, as from pleuritis or broken ribs, can result in abdominal breathing only.

Deeper breaths cause greater expansion of the lungs. If chest expansion is not possible or is painful, the animal breathes shallowly. Several shallow breaths are required for the same amount of gas exchange as one deep breath. Thus, the rate of respiration is elevated with shallow breathing. Shallow breaths without an increase in respiratory rate rapidly lead to hypoxia and cyanosis. Shallow breathing occurs with pain, nerve damage or pressure increases in the thoracic or abdominal cavity.

The depth of respiration is evaluated by observing the degree of chest expansion or rebreathing bag (on the gas anesthetic machine) expansion. Some animals naturally have a greater lung capacity than others and the amount of expansion varies with exercise, so judgement must be based on experience. Panting represents shallow breathing and deep breathing is seen after exercise, so keep this range in mind when making observations of depth of respiration.

The term Cheyne-Stokes breathing refers to breathing with a gradual increase then decrease in the depth of respiration in a cyclic pattern.

Pattern of Respiration

The pattern or rhythm of respiration can be varied voluntarily or involuntarily. The length of time for inspiration and expiration should be equal and any variation is an abnormality of rhythm (a slight pause occurs between them). Dyspnea (difficult, laborious breathing) can occur with lung and/or airway disease. On expiration, the normal lung collapses and airways narrow, so small obstructions can easily trap air. Inspiratory dyspnea (forced inspiration), with flaring nostrils and gasping can occur with loss of lung elasticity, fluid buildup in the lungs (pulmonary edema), upper airway obstruction, exercise or excitement. Dyspneic animals should be monitored carefully and the veterinarian notified regarding their condition. An animal with dyspnea extends its head and neck, dilates the nostrils, rotates its elbows away from the chest, may breathe through the mouth, and has exaggerated movements of the chest and abdomen, and pronounced respiratory sounds, especially grunting.

Respiratory Sounds

A variety of respiratory sounds may be heard in disease. Most fall into 2 groups; rales (moist, bubbly sounds) and rhonchi (dry, whistling sounds). Normal respiration is almost silent, though air flow may be heard in airways, so any especially obvious respiratory sound should be reported to the veterinarian. Coughing and sneezing are other signs of respiratory disease that should be monitored and their frequency noted.

Pain

Dorland's Medical Dictionary defines pain as a localized discomfort, distress or agony due to stimulation of nerve endings. In people, pain can be difficult to localize and may even be felt in a part of the body distant from an injury (referred pain). It can occur without a lesion (tissue defect), as pain in a "phantom" limb after amputation. Individual people can feel pain differently; the cause and prevention of pain are an area of intense medical study.

In veterinary medicine, the fact that animals feel pain is well established, though this was not always believed. Observing an animal react to the prick of a needle or a fractured limb has convinced most people the pain that animals feel is analogous to that in people.

The discomfort of pain can cause behavior abnormalities, delay recovery from injury or disease, lead to further self-inflicted trauma or cause disuse of a body part. For these reasons, as well as for reasons of compassion for any suffering organism, the recognition and alleviation of pain should be an important goal of all technicians.

Animals in pain may express it with a whimper, yipe or growl when an area is touched or moved. Causing this reaction may be necessary so the veterinarian can make decisions regarding the severity, type, treatment, etc, of an injury or disease. Because the animal's vocal response to stimulation may distress the client and further trauma to the injured area must be avoided, handling of an animal in pain should be minimized.

Often the expression of pain is nonvocal. Animals may refuse to eat or become withdrawn, anxious (alert and looks around constantly), irritable or restless. Large animals may struggle to get away or become aggressive when handled. Some animals endure pain stoically or seek human companionship. Limping on a painful limb, tilting an infected ear downward, holding an inflamed eye closed, lying on only one side, reluctance to stand, arching the back, abnormal tail carriage (especially in swine), etc, are all signs of pain. Knowledge of normal behavior and the ability to predict how an animal may react to pain are important. Use caution when handling potentially dangerous animals in pain by using restraint devices (*eg,* muzzle, kick bar, etc).

Relieving pain is a task involving nursing skill. Check casts and bandages to make sure they fit properly and are dry. Offer highly palatable food if the patient is not eating or thin it to a gruel if the painful lesion is oral. If the animal is withdrawn, a kind word or touch may help. If the animal is restless and cannot find a comfortable position in which to rest, bedding a stall deeper or adding padding to a cage may induce relaxation. Watch for self-mutilation or excessive licking of an injured area. There are a wide variety of analgesic (pain relieving) and antiinflammatory drugs available if needed. Surgical correction of a defect may give the animal relief from pain. In general, use common sense to meet patient needs on an individual basis.

Food and Water Intake

Any hospitalized animal should be monitored for food and water intake. A complete history should include the type, time and amount of food an animal is accustomed to eating. The change in environment when an animal is hospitalized may temporarily affect eating; if the patient has not consumed food and/or water for 24 hours, it should be brought to the veterinarian's attention. The amount of time an animal can go without eating depends on its activity level, size and body condition. A working, trim animal shows the effects of starvation more rapidly than a sluggish, overweight one. Refusal to drink liquids is of greater concern than loss of appetite (anorexia), as dehydration occurs more quickly than starvation.

Daily food and water intake should be recorded on the patient's chart. A standardized amount should be offered to each animal so the amount consumed can be estimated from the amount remaining.

Food

Canned foods for dogs and cats are usually more palatable than dry foods due to their higher meat and moisture content. Semi-moist foods fall in between them in palatability. Some animals, especially cats or small-breed dogs, eat only what they are accustomed to consuming, so a wide variety of foods should be stocked in the clinic. Mixing water or canned food with dry dog food and handling cat food with the fingers sometimes increases its acceptability to patients. Adding bottled baby food in meat flavors, cottage cheese, shrimp, meat broth or eggs may encourage animals to eat. For a docile animal, offering food by hand may start it eating. Dogs may want privacy when eating and typically consume their food in "meals." Cats are "snack" eaters and if dry food is left in the cage, they may consume it at night when the clinic is quiet. Uneaten canned food should be removed from the cage in several hours, as it spoils. If the animal still refuses to eat, forced feeding may be necessary.

Herbivorous animals (ruminants, horses) find sweet feeds and grains most palatable. Mixing these in with forage may encourage eating. Use of high-quality hay and a variety of feeds is desirable. Due to the larger capacity of the equine and bovine stomach, they can go for longer periods without eating than dogs or cats. Two days of fasting for an active horse or beef or dairy cow (where production is important) should be cause for concern, but up to a week without eating for a quiet pleasure horse in good condition is not dangerous to its health. Forced feeding by intubation may be required.

Correction of the underlying cause of anorexia is essential for its resolution. Drugs, including vitamins and steroids, may help stimulate the appetite.

Excessive consumption of food may also be a problem. A change in diet, especially from a dry to canned food, may stimulate an animal's appetite. The stimulus of seeing and hearing other animals eat may also encourage an animal to bolt down its food. Large volumes of food may upset the digestive system, causing vomiting and diarrhea. They may make the patient lethargic and obese. This is especially a problem if the animal's activity is limited by confinement and if "treats" are given by hospital employees.

Water

As the section on dehydration indicates, animals must consume water to maintain a normal physiologic environment. Typically, animals consume water at 45 ml/kg (20 ml/lb) daily, but the exact amount varies with environmental temperature, activity level, individual metabolism and the moisture content of feeds.

Water consumption can be encouraged by lightly salting the food, adding broth, or frequently setting out a fresh supply. Sometimes warming or chilling the water may increase intake. Adding water or broth to food or feeding succulent forage are other ways to increase liquid consumption.

A sudden switch in water source or adding medication to the water may have discouraged drinking and can be corrected. Most animals readily accept distilled water.

Using a wax pencil to mark the fluid level in the water bowl or bucket helps monitor intake. Only one person in the clinic should be responsible for filling water bowls or buckets and a standardized amount used. Spilled or evaporated water must be subtracted from the amount considered consumed and the daily intake noted on the patient's record.

If the animal refuses to drink, giving fluids by stomach tube or injection may be necessary.

Excessive fluid intake is also cause for concern. If an animal is using water internally, as for lowering body temperature or for metabolic processes, dilute urine is not produced. However, if the patient is drinking excessively (polydipsia) and urinating large volumes (polyuria), it is a sign of disease and should be reported to the veterinarian. Excited or bored animals may drink excessively, but if it happens continually, laboratory tests should be run to eliminate disease as a cause. Using ice cubes instead of liquid water slows water consumption of an excited patient.

Automatic watering systems should be checked on a regular basis for proper function. If an animal's intake must be monitored, water should be offered in a measured volume, or a flow meter should be installed in the line of an automatic watering system.

Urinary and Fecal Output

The waste products of an animal are a direct reflection of its internal conditions. Each species has a normal range of volume, content and consistency, and deviations from normal can be a sign of disease.

Feces

The digestive tract is actually a tube within the animal, in which food is digested and nutrients absorbed. This system protects the delicate internal environment from the foreign, nonsterile and possibly toxic material the animal consumes as raw material for body functions. Because the digestive system contacts substances from the environment, it is often a site of disease, and signs like vomiting and diarrhea are common. When describing feces, any abnormal color, odor, consistency, content or volume should be noted.

Color: Feces are normally brown to green, depending on the species, but they may range from white to black abnormally. Bacterial breakdown of yellow bile pigments (from worn-out RBC processed by the liver and excreted into the proximal small intestine) produces the normal brown color of small animal feces. If more RBC are broken down than normal, as from a blood parasite, the feces are yellowish, as more bile is present than the bacteria can process. This can also occur if bacteria are not present (*eg,* with antibiotic therapy) to break the bile pigment into the brown color.

Black, tarry stools indicate bleeding into the proximal digestive tract (esophagus, stomach, mouth, small intestine). The blood is partially digested as it passes down the tract, resulting in the black color. Fresh blood, mixed throughout the feces or present in flecks, results from bleeding in the distal digestive tract (distal small intestine, colon, rectum), as it has not been decomposed. Blood may not be visible (occult blood) and a laboratory test is required to detect it.

The color of feces depends on the diet of the animal. White stools may indicate the patient has consumed large numbers of bones (small animals) or excessive milk (calves). Consumption of plant material turns feces green due to chlorophyll and is normal for large animals.

Consistency and Content: Normal consistency of feces varies among species and before and after weaning. Become familiar with the normal consistency of feces for each species. If a patient is producing stools more liquid or dryer than is typical, note it on the animal's record. The degree the stool varies from normal and the duration of the abnormality are important.

Canine and feline stools should be firm enough to be picked up with a paper towel and leave only a small spot on the original surface. They should not be hard and dry. In cattle, normal feces are pudding-like and retain a flat shape with ridges after striking the ground. Normal equine feces are dry enough to break apart when disturbed.

Foreign material in feces, such as aluminum foil, plastic, cloth or bone chips, should be reported to the veterinarian. Excessive amounts of mucus give a jelly-like, transparent look to the stool. Small amounts of undigested food are no cause for concern, but significant quantities on a regular basis indicate the digestive tract is not functioning efficiently. Horses with teeth that need floating (filing down to a smoother surface) or that consume large amounts of water at meal time sometimes pass whole grain in their feces.

Odor: The odor of fresh feces also varies with the species. A putrid odor occurs when animal protein (meat) is digested and accounts for the difference in smell between the feces of carnivores (meat eaters) and herbivores (grain and forage eaters). A fetid odor, reminiscent of decaying flesh, may indicate the surface of the digestive tract is diseased and sloughing.

Volatile toxic materials, such as motor oil and gasoline, may impart their odor to feces.

Volume: Excessive volumes of feces are linked to large food intake, as one is not possible without the other. Inefficient digestion may force an animal to overeat to maintain itself. Poor digestion can result from a lack of the necessary enzymes or other substances to break down food (normally produced by the liver, pancreas, stomach and intestines).

Feces that contain excessive liquids also occupy greater volumes than normal. Ingesta (consumed food) is usually liquid when moving through the proximal digestive tract, but in the distal regions the liquid is absorbed and the feces compacted to their normal consistency. Liquid feces result when this function is lost, when food material is moving too fast for liquid to be absorbed or when nutrients are not absorbed into the body and they osmotically draw liquid from the tissues into the intestine.

Defecation: The way an animal defecates is determined by behavior and fecal consistency. Excessive straining or lack of straining when defecating is cause for concern.

Straining to defecate (tenesmus) may indicate constipation, a foreign body, inflammation or blockage of the distal intestine (in the proximal intestine, this causes pain rather than straining and in the stomach, it usually causes vomiting). Radiographs, palpation and/or rectal examination may be necessary for diagnosis. Laxatives, enemas or surgery are possible treatments.

Straining or not straining when passing liquid stools is an important diagnostic clue and should be noted on the record. Different diseases can produce different signs; for example, cattle with Johne's disease often do not lift their tails when defecating.

Urine

Urine is plasma (the liquid fraction of blood, or blood without proteins and cells) filtered by the kidneys and changed by adding and removing substances. Because urine originates as plasma, its composition is a reflection of internal conditions and its production is an indication of kidney function.

Volume: Loss of the ability to concentrate urine leads rapidly to dehydration. Dilute urine is normally produced when water intake is high. A water-deprivation test may be necessary to test an animal's ability to concentrate its urine. Familiarity with the volume of urine normally produced by different species is essential for detection of polyuria (see Appendix).

Damage to the kidneys, shock, low blood volume, cardiovascular abnormalities and obstruction of the excretory ducts (ureters, urethra) can all cause low or no urine production. This rapidly leads to accumulation of toxic waste products in the blood (uremia). A cat with a urethral obstruction (urinary duct leading out of the body) can become dangerously uremic in 24 hours. Thus, male cats that strain to urinate, visit the litter box frequently, or have an excessively full bladder should be treated as an emergency. Obstruction of the ureter (duct leading from the kidney to the bladder) can result in kidney damage.

The rate at which urine is produced is an indication of blood flow and kidney function (glomerular filtration rate, GFR). The bladder can be catheterized and urine production monitored by watching the drops/minute produced. Most animals produce urine at 20-50 ml/kg (10-20 ml/lb) in a day, which averages to about 1.5-2 drops/minute in a medium-sized dog. Faster urine production than this is not a problem, but slower or no urine formation should be called to the veterinarian's attention.

Physical Characteristics: The odor, color and consistency of urine vary with the animal's diet, species and metabolism. For example, horses typically produce thick, opaque urine, and male cat and goat urine has a pungent smell.

Normal urine color ranges from pale to dark yellow, depending on its concentration. Red, cloudy urine indicates the presence of blood (hematuria), whereas clear, red urine (port wine colored) indicates the RBC in the urine have lysed (broken open) and released their hemoglobin (hemoglobinuria). Some drugs excreted in urine may color it.

Urea (from the breakdown of protein in the body) in urine is degraded by bacteria into ammonia when urine is left standing after it has been excreted or if there is a bacterial infection in the bladder (cystitis). A ketone smell (like nail polish remover) indicates an energy imbalance in the body (excessive fats being degraded). Some toxins produce a "chemical" odor in urine.

Urine can appear cloudy due to the presence of yeast, crystals, molds, pus, mucus, or contaminants from cage surfaces and fecal material. Crystals normally thicken horse, rabbit and rodent urine. The cause of increased urine turbidity can be determined by microscopic examination and other laboratory tests.

Vomit

Vomiting may be caused by pain, toxins, drugs, distasteful odors, foul tastes, metabolic disorders, throat irritations, neurologic problems and motion sickness. It may be preceded by restlessness, salivation, swallowing, nausea and retching in dogs, cats and swine. The length of time between eating and vomiting or regurgitation may help indicate the cause. If it occurs immediately after eating, it is termed regurgitation and the esophagus is implicated; if 30-60 minutes after eating, the stomach may be involved; and if 3-4 hours have passed since eating, the lesion may be in the small intestine. Problems in the large intestine do not usually cause vomiting. Vomiting related to specific foods may be related to changes in diet, spoiled food, meals consumed too hot or cold, gulping food, or food allergies.

Vomiting not related to food intake may be caused by systemic (generalized) infection, poisons and metabolic or neurologic abnormalities. Chronic digestive problems may cause continual vomiting. Intermittent vomiting can be due to an obstruction or other interference with digestive function. Obstructions closer to the mouth than the small intestine result in regurgitation and recognizable food material.

The volume of vomit decreases with the number of times the animal has vomited after a particular meal. If retching is severe, bile from the small intestine and liver stain the vomitus yellow to green. Protracted vomiting can lead to dehydration and electrolyte imbalances that can be fatal. Nerve receptors that send impulses to the vomiting center in the brain are found throughout the abdominal organs and may be activated by pain, infection, etc.

Projectile vomiting occurs when the stomach contents are ejected with force and is not preceded by retching and nausea. It can be seen with cranial (head) trauma or obstructions of the stomach or esophagus.

Fresh blood in the vomit is associated with bleeding from the mouth, pharynx or esophagus. Partially digested blood appears as brown flakes resembling coffee grounds.

Horses and cows do not vomit unless they are very ill, due to the anatomy of their digestive tract. Horses vomit through their nose, rather than the mouth, inhale the vomit and usually die of aspiration pneumonia due to the inhaled particles.

Regurgitation occurs when undigested food is brought up without retching. It happens normally in cattle when they ruminate (chew their cud). It may be due to overeating, hairballs in cats or disorders of the stomach and/or esophagus.

The frequency, character (color, consistency, odor, content) and volume of vomit, and severity of retching should all be communicated to the veterinarian as they may provide clues regarding the origin of the disorder.

Nervous System

Head and spinal cord injuries can result in coma, spasm, convulsion, incoordination, and changes in pupil size and response to light.

Progressive worsening of these signs indicates increasing pressure on the brain, a low brain O_2 level or other defects.

The animal's state of consciousness is evaluated by response to its name, painful stimuli (such as pricking its rump with a needle), change in position, etc. The patient may be alert, depressed, confused (animal is aware of its surroundings but does not react normally to stimuli), delirious (animal moves and may make sounds but is not aware of its surroundings), semicomatose (animal is unconscious but reacts to pain) or comatose (animal is unconscious and cannot be aroused).

Pupils that are dilated in bright light, constricted in low light or asymmetric (one dilated and one constricted) indicate a brainstem injury. Pupillary response to light is usually evaluated by shining a light in the eyes and observing the response of the pupil and comparing the response of one pupil against the other. Nystagmus (eyes rhythmically move back and forth horizontally or vertically) may indicate a skull fracture, bruising of the brain, or high intracranial pressure (inside the skull).

Any abnormal posture (head tilt, leaning), paralysis, rigid limbs, incoordination, loss of ability to flex the limbs, etc, should be reported to the veterinarian.

Convulsions should be brought to the doctor's attention immediately as they can be fatal if protracted or if they affect the heart, certain blood vessels or the respiratory system (see Chapter 1).

Miscellaneous

Blood or pus exiting the anus, mouth, mammary gland, eyes, nose, ears or wounds may be significant and the veterinarian should be alerted. Excessive matter in the eyes, ears or nose may indicate disease. Lymph nodes are easiest to palpate (feel) when enlarged. Typically the easiest places to palpate them are below the ear, at the angle of the jaw, behind the knee, and where the neck joins the shoulder. Fluid accumulations in body tissues or cavities are also important. Breath that smells like spoiled fruit may indicate diabetes mellitus. Ammonia breath occurs with uremia. A musty smell on the breath of a comatose animal can indicate liver disease.

Conclusion

Recognition of when an animal is in difficulty is the first step in monitoring a critically ill animal. This may not be easy, and seemingly inconsequential findings may precede disaster. Changes may be subtle even though one or more body systems are near collapse. An abnormal finding may easily be dismissed as due to an unimportant cause, but such thinking can lead to deterioration in a patient's condition before the signs are taken seriously.

All clinical signs are interrelated. Any disturbance in the natural harmony of the body is often reflected in several abnormal signs. Thus, it is essential that all body systems be checked each time an animal is examined.

ELECTROCARDIOGRAPHY

Muscles contract in response to electrical stimulation. The pacemaker of the heart is the sinoatrial node (SA node), located in the top quarter (end opposite the pointed apex) of the right side of the heart. Other areas of the heart can produce impulses, but the SA node sets the pace for the heart beat. The electrical impulse it generates is conducted through the heart by specialized fibers. This allows contraction in a specific sequence, so blood is "milked" from the heart rather than with a uniform, simultaneous contraction, which is not efficient in pumping blood.

The heart is responsive to hormonal (*eg,* epinephrine) and nervous stimulation. It normally pumps all of the blood delivered to it by the veins and, like any muscle, enlarges in response to increased work loads. Contraction rate and/or strength can increase or decrease as tissue needs change.

The electrocardiogram (ECG) measures electrical activity on the surface of the body, resulting from impulse flow through the heart. The electricity travels in all directions away from the heart but is measured in a standardized way.

The pattern of electrical flow through the heart is irregular with cardiac arrhythmias (irregular heart beats), is prolonged with heart enlargement due to a greater muscle mass to stimulate, and is abnormal when the heart muscle is diseased or affected by metabolic problems. The ECG is useful in diagnosing any of these conditions, detecting electrolyte imbalances, determining response to therapy for heart disease, monitoring the patient's condition during anesthesia and in establishing a prognosis for cardiac abnormalities.

Making an ECG

The ECG machine consists of leads (wires) that attach to the animal, a terminal that interprets the electrical impulses and a device that displays the impulses on paper or a screen.

The leads are color coded. The black lead attaches to the left front leg, the white to the right front leg, the green to the right rear leg and the red to the left rear leg. The leads are composed of plastic-coated wires with alligator clips, plugs or sticky pads on the free ends. The clips are clamped to the skin over the elbows and stifles of the patient. Good electrical contact between the animal's skin and the clips is essential so that the electrical impulse can be transmitted to the machine. Contact is enhanced by wetting the skin with alcohol, water or electrode jelly where the clips attach. Some machines have an extra lead (chest lead) that is attached to different sites on the animal. Sticky pads are used for long-term monitoring of the heart and must be used directly on the skin (hair is shaved off).

Contraction of muscles other than the heart also generates small electrical impulses, so the patient must remain immobile for a good ECG reading. Tranquilization and anesthesia affect the rate and rhythm of the tracing (pattern of the impulse on the ECG paper). Most animals are quiet enough for a good reading if patience and mild restraint are used.

In large animals, an ECG is performed with the patient standing, but small animal patients are usually held recumbent on their right side, with the legs parallel to each other and perpendicular to the body (Fig 6). Cats, severely ill patients or animals that resist being held in lateral recumbency may be allowed to rest in sternal recumbency (on their breast bone), but this position is not as desirable as lateral recumbency. The technic should be standardized for all patients. A wooden, Formica-topped or rubber-insulated table should be used to prevent impulse conduction to the table surface.

The machine traces the electrical flow on a piece of graph paper (electrocardiographic paper) and/or a screen. Paper speed is 25 mm/second or 50 mm/second. The faster paper speed (50 mm/second) spreads out the tracings so they are easier to read.

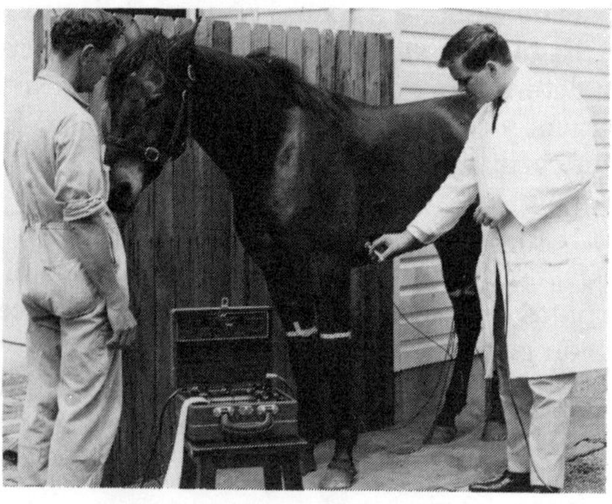

Fig 6. Recording an ECG on a horse.

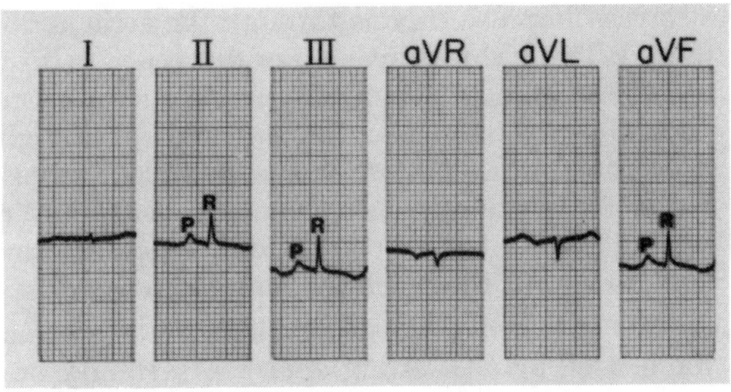

Fig 7. Normal ECG tracings from a cat, using the various leads.

Leads detect electrical activity in different planes through the animal's body and are called I, II, III, aVR, aVL and aVF (Fig 7). Lead I records electrical activity from the left front leg to the right front leg, lead II from the left rear leg to the right front leg, III from the left rear leg to the left front leg, aVR (augmented vector right) from the right front leg to the left limbs, aVL (augmented vector left) from the left front leg to the right front leg and left rear leg, and aVF (augmented vector foot) from the left rear leg to the front legs. As previously mentioned, some machines have a movable chest lead and recordings are made at 4 standard locations (over the 7th thoracic vertebra, at the 5th and 6th intercostal spaces near the edge of the sternum and at the 6th costochondral junction). By recording the electrical flow between each of these locations, a composite picture can be formulated of the heart's activity.

Recording the ECG is simple. After the paper speed is set (usually 50 mm/second for small animals and 25 mm/second for large animals), about 6-12 beats of the heart are recorded at each lead setting. In addition, 20-60 beats on lead II are recorded to evaluate the heart's rhythm.

If the tracing is too high for the paper width (pen moves higher or lower than the paper width), the sensitivity of the machine may be reduced. If the tracing is too small to be easily read, the sensitivity can be increased. Machines with the capacity to change the sensitivity have a control marked "½, 1, 2" to double the height of the reading (2) or halve it (½). The center of the tracing (baseline) should be in the middle of the paper and maintained there by adjusting the pen (stylus) position throughout the recording. The baseline changes with respiration and other muscular movements.

Interpreting the ECG

The mammalian heart is composed of 4 chambers: 2 atria and 2 ventricles. The first small peak on the ECG tracing is formed as the electrical impulse travels through the atria and is called the P wave (Fig 7). The stylus moves up or down and returns to the baseline to record the impulse. The QRS complex is the second and highest peak and is formed by passage of the impulse through the ventricles. The R fraction of the complex is a large spiked wave. The final deflection is the T wave and results when the ventricles "recharge" (return to resting state after depolarization). Tracings may contain additional landmarks but these are the major waves of diagnostic interest.

The P, R and T waves should be clear on tracings from each lead for a useful ECG. Additional beats should be recorded if patient movements and other artifacts obscure the tracings.

Many technicians read tracings to free the veterinarian's time for other tasks. Reading the ECG involves measuring wave height and width, intervals between waves, and the heart rate.

At a paper speed of 50 mm/second, the large grids on the calibrated ECG paper are 0.1 seconds wide and 0.5 millivolt high (Fig 8). The small grids are 0.02 seconds wide and 0.1 millivolt wide. There are small lines (hash marks) on the top of the paper every 1.5 seconds at a paper speed of 50 mm/second and every 3 seconds at 25 mm/second (the lines are 7.5 cm apart). Counting the number of beats (P, QRS and T waves combined) between several lines and multiplying by the time in which the beats occurred determine the heart rate.

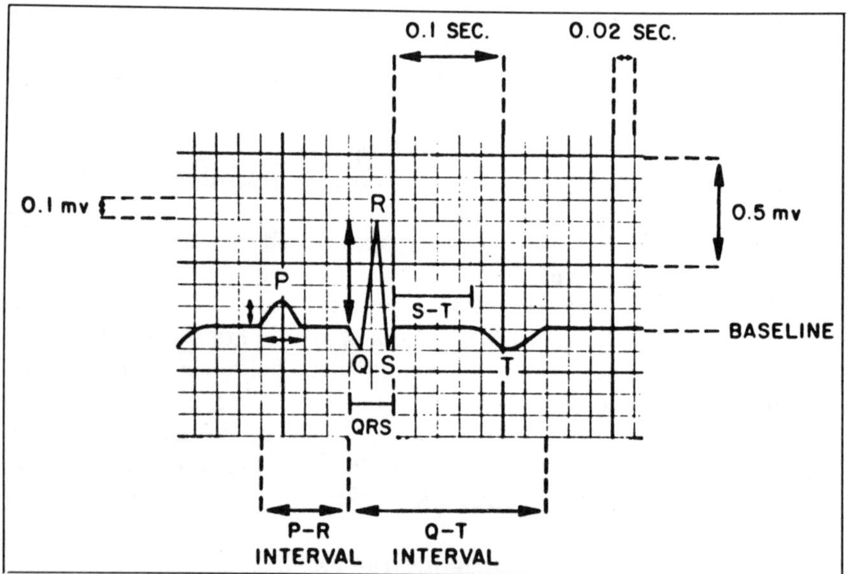

Fig 8. A normal lead II ECG tracing. (Courtesy of C. V. Mosby)

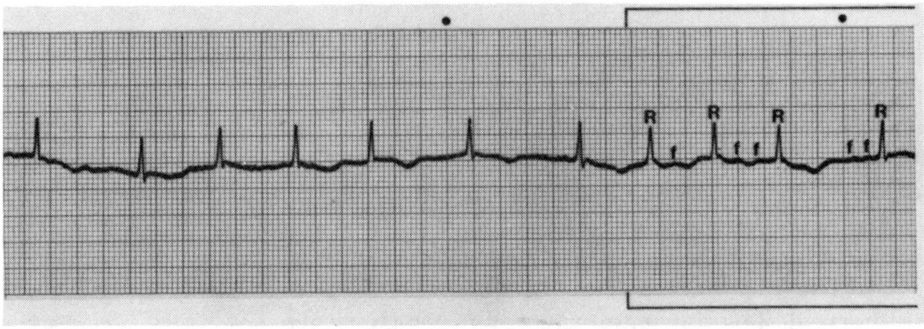

Fig 9. ECG tracing from a cat with atrial fibrillation. (Courtesy of C. V. Mosby)

Measurements of wave heights and widths, and intervals between waves is done on the long lead II strip (Fig 8). Upward (positive) deflections are measured from the upper edge of the baseline to the peak of the wave and downward (negative) deflections are measured from the lower edge of the base line to the lowest wave point. The width of the wave and intervals between waves are measured from the beginning to the end of the deflection. Measurements usually include the width and height of the P wave, QRS complex, T wave and ST segment. The lengths of the PR and QT intervals are also measured. Calipers and special ECG rulers are useful in measuring the tracing. Results are recorded in seconds or millivolts. It is a good idea to check all measurements twice.

Interpreting the ECG is a complex skill involving knowledge of cardiac structure and function, familiarity with species and breed variations, and an idea of how a given disease can affect the heart. The technician's function is to provide the doctor with readable tracings and measurements for medical analysis, not to interpret the tracings. Some veterinarians may refer tracings to specialists or use a system where the ECG is telephonically transmitted to an expert for interpretation.

Abnormal Tracings

Though interpreting ECGs is complex and should be left to the veterinarian, there are some potentially fatal conditions the technician should be able to recognize, so the veterinarian can be notified immediately. The following questions should be considered in a quick inspection of the tracing: Is there a P wave for every QRS complex? Is there a QRS complex for every P wave? Is the distance between P and R waves consistent? Are all of the QRS complexes alike and normal in shape? Do the beats occur regularly and at a normal rate?

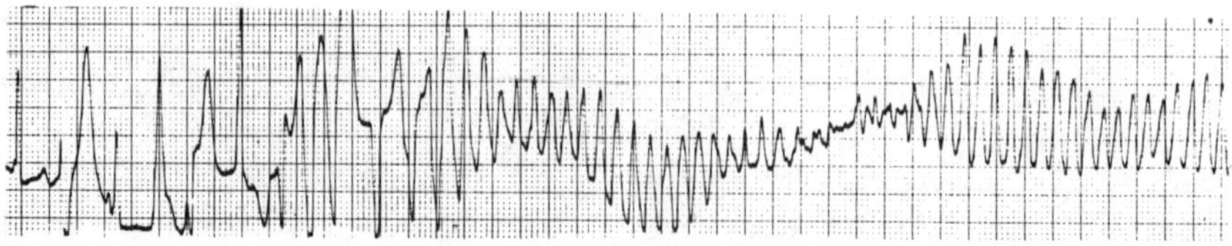

Fig 10. ECG tracing from a dog with ventricular fibrillation.

If the answer to any of these questions is "no," the tracing may be abnormal. The more negative answers there are, the more serious the patient's condition and the quicker the veterinarian should be alerted.

Atrial fibrillation occurs when multiple areas in the atria generate electrical impulses (rather than just the SA node). The resulting irregular beat causes inefficient pumping of blood. The ECG shows a fast, irregular heart rate, with the P wave replaced by multiple waves of various sizes (they may be very short), and a normal or wide and bizarre QRS complex (Fig 9). A normal QRS usually follows a group of ripples that represent the P wave.

Ventricular fibrillation is similar to atrial fibrillation but is fatal in a very short time, as the heart pumps almost no blood. The tracing appears as waves of varying heights and widths (large and coarse or small and fine). Individual P, QRS and T waves cannot be recognized (Fig 10). The abnormal waves progress to a wavy or straight line as cardiac arrest occurs.

Ventricular premature contractions (VPC) occur when the ventricles beat separately from the pacemaker (SA node) impulse. It is a common arrhythmia of dogs. With VPC, the P waves are normal but may precede, be within or follow the QRS complex. The QRS complex may be bizarre, wide and deflected in a positive and/or negative direction (Fig 11). The typical VPC appears as 2 wide, tall waves close together and pointed in opposite directions. A succession of 3 or more VPC in a row is called ventricular tachycardia (fast heart beat).

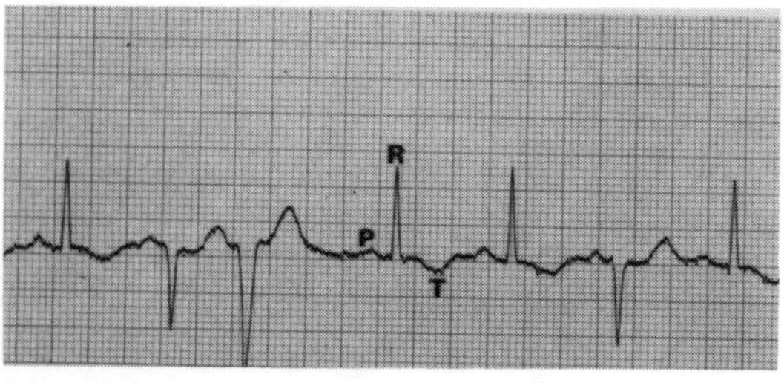

Fig 11. ECG tracing from a cat with premature ventricular contractions. (Courtesy of C. V. Mosby)

ECG Artifacts

Artifacts in the ECG are distortions that are not due to cardiac abnormalities and interfere with ECG interpretation.

Electrical interference occurs as 60 sharp waves/second. If it is present, check to see that the machine is plugged into a properly grounded (3-prong) outlet, that the leads are well attached to a fleshy part of the limb (not a large fold of skin), that the leads are clean and not saturated with alcohol, that the leads are not touching each other and the clips well fixed to them, that all other electrical equipment in the room is unplugged (*eg,* x-ray machine), that fluorescent lights are turned off, that the table is moved away from walls with electrical wiring in them, that nothing is touching the clips (other than the patient), and that the table is properly grounded. Many ECG machines have a ground wire affixed to a cold water pipe in the clinic.

Body movements or respiration can produce ECG interference. To minimize it, discourage purring in cats, make sure the animal is comfortable, apply moderate pressure with a hand on the chest to reduce muscular tremor (nervous or cold shivering), or lower the sensitivity of the ECG machine. Television and digital watches (electronic) may also produce artifacts in the tracing.

POSTOPERATIVE CARE

Surgery, by its invasive nature, unavoidably injures and stresses the patient. During recovery from anesthesia, the patient's normal response to environmental stimuli and ability to protect itself from harm are depressed. The technician must assume responsibility for the patient's well-being in this helpless state and be especially diligent in monitoring body functions.

Immediately after the end of surgery, determine the rectal temperature, pulse and respiration rates and mucous membrane color, and inspect the incision site. If the animal's temperature is below 100 F (38 C), cover it with a blanket, towel or newspapers. Insulation beneath the patient is especially useful in conserving body heat. If the temperature is below 98 F (37 C), some external heat supply should be used, such as a heating pad, hot water bottle or infrared light. An unconscious animal cannot move if the heat source is too hot, so do not place heating devices in direct contact with the animal's skin; check the skin temperature frequently. Pale mucous membranes can indicate blood loss or shock, and cyanosis an inadequate oxygen supply. Administering pure O_2 for about 10 minutes after gas anesthesia has been discontinued speeds elimination of the anesthetics and the animal's recovery.

If the incision site is bleeding, direct digital pressure (with fingers and a gauze pad) or application of a cold, dry compress can be used to stop it. A small amount of seepage for a short time is normal. The veterinarian should be notified immediately of excessive incisional bleeding. Remove dried blood from the skin around the wound with 3% hydrogen peroxide. In some cases, a bandage to support the incision, prevent contamination or reduce joint motion may be useful.

Always deflate the cuff of the endotracheal tube before it is removed. Most veterinarians prefer to untie the tube from the animal's jaw for quick removal when the swallowing reflex returns; however, the tube may slide down the trachea and block an airway, so this practice is not recommended. Tying the tube with a quick-release knot is a safer method.

Once the animal's vital signs (pulse, temperature, respiration) are in the normal range, it can be moved to a recovery area with a cart, stretcher or small tractor ("bobcat" for large animals). When transporting the patient, do not stretch the incision site, and protect appendages and the head from banging against objects. Room temperature in the recovery room should be 68-72 F (20-21 C). The area should be dark and quiet but easily accessible for observation of the patient.

Small animals are usually placed in an empty cage, with adequate insulation from the cold cage bottom and the surgical site up or not in contact with the cage bottom. The animal's tongue should be drawn out of the animal's mouth so it does not lodge in the back of the throat and obstruct respiration. The exposed tongue is also a convenient monitor for cyanosis. Urinary catheters, chest tubes, IV drip lines and so forth should be firmly affixed to the animal to prevent dislodging during recovery from anesthesia.

Large animals may be placed in a padded stall or an open field during recovery from anesthesia. They are watched from a safe distance and kept as quiet as possible. An alternative method involves kneeling at the animal's head (with one knee on its neck) and holding the muzzle flexed slightly back along its neck. As the patient begins to recover consciousness and struggle, one person holds onto the animal's halter (while standing directly in front of the patient) to stabilize the head, and another holds onto the tail to stabilize the rear end. They assist the patient in standing and balance it until recovery is complete. Never approach the legs and feet of an anesthetized large animal.

Check the patient's vital signs at least every 15 minutes. Irregular heart beat, difficult breathing, cyanosis, signs of shock, and/or a very low temperature are cause for concern, and require appropriate therapy (see Chapter 1) and notification of the veterinarian.

The time required for recovery from anesthesia depends on the type and duration of anesthesia used and the patient's metabolism. An unconscious animal cannot respond to most stimuli and is unable to swallow or blink its eyes. Do not slap, yell or try to arouse the patient quickly, as a true recovery from anesthesia requires elimination of the drug by the body and cannot be speeded in this way.

Turn (roll over) the patient every 30 minutes to prevent pooling of blood in the lungs of the dependent (down) side; the larger the animal is, the more important this is. Support the incision site carefully while turning the animal. Inspect dressings, bandages and bedding for signs of bleeding. Fresh blood is bright red, while old blood is dark red to brown. Palpate the toes, ear tips, etc. extending from bandages and casts for coolness or swelling, which may be evidence of improper application or constriction of blood vessels. A tight bandage interferes with blood circulation, causing cold, swollen and/or cyanotic toes or ear tips.

When the animal begins coughing and swallowing, remove the endotracheal tube by pulling ventrad (down) and out gently. The cuff on the tube must be deflated before the tube is removed. The endotracheal tube should never be removed before the animal can swallow, as vomiting may lead to aspiration of vomitus and subsequent pneumonia. In addition, the unconscious animal may need O_2 therapy, using the endotracheal tube.

A semiconscious animal can respond to pain, has reflexes and can move somewhat but does not respond to verbal commands. If the patient is thrashing and may injure itself, pad the recovery area. Howling, whining and other noises do not necessarily indicate the animal is in pain; however, if they continue for more than 30 minutes, call it to the doctor's attention. Many animals have a dry mouth after surgery and rinsing it with a small amount of water may have a quieting effect. Keep the head below the level of the chest while rinsing so any excess water runs out of the mouth not back into the lungs.

Soiling of the recovery area with urine, feces or vomit should be cleaned immediately as the animal can easily roll in it. Shivering and uncontrolled movements are not uncommon, but persistent coma, convulsions, widely dilated, fixed pupils (do not respond to light), pupils of unequal size or rigid limbs are indications of a problem.

Semiconscious large animals should be approached with extreme caution. They should be provided with secure footing when attempting to rise so they do not injure themselves by slipping. A dimly lit, quiet recovery area may make recovery from anesthesia smooth.

The final stage in recovering from anesthesia is disorientation. Here, the patient responds to stimuli but is confused about where it is. Slow walking of horses during this stage may steady them.

A fully conscious animal is alert and able to appropriately respond to all stimuli.

Recovery from Surgery

A rectal temperature elevation of 1-2 degrees often occurs for up to 48 hours after surgery. A persistent or higher fever could be a sign of infection, especially if respiratory distress, vomiting or other signs accompany it. Animals that have had catheters inserted, those that are debilitated, those that have lain on one side for long periods, or those that have had GI contents spilled into their peritoneal cavity are particularly prone to infection.

Check the incision site at least twice a day for inflammation (redness, heat, swelling, pain and/or a serous or purulent exudate) around a suture or line of sutures. Soreness and inflammation associated with incisions normally decrease daily.

Dehiscence (opening of the incision) can occur in debilitated animals, regardless of the surgeon's skill. Coughing, vomiting, strenuous exercise, infection, licking at the incision, and an inadequate diet all predispose wounds to dehiscence. Evisceration (spilling of bowels or other internal organs through a broken incision line) is frightening but seldom fatal if organs are protected from soiling and damage, and the wound is closed again in a short time. A watery, pink discharge from the wound is a forerunner of dehiscence. If this is seen, bandage the wound firmly and alert the veterinarian. Most incision separations occur 6-8 days postoperatively.

Patients wearing an orthopedic device (cast, splint) may require 2-3 days to learn to rise and walk with it.

Because animals heal at different rates and the trauma produced by surgery varies, suture removal times may differ. The key to recuperation is rest and a proper diet. For large animal patients, drug administration, stall cleaning and patient examination should all be done at the same time so the patient can have long periods of uninterrupted rest. Overexertion and exposure to harsh environmental conditions should be avoided during the postoperative period.

Early ambulation (patient walking) usually is desirable to prevent joint stiffness, improve circulation and exercise muscles. It also encourages patients to urinate and defecate.

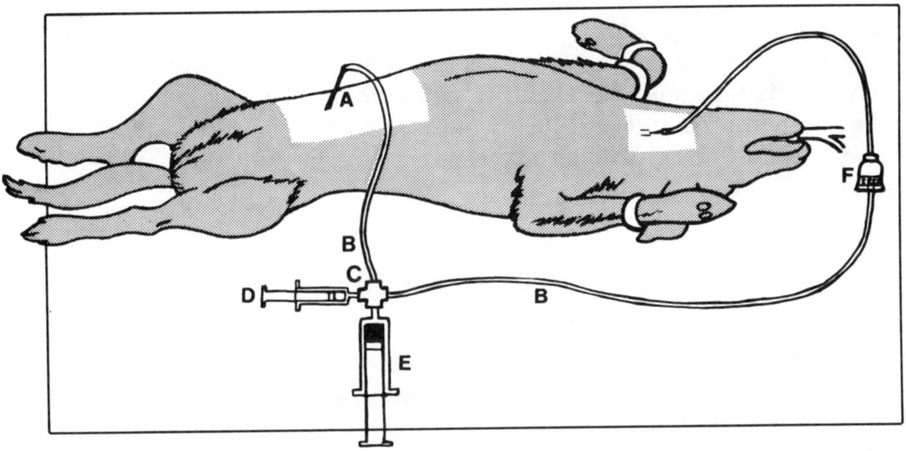

Fig 12. Autotransfusion. In this dog with severe abdominal bleeding, a dialysis catheter (A) is used to transfer blood, via IV tubing (B), to a 4-way stopcock (C) attached to a 3-ml syringe (D) and a 60-ml syringe (E). The large syringe is used to aspirate blood from the abdomen and then to force it through a filter (F) and into the jugular vein.

Licking and biting at incision sites and bandages should be strongly discouraged by using bitter-tasting compounds, Elizabethan collars, etc (see Chapter 2).

Flies can be a problem in the spring and summer. Wound exudates attract them and they may bite, lay eggs (which hatch into maggots that burrow into and liquefy tissues) and irritate the patient. Bandages, repellents and/or insecticides should be applied if flies have access to the patient.

Patients that cannot walk or that require long-term postoperative care should be treated as debilitated animals.

MANAGEMENT OF SHOCK

Shock is a state of circulatory collapse that can be fatal if untreated. It is precipitated by blood loss, pooling of blood in body vessels or cavities, or cardiac dysfunction. Causes of shock include endotoxins (from bacteria), CNS trauma, acute allergies (anaphylaxis), poisoning and severe injury.

Supportive care is aimed at maintaining the circulating blood volume with fluid therapy (except in neurogenic shock, where fluid therapy may increase intracranial pressure dangerously). Various types of fluid are given IV, including whole blood, plasma, saline or Ringer's solution, and blood volume is monitored with the PCV.

Blood or plasma pooling in body cavities may be removed and reintroduced into the cardiovascular system (autotransfusion) (Fig 12). Oxygen therapy may be useful in cyanotic animals. If the kidneys have been injured and the blood volume is normal, diuretics are given to encourage urine production. Heart function may be monitored with an ECG.

SUPPORTIVE CARE IN SPECIFIC DISEASES

Respiratory Disease

There are 3 phases of normal respiration. The lungs must fill with air and empty, the blood must flow through the lungs, and tissues must pick up and discard gases. A common sign of respiratory disease is dyspnea (difficult breathing). Exaggerated respiration is normal after heavy exercise, but not at rest. Dyspnea is commonly associated with hypoxia (low O_2), hypercapnia (high CO_2) and acidosis (low blood pH).

In all respiratory diseases, the patient should be kept quiet and at a comfortable temperature to minimize respiratory stress.

Nosebleed

Epistaxis (nosebleed) is caused by trauma to the nose, nasal tumors, coagulation (blood clotting) disorders, poisoning (warfarin or sweet clover poisoning), and racing in some horses. Bleeding can originate in any part of the respiratory system, not necessarily the nasal passages.

Supportive care can involve decreasing the blood volume (and blood pressure) with diuretics or excessive protein in the diet and use of agents that encourage clotting, such as vitamin K. Bleeding originating in the nasal blood vessels is treated by direct pressure using a tampon or packing the nose with gauze, decreasing blood flow to the area with cold packs, elevating the head, or use of epinephrine or cocaine.

Free blood in the lungs may interfere with breathing, lead to pneumonia, and cause shock due to blood loss.

Exudates

Exudates can be serous (clear and watery), mucoid, mucopurulent (mucus mixed with pus), purulent (pus), serosanguineous (watery blood) or hemorrhagic (bloody). Exudates can be caused by viral, bacterial or fungal infections, foreign bodies (*eg*, grass awns), tumors, irritants (gasoline or ammonia) and allergies (pollen, dust, etc).

Discharges may exit one or both nostrils, depending on the area involved.

Supportive care may involve use of hot packs (to break up mucous obstructions and stimulate circulation), antibiotics, nose drops, vaporizers (humidifiers), nebulizers (see Chapter 4), O_2 therapy, or bronchodilators.

Inspiratory Noise

The upper airways narrow on inspiration, whereas the lower tract expands. Thus, narrowing of an upper airway causes increased noise on inspiration. The narrowing may be caused by a foreign body, exudates, tumors, enlarged or constricted normal structures (elongated soft palate, hypoplastic trachea, etc), paralysis (toxic, infectious, traumatic), or impingement on airways (tumors).

Supportive care involves use of decongestants, antihistamines, and/or antiinflammatories to help clear the airways. Surgery to correct structural defects or remove occluding structures may be necessary.

Coughing

Coughing occurs with irritation and stimulation of cough receptors in the pharynx, larynx (voice box), trachea, bronchi (primary and secondary), pleura, pericardium and diaphragm. Many diseases cause similar coughs. Coughs can be categorized as wet or dry. Wet coughs are productive, that is, they sound like material is being expelled from the respiratory system, usually into the pharynx to be swallowed. Dry coughs are harsh and may be followed by a gag at the end. Coughs may also be loud, soft, paroxysmal (several in quick sequence), intermittent, accompanied by expulsion of blood (hemoptysis) or caused by eating or drinking. A description of the character of the cough provides diagnostic clues to the veterinarian. Coughs may be caused by parasites, foreign objects (*eg,* hairballs), tumors, heart disease, allergies and other factors.

Supportive care involves use of expectorants if the cough is wet, or antitussives (cough suppressants) if the cough is dry (wet coughs usually should not be suppressed). Most coughs resolve if the underlying cause is removed.

Sneezing

Sneezing is associated with disease of the nasal cavity and sinuses, though it may be associated with concurrent disease of the lower respiratory tract. Sneezing is a reflex initiated by irritation of the cilia of the upper respiratory tract. It is usually accompanied by a nasal discharge that may vary in character. Causes include infection, foreign objects, allergy, tumors, trauma and parasites. Supportive care involves elimination of the underlying cause. The reverse sneeze is a sudden, deep snort (or snore) on inspiration.

Expiratory Noise

Pulmonary emphysema, an abnormal accumulation of air in the lungs due to pathologic processes, is a cause of expiratory noise. Emphysema may be due to loss of lung elasticity or destruction of the walls separating the alveoli (air sacs). Causes include infection, allergy, irritant gases and parasites.

Supportive care usually involves rest, decreasing the amount of environmental dust (moisten feed or the stall floor for large animals), and use of decongestants, antihistamines and/or bronchodilators.

Pneumonia

Inflammation of the lung tissues (pneumonia) can be a direct result of microbial action or secondary to other disease or injury (*eg*, parasites or inhaled foreign materials) that allows invasion. It is especially severe in young and very old animals, and may be caused by bacteria, viruses, fungi, parasites, allergies or toxins. Systematic signs are also often seen (fever, depression, etc).

Supportive care generally requires antibiotics, antitussives (cough suppressants), expectorants, antihistamines, decongestants and O_2 therapy.

Circulatory System

Diseases affecting the heart and blood vessels involve all other systems in the body because adequate circulation is required by all tissues. The technician must be especially diligent in monitoring the cardiovascular status.

Inadequate circulation causes loss of cells due to hypoxia, resulting in myocardial infarction, cerebral aberrations, syncope (fainting), stroke or death. Care of chronically affected animals is rarely attempted in food animals, as their value is in production of meat and milk. Companion and performance animals are the primary recipients of nursing care. Affected animals are first stabilized and then maintained in a manner to reduce further damage (*eg*, as from pulmonary edema) while working toward rehabilitation of this vital system.

Venous Engorgement

Engorgement (especially of the jugular vein) is seen when the central venous pressure is elevated (Fig 13). Inadequate cardiac output

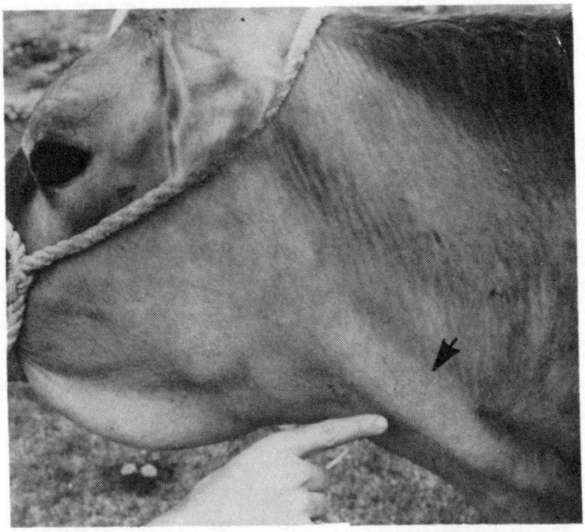

Fig 13. Jugular vein distention in a cow, caused by traumatic reticulitis and atrial fibrillation.

causes blood to collect in the vessels. Causes include congestive heart failure, hypernatremia (excessive sodium in the blood), renal failure, vasoconstrictive shock, pericarditis, myopathy (as in selenium deficit), or impingements (*eg,* tumors) or constrictions of major arteries (stenosis).

Supportive care includes reduction of dietary sodium (salt) intake and use of diuretics or bleeding to reduce blood volume. Some drugs (furosemide, digoxin) are effective in long-term therapy.

Fibrillation

Fibrillation (flutter) in the upper chambers of the heart (atria) may not result in signs of disease, but fibrillation of the larger, lower chambers (ventricles) may cause death. Causes of fibrillation are hypoxia, electrocution and toxins.

Chronic care usually involves use of precisely timed doses of cardiac drugs (digitoxin or quinidine) and restriction of activity.

Bradycardia

Bradycardia (abnormally slow heart rate) is normal in athletic animals at rest but is a sign of disease in unconditioned animals. Many toxins and depressant drugs (anesthetics, hypnotics) slow the heart and can cause circulatory collapse or shock. Consider the condition and activity level of the patient before deciding if the veterinarian should be alerted to a slow heart rate.

Supportive care involves use of fluid and O_2 therapy, stimulants or hormones.

Cyanosis

A blue cast to the tongue and other mucous membranes indicates a large amount of the animal's hemoglobin is not carrying O_2. Arterial blood O_2 has been reduced by high cell demand for O_2, inadequate exchange of gases in the lungs or low pulmonary blood supply (perfusion). Causes for cyanosis include airway obstruction, a barrier to diffusion of O_2 from lungs to blood (emphysema, allergy), hypoventilation or mismatched ventilation:perfusion ratio. Anemia does not cause cyanosis, as the hemoglobin is fully saturated with O_2 though reduced in amount. Reduced ability of the blood to carry O_2 can also prevent normal mucous membrane color (*ie,* blood drawn into a tube remains brownish when shaken), as in cyanide poisoning. Cyanosis is a sign requiring immediate notification of the doctor. Transfusions, fluid and O_2 therapy, and antiinflammatory drugs may be used to correct cyanosis.

Syncope

Syncope (fainting) may be caused by circulatory or neurologic impairment, hypoxia, hypoglycemia, toxins, epilepsy, narcolepsy and metabolic disease.

Supportive care for syncope depends upon the cause. Protecting the animal from injury (removing obstructions from the area) and use of circulatory or nervous system stimulants are beneficial.

Tachycardia

Tachycardia is an abnormally high heart rate. Disease occurs when the heart rate is so rapid as to prevent effective pumping of blood. Mild to marked increases in heart rate are normal during fear, heavy exercise and excitement. Impaired circulation to the brain or skipped beats may be dangerous to the animal's health. Causes include intoxications, pain and heart disease.

Supportive care is directed at maintaining an adequate supply of blood to the body tissues, especially the brain, and reducing the heart rate. Adjustments in environmental conditions (reducing stress), and analgesics or mood-altering drugs are used in therapy.

Neurologic Disease

The nervous system is a communication network for response to stimuli and coordination of internal and external body functions.

The center of the nervous system is the brain and spinal cord (central nervous system or CNS), which are involved in conscious thought, processing sensory information and maintaining autonomic functions. Specific areas of the brain are devoted to different tasks. The brain and spinal cord are enclosed in a fluid medium (cerebrospinal fluid or CSF) much like plasma, for protection. The CNS is richly supplied with blood vessels, but the capillaries are not as freely permeable as elsewhere in the body and form a barrier between the blood and CNS (blood-brain barrier) that helps keep microorganisms, toxins, etc, out.

The spinal cord is a collection of descending tracts from the brain and ascending tracts from the periphery of the animal. Major nerve trunks exit and enter between the vertebrae (spinal column). The spinal cord terminates as a bundle of nerves supplying the tail and rear quarters of the animal.

The peripheral nervous system is composed of all nervous tissue not in the CNS and includes spinal nerves for sensory input and motor (muscle or organ action) output. The autonomic system, a part of the peripheral nervous system, has sympathetic and parasympathetic components that control visceral (organ) functions of the body not under conscious control, such as the cardiovascular, respiratory and digestive systems.

The nervous system is highly complex and neurologic damage may result in various abnormalities. Nervous diseases may be treated medically; however, most nervous system tissue does not regenerate or regenerates very slowly. The nervous system is evaluated by a systematic neurologic examination done by the veterinarian.

The brain is divided into 3 main parts: the cerebrum (main part of the brain, involved in thought, sensory integration, etc); the cerebellum (involved in coordination of incoming and outgoing impulses); and the brainstem (cranial nerve and autonomic nervous system function control). Lesions in the cerebrum can be manifested as behavior and/or personality changes, such as loss of housetraining, atypical aggression or docility, disorientation, avoidance of a favorite pastime, failure to recognize people, aimless wandering, loss of interest in life, head pressing, excessive excitement, abnormal performance of a learned task and hiding.

Seizures may occur with bursts of electrical activity from the brain, resulting in uncoordinated muscular contractions. Epilepsy, characterized by repeated seizures, usually responds well to drug therapy.

Stupor (animal requires a painful stimulus to arouse it), semiconsciousness or coma (animal cannot be aroused) may occur with lesions of the cerebrum. Pain occurs with certain cerebral diseases or when the membranous coverings of the CNS (meninges) are inflamed.

Delicate tremors and inability to correctly judge distances are signs of cerebellar disease.

Cranial nerve deficits may indicate brainstem injury or peripheral damage of the cranial nerves. Involvement of more than one cranial nerve or abnormal autonomic function is a more definite indication of brainstem disease.

Brain injuries should be handled as emergencies, especially if the signs progressively worsen. A common result of brain injury is edema (due to increased production of CSF, hemorrhage or obstruction of CSF outflow tracts). Because the brain is encased in the skull, it cannot swell (as other tissues do when they are inflamed) without the increased pressure permanently damaging nervous tissue. Progressively worsening signs indicate continuing brain damage and warrant immediate attention.

Supportive care for neurologic disease may include use of osmotic agents (*eg,* mannitol), antiinflammatories, cage or stable rest, fluid therapy, and antimicrobials that can cross the blood-brain barrier. Given time, the brain has an amazing capacity to recover from injury, and certain types of neurologic surgery have been very successful.

Vestibular Apparatus

The vestibular system is part of the inner ear and functions to maintain balance and the animal's perception of its orientation in space.

Signs of vestibular damage may include loss of balance, a head tilt, walking in tight circles, falling or rolling, dizziness or vertigo (animal appears disoriented, excited or restless), nystagmus (eyes move rhythmically from side to side, up and down or in a circle) and/or nausea (like "sea sickness").

Vestibular disease may result from trauma, severe ear infections, stroke, tumors, intracranial infections or damage to the eighth cranial (vestibulocochlear) nerve.

Supportive care may involve use of antiinflammatories, antimicrobials and diuretics. Animals should be protected from injuring themselves (remove protruding objects and confine in a safe area) and assisted with normal body functions (eating, urination, etc) with gentle support.

Cranial Nerves

Olfactory: The first cranial nerve (olfactory) is involved with the sense of smell. An animal's sense of smell is difficult to evaluate, but anorexia, refusing some foods, and a decrease in sniffing behavior may be clues. Conditions causing loss of the sense of smell may be canine tooth abscesses, tumors, upper respiratory infections and damage to the olfactory nerve.

Optic: The second cranial nerve (optic) is necessary for vision. Animals with optic nerve damage may bump into things or fail to avoid objects introduced into their path. Other causes of blindness include damage to the retina (light-sensitive lining of the eye), intraocular infection, brain damage, tumors and congenital (birth) defects.

Oculomotor: The third cranial nerve (oculomotor) and the sympathetic nervous system control the size of the pupil. Abnormal pupillary dilation or constriction, lack of response to light, and unequal pupil sizes (anisocoria) are signs of cranial nerve or brain damage and should be reported to the veterinarian.

Trochlear, Abducens: With the third cranial nerve (oculomotor), cranial nerves IV (trochlear) and VI (abducens) control eye position and movement. The position of the pupils can be used to determine if the eye is tilted.

Trigeminal: Damage to cranial nerve V (trigeminal) may result in a dropped jaw, inability to chew, a protruding tongue, drooling, shrinking (atrophy) of some of the cranial muscles, loss of skin sensation to the ear, eyelid and/or lower lip, and food impaction in the cheeks.

Facial: Cranial nerve VII (facial) innervates the muscles of facial expression, the tear glands and certain salivary glands. Drooping of the ear, eyelid and/or upper lip and drooling are signs of facial nerve damage.

Vestibulocochlear: The vestibular apparatus and sense of hearing are supplied by cranial nerve VIII (vestibulocochlear). Loss of hearing is difficult to assess in animals unless both ears are involved. Severe inner ear infections and space-occupying masses may also cause loss of hearing.

Glossopharyngeal, Vagus, Accessory: Cranial nerves IX (glossopharyngeal), X (vagus) and XI (accessory) are all involved in innervation of the throat. Dysphagia (loss of swallowing ability) and/or a change of voice occur when they are damaged. The vagus nerve also innervates the heart and viscera.

Hypoglossal: The tongue musculature is innervated by cranial nerve XII (hypoglossal). Injury to the hypoglossal nerve results in loss of muscle tone and impaired movement of the tongue.

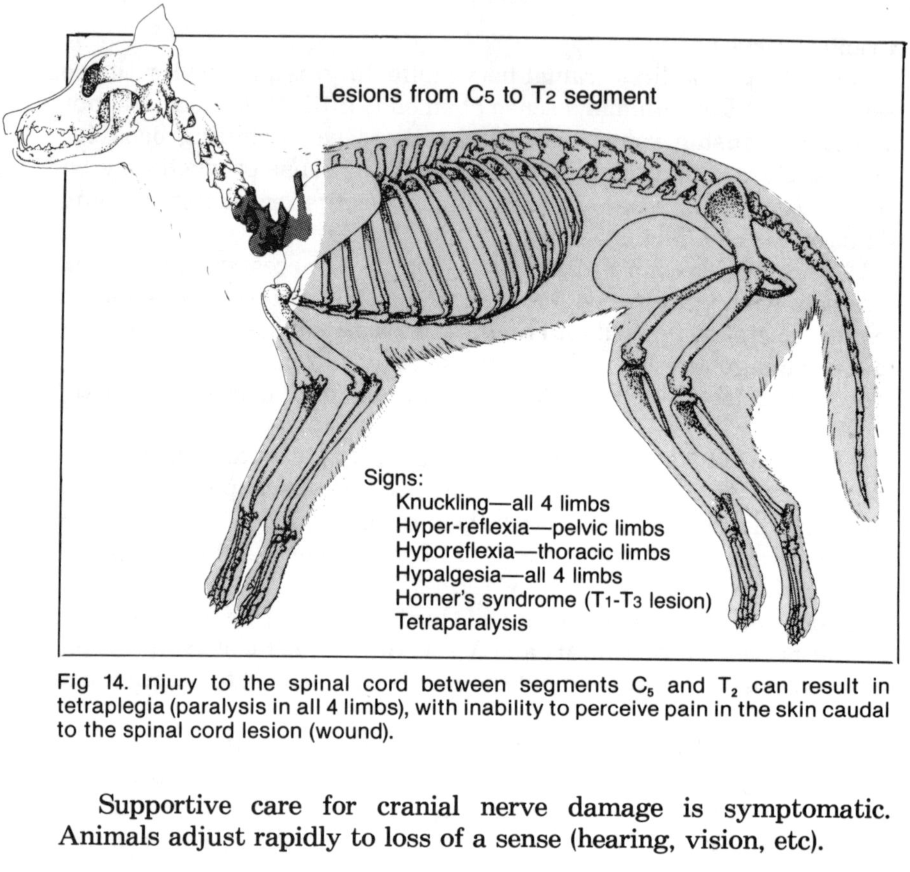

Fig 14. Injury to the spinal cord between segments C_5 and T_2 can result in tetraplegia (paralysis in all 4 limbs), with inability to perceive pain in the skin caudal to the spinal cord lesion (wound).

Supportive care for cranial nerve damage is symptomatic. Animals adjust rapidly to loss of a sense (hearing, vision, etc).

Spinal Cord

Damage to the spinal cord is manifested as a neurologic abnormality caudal to the lesion. Signs include limb paresis (weakness), paralysis (inability to move), rigidity or pain, loss of proprioception (ability to determine position in space), urinary or fecal incontinence (inability to control urination or defecation), ataxia (poor coordination in moving the limbs and body), and cutaneous anesthesia (loss of perception of pain in the skin) (Figs 14-16).

Spinal cord damage can result from compression of the cord due to intervertebral disc herniation, space-occupying masses (tumors), swelling due to inflammation, edema or hemorrhage, and bruising or tearing of the cord from trauma (*eg,* spinal fracture).

Supportive care involves restricting movement of the animal and use of antiinflammatory drugs or surgery to reduce pressure on the cord. Many animals with spinal cord injury cannot voluntarily urinate or defecate. In such cases, the bladder should be manually expressed 2-3 times a day (even if the animal dribbles) and enemas administered as needed. Animals should be cared for as if debilitated.

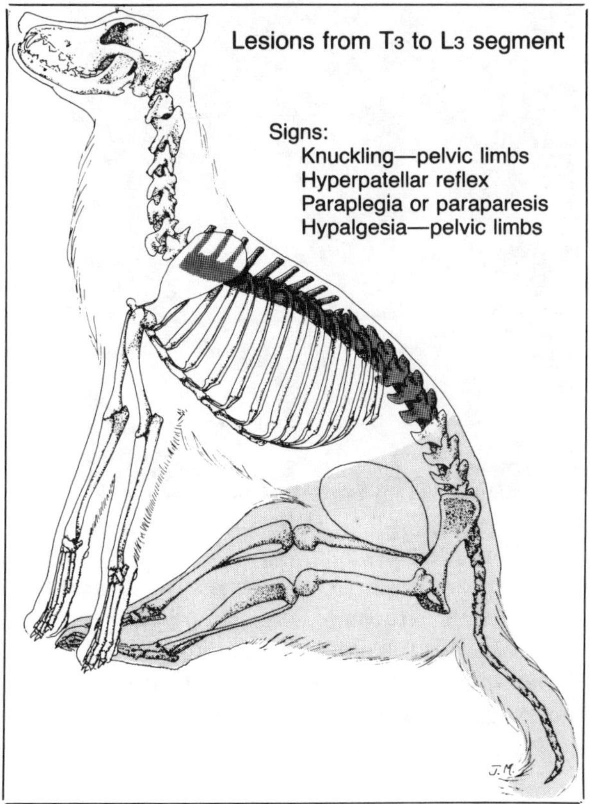

Fig 15. Spinal cord injuries between segments T_3 and L_3 usually cause hindlimb paralysis and decreased skin sensation. Respiration and urination may also be affected.

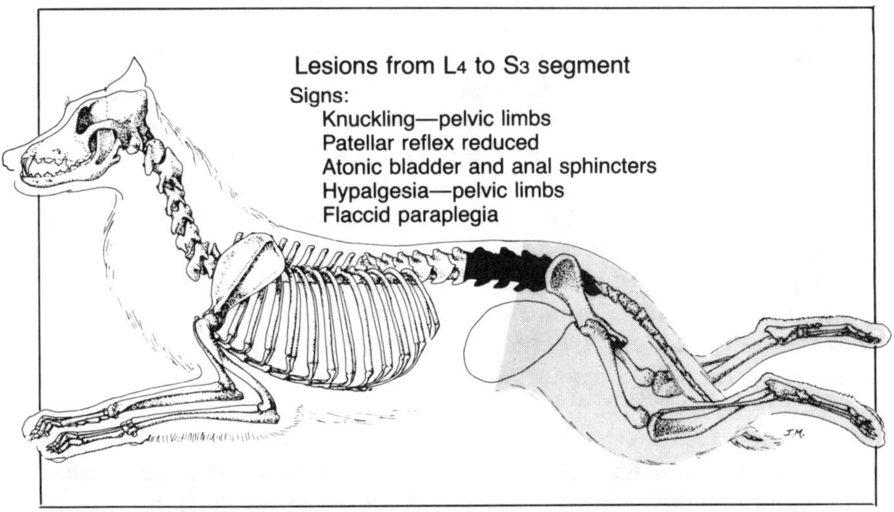

Fig 16. Spinal cord damage in segments L_4 to S_3 causes paraplegia (rear-limb paralysis), with the possibility of inability to urinate and loss of anal sphincter function and skin sensation.

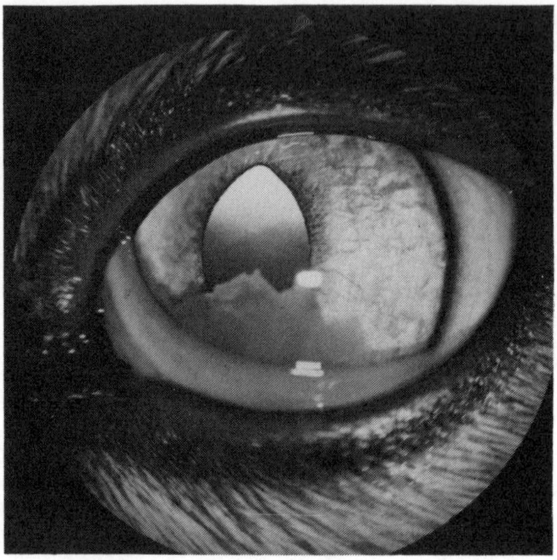

Fig 17. Anterior uveitis in a cat's eye.

Peripheral Nerves

Damage to peripheral nerves, as from trauma or improper injections, results in loss of sensation and/or loss of function. The affected area becomes flaccid (limp) and atrophied (muscles shrink with time). Supportive care includes protection of the limb from damage (self-mutilation, dragging on the ground, etc), physical therapy and surgery.

Ocular Disease

Inflammation

Eye inflammation, either on the surface or inside the eye, can manifest itself as redness, pain (seen as tearing or rubbing the eyes) or an ocular discharge (may be watery or thick and yellowish, gray or white). Inflammation can be due to infection (*eg,* canine distemper, *Chlamydia,* etc), allergy, parasites (*eg, Thelazia californiensis* or flies), chemicals, drugs, trauma or other eye diseases. Thick, purulent (pus) discharges indicate infection.

Supportive care may include flushing the eye and use of antimicrobial or antiinflammatory ointments. Application of an Elizabethan collar or neck cradle may be necessary to prevent the animal from rubbing its eyes.

Ocular Opacity

Opacification (cloudiness) of various parts of the eye (*eg,* cornea, lens) can prevent the light transmission necessary for vision. The cornea may become dry, cloudy and ulcerated, the lens may gradually become cloudy with age (cataract), and the normally transparent fluid between the lens and the cornea (aqueous humor) may fill with debris due to inflammation (anterior uveitis) (Fig 17). Treatment for corneal lesions includes topical application of antimicrobials and antiinflammatories. Cataracts can be removed surgically. Anterior uveitis is often treated with topical atropine and corticosteroids.

Glaucoma

The eye is a fluid-filled structure, with intraocular pressure maintained within close limits by various physiologic mechanisms. A group of diseases, collectively called glaucoma, result in an elevated intraocular pressure with resultant damage to the delicate internal structures necessary for vision. Certain breeds are prone to glaucoma. The condition can occur secondary to trauma or infections.

Acute glaucoma is an emergency that must quickly be treated with drugs to decrease intraocular pressure and so reduce pain. Glaucoma commonly results in blindness, regardless of the treatment.

Urogenital Disease

Diseases of the reproductive and urinary tracts are closely linked and result in a variety of problems, from reduced fertility to death due to systemic accumulation of metabolic wastes.

Persistent Hymen

The hymen, which normally covers the opening into the vagina in females that have never been bred, may be retained and so result in vaginitis or failure to breed. Pathogenic organisms may penetrate the cervix and cause infections that may lead to permanent sterility. Surgical correction is usually simple and supportive care involves treating any infection with antimicrobials.

Masculinization in Females

Masculinization of females involves an imbalance of sex hormones. It can occur with male and female twin calves, due to masculinization of the heifer calf by the bull calf's sex hormone (testosterone). Such masculinized heifer calves are known as "freemartins." Masculinization can also occur as a side effect of various drugs (*eg,* anabolic steroids) and in some forms of neoplasia (cancer).

Supportive care involves therapeutic use of estrogen. Use of estrogen (female hormone) and related compounds, such as diethylstilbestrol (DES), may be helpful but often requires long-term medication to maintain the effect and does not reverse all masculine changes. Surgery may be necessary to remove a masculinizing tumor.

Nymphomania, Satyriasis

Nymphomania and satyriasis refer to an excessive degree of sexual desire in females and males, respectively. They are expressions of abnormally high levels of sex hormones that may come from drug therapy, or ovaries that contain abnormal or cystic follicles. Affected females continually display signs of estrus (heat) and stand for repeated matings. Affected males attempt to copulate excessively or with inappropriate objects (masturbate).

Care involves reducing the level of sex hormone by surgical, mechanical (rupture of cystic follicles) or hormonal means.

Homosexuality

Homosexuality (sexual attraction between animals of the same sex) is "normal" in male populations with limited or no access to females. It is also an expression of dominance between alpha (socially high ranking) males and submissive males. "Bulling" occurs when cows mount each other and is used by herd managers to detect heat. Endocrine disturbances may influence homosexual behavior but are not a consistent cause. Homosexuality in breeding males is undesirable because it leads to a reduced sperm count.

Retained Placenta

The placenta may be retained when the afterbirth does not detach from the uterus during parturition (birth). It may protrude through the cervix or be held in the uterus. Placental retention may result from infection during gestation, scar tissue from a cesarean section, abortion, mummified fetuses (dead, dehydrated and partly resorbed), or poor uterine tone. Natural detachment may occur in a few hours or days, or may be accomplished mechanically (rectally in large animals and surgically in small animals), with infusion of hypertonic solutions of salt, or with hormones (*eg,* oxytocin, estrogen).

Prolonged Gestation

Endocrine imbalances in the dam or fetus can result in an abnormally long gestation period (duration of pregnancy) (breeding date must be known). Other causes include an overly large fetus, fetal death, fetal monstrosities (congenital defects), and adverse drug reactions.

Supportive care involves isolation of the dam in a comfortable environment similar to that for normal parturition. Often this alone relaxes the dam enough so that parturition occurs without assistance. Use of drugs to induce labor, or cesarean section may be necessary.

False Pregnancy

Pseudocyesis (false pregnancy) is not uncommon in the bitch and is often recurrent and associated with endocrine disturbances. The female may display various signs of pregnancy, including a watery (serous), milk-like secretion from the mammae. Affected females often seek isolation, build nests and may "adopt" toys as offspring.

Treatment is normally with ovariohysterectomy (spay) or use of hormones.

Vaginal or Uterine Prolapse

Protrusion of the vagina and/or uterus through the vulva usually occurs after dystocia (difficult birth) (Fig 18). Replacing the organs or surgical removal is required.

Supportive care involves keeping the tissue clean and protected. Antimicrobial and antiinflammatory drugs are used during convalescence.

Abortion

Expulsion of a fetus at less than the full term of pregnancy is called abortion. Abortion can be induced with drugs or instruments to terminate any unwanted pregnancy. Abortion indicates an immunologic incompatibility between the dam and fetus or infection by viral

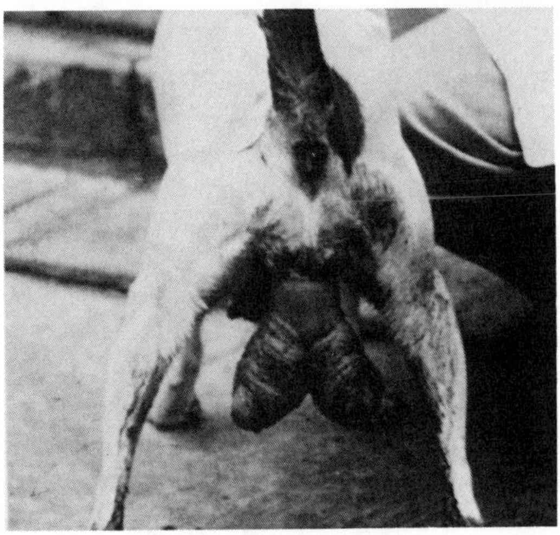

Fig 18. Uterine prolapse in a bitch.

(IBR, BVD), chlamydial (foothills abortion), bacterial (*Brucella*, *Campylobacter*) or protozoal (*Toxoplasma*) agents. Toxins and drugs (locoweed, corticosteroids) may also cause abortion.

Preventive care is aimed at keeping the fetus, if viable, and the mother healthy. The dam may also be isolated, rested and protected from stress. Nutrition may be critical, especially if the dam is starved or dehydrated from disease.

If an abortion has already occurred, supportive care is directed at returning the uterus to normal. Drugs that help clear out the uterus (prostaglandins, oxytocin, estrogen) and antimicrobial therapy may be started.

Savaging of Offspring

In some species the dam (mother) may destroy ill or deformed offspring; however, savaging (attacking and perhaps killing) normal offspring is abnormal and undesirable. Restraint and mild tranquilizers may quiet the dam, but if the dam still refuses to care for her young, they must be raised as orphans or placed with a foster dam.

Mastitis

Mastitis (mammary gland inflammation) is a serious problem in the dairy industry as it reduces profit (loss of milk sales) and can increase death losses of the newborn animals. Mastitis is frequently manifested as an unusual milk consistency and content (clots, fibrin shreds, mucus) and abnormal color (pinkish, greenish, etc) or odors (ketones).

Causes for mastitis are often related to milking management. Keeping milking machines properly adjusted (correct vacuum and pulse ratios), scrupulous attention to hygiene (use of teat dips, hand washing, etc), and good bedding practices all are necessary to control the primary or secondary microbial invaders of mammary tissue. Trauma is another cause, as from the teeth of the young (milk teeth in piglets) or being trampled. Milk from cows with mastitis is unfit for human consumption. If infectious organisms (*Salmonella*, coliforms, *Staphylococcus*) are present, the milk should not be fed to calves.

Supportive care in mastitis should be directed toward prevention. Repeat infections may occur in a herd as most animals in a given herd are managed similarly. Sanitation, antimicrobial therapy, elimination of irritants and toxins, and use of soothing or cooling applications are beneficial.

Penile Problems

Phimosis (inability to extrude the penis from the sheath) or paraphimosis (inability to retract the penis into the sheath) may be caused by penile inflammation (stallion kicked while breeding or dog with fractured os penis), or the opening into the sheath may be too small (pizzle rot of sheep). Inflammation, infection and fly strike (maggots in the sheath) may complicate these problems.

Repeated application of cold packs or soaking the penis in cold water, cleaning the area scrupulously or surgical measures (splitting the sheath) may aid the animal. Paraphimosis is an emergency, as the penis quickly dries and becomes inflamed.

Vulvar Discharges

Discharges from the female reproductive and urinary tract may be normal (estrus) or due to disease. Causes for abnormal vulvar discharges include infection, trauma, tumors, foreign bodies and cystitis.

Supportive care includes reducing damage to the reproductive tissues with cleansing and disinfecting solutions. Active lesions may be cauterized (chemical or heat) or surgically removed.

Udder Edema

Fluid accumulation (edema) in the udder may be due to ascites (see Digestive Disease), mastitis or a genetic condition. Some females produce milk and develop udder edema before parturition and may have to be milked to reduce the pressure.

Other supportive care may include massage, a reduction in fluid intake, use of diuretics to increase urine production, and use of corticosteroids to decrease any inflammation.

Agalactia

There are many causes for agalactia (failure to produce milk), including hormonal imbalances, surgery, stress, toxins (ergot), and low blood calcium levels (eclampsia). In some cases (mostly swine), the cause is unknown.

Offspring should be raised as orphans or placed with a foster mother. Nursing and handmilking may encourage milk production, but oxytocin administration has no effect on milk production.

Incontinence

Inability to control urination or defecation is called incontinence. The usual sign reported is wet spots where the animal sleeps, but dribbling and dropping feces are also seen.

The causes are varied and in some cases poorly understood. Low levels of estrogen, loss of reflex control of the sphincters (spinal cord damage), masses (tumors) impinging on the bladder, developmental defects or behavior problems are causes.

Supportive care is directed at keeping the diet and fecal and urinary output as normal as possible, modifying inappropriate behavior and providing ample opportunities to void. Debilitated and old animals may lose control of elimination and require nursing care, such as providing deep bedding, frequent turning if recumbent (as often as every 30 minutes), or catheterization.

Urination Problems

When an animal assumes the posture of urination without producing urine, remains in position long after urine flow has stopped or urinates in inappropriate places, there may be a problem with urine passage.

In the normal urination posture for horses, the animal presses forward, slightly spreads its legs and either drops its penis (stallions, geldings) or lifts its tail (mares). Mild groaning is not a sign of pain. Recumbent horses do not urinate. Mares in heat urinate frequently.

Normal cows arch their backs and draw their legs up under themselves to urinate. Bulls and steers may dribble or produce short pulsations. Cattle are not particular where they urinate and, unlike horses, void while walking, eating or lying down.

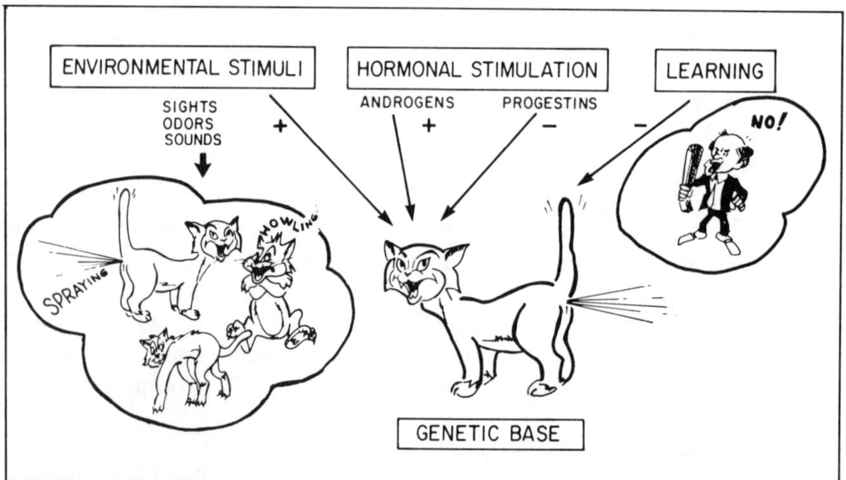

Fig 19. Spraying of urine by male cats is genetically based behavior, the expression of which is influenced by numerous stimuli. (Courtesy of the *California Veterinarian*)

Normal sows urinate in a posture similar to that of cows, but young pigs and boars may pulse or spray urine to the right or left.

Normal cats squat to urinate, though sexually active males and females may spray urine behind them to mark objects (Fig 19). The tail quivers and the hind legs tread up and down during spraying.

Female dogs also squat to urinate, but void only small volumes each time if they are in estrus. Adult male dogs raise one leg to direct a stream of urine against an object. Male puppies squat, but as they mature, gradually begin to lift their legs (males neutered early may always squat to urinate).

Causes for unusual urination behavior include cystitis (bladder infection), calculi (stones) or tumors blocking the urinary tract, and kidney disease (nephritis, renal failure). Additional causes or contributing factors include a high-mineral diet, use of certain drugs (cyclophosphamide) and various developmental anomalies (patent urachus in foals).

Treatment involves ensuring urination by catheterization, cystocentesis or surgical correction of the cause, and maintaining the animal with an appropriate diet and/or IV fluid administration.

Polyuria

An increased volume of urine (polyuria) or frequency of urination may signal a problem. Urine production normally reflects fluid intake; however, regardless of fluid intake, diuretics and some diseases can cause polyuria, including diabetes (insipidus or mellitus), and renal, liver, adrenal, uterine or thyroid disease.

Supportive care is directed toward balancing body fluids, electrolytes and pH. Any losses of protein (albuminuria) and glucose (glycosuria) are also considered in selecting treatment. Maintaining hydration and meeting caloric requirements may be difficult in patients losing protein or glucose.

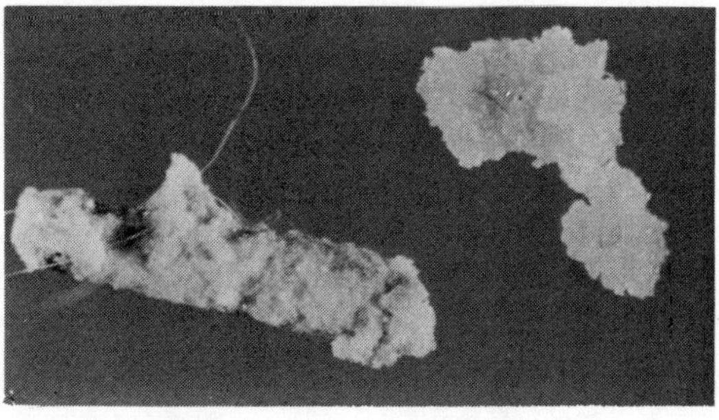

Fig 20. Obstructive debris removed from the distal urethra of a male cat with the feline urologic syndrome.

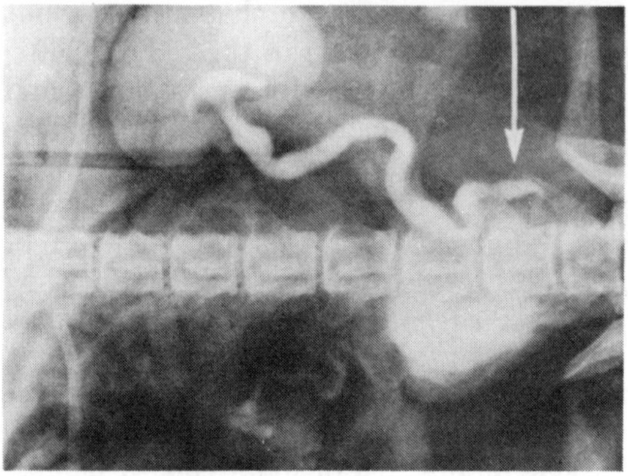

Fig 21. Urogram in a dog reveals a distended ureter, obstructed by a ureteral calculus (arrow).

Anuria

Anuria (lack of urine production) and oliguria (production of only a small volume of highly concentrated urine) are caused by dehydration or low renal blood flow (perfusion) due to heart failure, shock, acidosis (excessive levels of acids), hyperkalemia (high blood levels of potassium) and a variety of infections. Obstructions in the urinary system can cause renal failure if not corrected rapidly (Figs 20, 21). Accumulation of waste products in the blood (urea, creatinine, etc) causes toxic signs, such as vomiting and diarrhea (uremic syndrome).

Supportive care depends on the duration and severity of the problem. Acute episodes can usually be managed by providing wholesome drinking water and use of diuretics. Chronic cases may require extended, aggressive fluid therapy and dialysis or surgical measures.

Abnormal Urine

Red to brown urine may be due to whole RBC, hemoglobin or the muscle pigment, myoglobin (Monday morning sickness in horses).

Because normal urine may turn brown (horse) or cloudy upon standing at room (or lower) temperatures, gross observations should be made on freshly voided urine. Some drugs (methylene blue, epinephrine) cause production of colored or highly concentrated urine that appears cloudy. Mucus and excessive numbers of cells (WBC in bladder infections) result in thick, translucent urine.

Supportive care involves maintaining urine output and hydration status. Antimicrobial drugs may be given, but long-term use may allow resistant organisms to overgrow.

Digestive Disease

Failure To Eat

Failure to eat is a common sign of digestive tract disease and results in progressive starvation. It may be caused by dental problems (sharp teeth, teething, misalignment, etc), anorexia (inappetence) foreign objects, pain or systemic diseases.

Supportive care involves management of any wounds, correcting dental problems, providing a soft, palatable diet, appetite stimulation, and general attention to the animal's overall health (parasite control, foot care, etc).

Dysphagia

Dysphagia (failure to swallow) may be a signal of paralysis of the throat due to nerve damage, infectious disease (rabies) or poisoning. It also is associated with pharyngeal and/or esophageal trauma caused by foreign objects or caustic chemicals (*eg,* bone slivers, lye) and may produce excessive salivation. Animals with suspected infectious disease should be quarantined for observation.

Failure To Ruminate

Failure to ruminate ("make cud") is cause for concern in any mature ruminant. Various drugs, infection, foreign bodies, bloat, eclampsia (hypocalcemia), ketosis or GI obstruction reduces rumination. Ingestion of low-fiber feeds lowers the frequency of rumen contraction but does not totally eliminate rumination.

Supportive care involves meeting fluid and energy needs, and correcting any deficits in muscle activity with drugs. Transfaunation, usually done after antimicrobial therapy or starvation has killed off the normal rumen flora, involves transferring rumen contents or a cud from a normal animal to the nonruminating patient. Once the microflora in the rumen return to normal, the rumen resumes its role in digestion. Increases in digestible protein and energy in the feed should be considered in long-term management of poor rumen activity.

Regurgitation and Vomiting

Vomiting (expulsion of stomach contents) can be caused by GI inflammation, infection or obstruction, uremia, motion sickness, and a variety of other conditions. Vomiting is preceded by retching, whereas regurgitation is not. Continual vomiting results in alkalosis, dehydration and electrolyte imbalances. Regurgitation (expulsion of undigested food) may be caused by esophageal malformation or stricture and neurologic damage. Inhalation pneumonia is often a result.

Supportive care is directed at stopping the losses of body fluids and electrolytes, and compensating for the lack of nutrition. Protectants (Kao-Pectate, Pepto-Bismol), antiemetics and lubricants (for hairballs) may be used to soothe gut tissues. Because vomiting is an early sign of many infectious diseases, the animal should be monitored for other signs of disease.

Bloat

Bloat is distention of the GI tract with gas and is caused by excess gas production or an inability to eructate (belch). Ruminal tympany (bloat) is common in ruminants on lush spring pastures or in some feedlot operations.

Monogastric animals (nonruminants) can have the signs of bloat when the gut twists (torsion) or telescopes back on itself (intussusception), allowing accumulation of gas and causing great pain.

Prevention of bloat involves prefeeding animals turned out to pasture, limiting access to grain or water, top-dressing rations with oils and feeding antifoaming agents (poloxalene). A plastic one-way valve can be placed in the rumen of chronically affected animals to allow gas to escape.

In nonruminants, avoiding heavy meals before strenuous exercise, good parasite control and soaking dry feeds with water help prevent GI distention.

Maldigestion

Maldigestion, manifested as recognizable food material in feces, results in poor feed efficiency, malnutrition, and poor growth rates or performance. Unground or otherwise unprocessed grains are found in the feces of normal animals, but passage of normally easily digested materials (meat fiber, starches, etc) signals a problem. Hypermotility of the gut is a common cause and may be associated with toxins, infections (*eg,* parvovirus infection), parasitism (*eg,* coccidiosis) or allergy.

Supportive care involves meeting the animal's caloric and nutrient requirements, generally by IV injection. Adequate water and electrolyte balance is critical as usually the patient has been off food and water for a day or more. Protection of the gut and reducing hypermotility are primary goals. Frequently feeding small amounts of high-quality food may help restore normal gut activity. The normal microbial population may be augmented by feeding yogurt or a commercial bacterial culture (some are freeze dried). Long term use of digestive enzymes may be needed in some cases.

Malabsorption

Malabsorption has many of the characteristics of maldigestion. The food is digested but the nutrients are not absorbed from the gut, resulting in progressive loss of weight, condition and performance. The main signs of malabsorption are a foul fecal odor, fat, mucus or glycogen in the stool, and unusually colored feces. Causes of malabsorption include bile duct obstruction, allergies, a poor diet and chronic intoxications (paint, molds, etc).

Treatment is often only supportive. The animal's nutritional needs must be met, usually by artificial means, until the problem is resolved. Predigested foods, digestive enzymes (trypsin, etc) and vitamin-mineral supplements are used when indicated.

Ascites

Ascites (accumulation of fluid in the peritoneal cavity) is seen in a variety of disorders and is usually a sign of an underlying problem in fluid balance. Hypoproteinemia, electrolyte imbalances, infection, toxic conditions (endotoxic shock, etc), migration of parasite larvae, congestive heart failure (due to stenosis myopathy, anemia, etc), neoplasia, trauma and septicemia (bacteria in blood) are common causes of ascites. Overtransfusion or overhydration is usually noted first as pulmonary edema but may subsequently cause ascites.

Supportive care involves maintaining hydration while preserving the osmotic balance between the tissues, body cavities and vessel spaces. Blood protein levels and the PCV can be monitored and fluids and/or colloids given accordingly.

Flatulence

Excessive gas in the GI tract (flatulence) can be rather uncomfortable but is rarely of concern. It is caused by feeding highly fermentable feed or upsets in the intestinal microbial populations. Bicarbonates in feed can increase intestinal gas production.

Management is directed at a gradual diet change, feeding bacterial cultures, such as yogurt, and use of certain drugs.

Diarrhea

Diarrhea (abnormally frequent defecation or abnormally liquid feces) can be caused by inflammation (enteritis, gastritis, etc), infection, parasitism (hookworms, coccidia, strongyles, etc), allergies (*eg*, milk) and irritants. A variety of drugs and toxins adversely affect the gut, including lead, bacterial enterotoxins (*eg*, from *Clostridium perfringens*), digitalis, and some antibiotics (tetracycline, ampicillin, neomycin).

Abnormal stool color may be due to feed additives (*eg,* artificial colors in some pet foods), drugs, bile, GI bleeding, and some diseases (*eg,* pancreatitis may cause tan stools). Normal neonatal (newborn) animals may have a yellow to orange stool.

Supportive care starts with replacing the fluids and nutrients lost from the intestine. Mild diarrhea may resolve when food intake is reduced or eliminated for 8-48 hours to rest the gut. Increasing the dry matter content of the feed may aid long-term management of diarrhea. More severe or chronic cases may require a complete evaluation of the animal's condition. Anticholinergic drugs (Lomotil, atropine) or manipulation of the microflora (with antibiotics, antifermentives or live cultures) have been used with mixed success. In many cases, continuous use of protectants and absorbents is impractical for chronic care. Use of bland diets (Hill's i/d or rice, cottage cheese and chicken mixtures) after the intestine has been rested and then gradually returning the animal to normal feed are most often successful.

Anal Irritation

"Scooting," or rubbing and licking the anus is often caused by distention of the anal sacs, on either side of the anus, in dogs and cats. *Oxyuris equi,* the equine pinworm, can cause mild anal irritation and provoke tail rubbing. Diarrhea can cause anal irritation but does not last long after defecation.

Supportive care is limited to care of the perianal region, including cleansing and lubricating, and increasing the roughage content in the diet of affected dogs and cats. Horses with pinworms should be dewormed. Surgical intervention may be needed to remove anal sacs, obstructions, serious impactions and tumors (Fig 22).

Constipation

Constipation (infrequent or difficult passage of dry feces) is frequently accompanied by straining (tenesmus). The posture of the animal may be the same as in animals with cystitis. Causes of constipation include dehydration, gut hypomotility (slow rate of fecal passage), or bowel obstruction. Meconium (first stool of neonates) impaction, especially in foals, may necessitate use of enemas to clear the bowel. Other causes of constipation are use of certain drugs (diuretics, anticholinergics), toxins (*eg,* nightshade) and intestinal problems (colic). Some house-trained dogs become constipated if confined in a cage for long periods.

Treatment of constipation may require long-term care. Changes in feed (type, amount of moisture) and feeding frequency may be helpful.

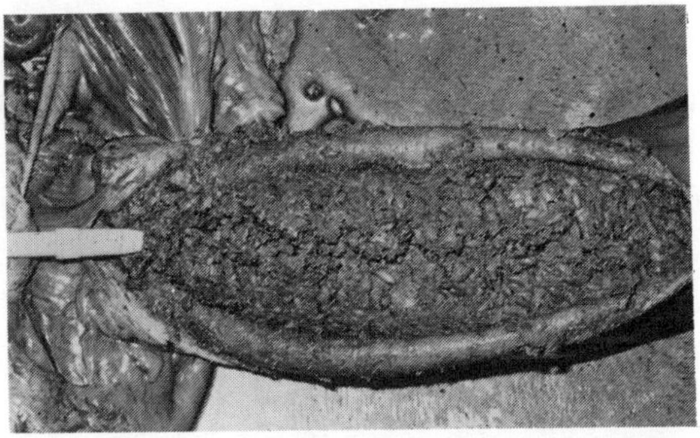

Fig 22. Intestinal impaction in a horse, caused by ground corn cobs.

Agents that promote evacuation of the bowel include Epsom salt, bran, mineral oil and petroleum jelly.

Mechanical removal of stools per rectum, colotomy (colonic surgery), anorectal massage and repeated enemas may be necessary in severe cases.

Skin Disease

The largest organ in the body is also the most easily observed, accounting for the high number of skin conditions treated. The skin reflects both the general state of health (glossy, plush coat over supple, flexible skin) and specific disease processes. Some infectious diseases cause specific skin lesions (*eg,* diamond-shaped lesions in swine erysipelas), but most cause nonspecific lesions. The skin is covered with opportunistic organisms that, upon injury to the skin, can gain entry to deeper tissues to cause infection.

Pruritus

Pruritus (itchiness) is usually a sign of inflammation but also may be behavioral in origin. It can be due to allergies (flea-allergy dermatitis) or central nervous system disorders (scrapie of sheep).

Supportive care involves use of soothing baths, soaks, flushes or topical medication (lotions, salves). Reducing the perception of itchiness with drugs (narcotics, sedatives) helps prevent self-trauma but may mask a systemic problem.

Eruptions

Any change in surface skin may be considered an eruption, including blisters (vesicles), crusts (scabs), abscesses (pustules), masses (warts) or fluid pockets (hematomas, seromas). Each eruption should be classified as to the area affected and extent, and this information added to that obtained from the history and physical examination.

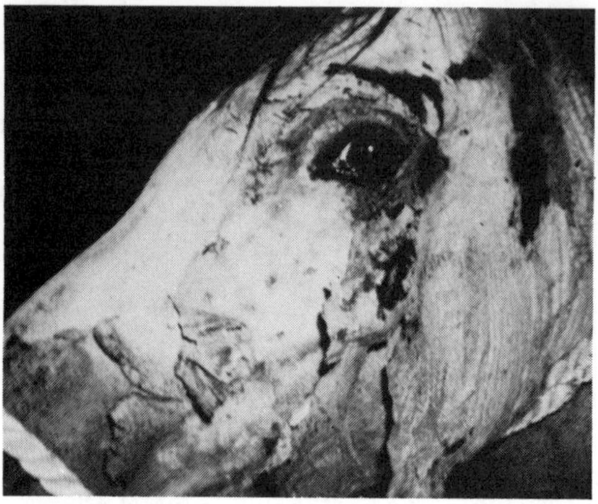

Fig 23. Sloughing of skin in a horse with severe photosensitization.

Causes for eruptions include allergy (fleas, bee sting, plants) hormonal imbalances (hypothyroidism), infections (foot and mouth disease, erysipelas), chemical irritations (battery acid), parasites (bots, warbles), photosensitivity (phenothiazines) and acne (Fig 23).

Supportive care is directed at removing the cause and symptomatic treatment, such as removing hair, debriding and flushing or bathing. Various drugs (antihistamines, antiinflammatories) are used for specific skin disorders. Surgical, chemical or thermal (cautery, cryosurgery) removal of affected tissue may be necessary.

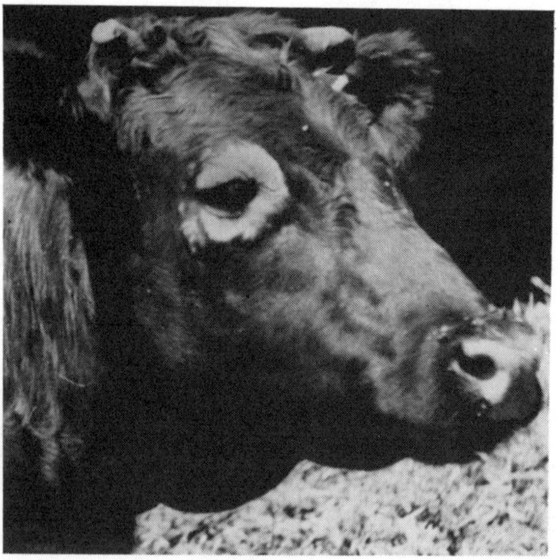

Fig 24. Ringworm lesions around the eye of a steer.

Alopecia

Alopecia (hair loss) is a common problem in animals. The causes are sometimes obscure, but infections (ringworm, bacteria), parasites (fleas, mites, ticks), toxins (heavy metals, molds), and nutritional deficiencies may be involved (Fig 24).

Supportive care may include a dietary change, medicated baths and drug therapy (parasiticides, corticosteroids).

CARE OF OLD OR DEBILITATED ANIMALS

Senile changes (changes associated with aging) involve all body systems. Specific changes in the function of the nervous system include reduced sensation (taste, smell, sight), altered sleep patterns, and reduced intelligence and coordination. Changes in the pulmonary and cardiovascular systems reduce pulmonary gas exchange and perfusion, vascular elasticity and cardiac output. Control of blood pH, renal filtration and liver function may also be impaired. In the GI tract, the ability to digest proteins and absorb calcium is reduced. Metabolic changes hinder the animal's ability to respond to its environment and to resist disease. This is most evident in the immune system, in which impaired function results in an increased incidence of neoplasia and reduced resistance to infection.

Activity decreases with age due to reduced musculoskeletal function. Moderate exercise is beneficial as it slows senile changes and increases longevity. Because older patients do not adapt to environmental changes as well as younger animals, their environmental temperature and humidity should be kept within the optimum range. The decline in the appearance of some old animals may decrease the amount of attention they receive and can result in personality changes. Owners should be advised to make play and affection time available to old animals that are dependent on them.

Debilitated and aged animals have many similar needs. A balance should be struck between the patient's need for rest and its requirement for exercise. Both are necessary and movement of body parts is essential, even if it is passive physical therapy (see Chapter 4). Pain relief aids healing and rehabilitation and should be provided from a humanitarian viewpoint. Bedding should be thick and clean. Frequent turning is necessary for recumbent animals, and the environment comfortable and draft free. Most debilitated animals require extra warmth.

Because debilitated animals may refuse to eat their usual ration, increasing the palatability (top-dressing hay with molasses or adding flavoring agents) and aroma (adding onion or garlic) of their feed may stimulate their appetite. The ration should be nutritious, easy to digest and geared to the patient's special needs. Geriatric animals should have a diet with high-quality protein and increased calcium content. Fluid and electrolyte levels should be monitored carefully, as debilitated animals rarely drink adequate amounts.

Moistening the ration can aid both food and water intake. Supplemental forced feedings may be required in some cases. Because debilitated or geriatric animals may lose control of urination and defecation, they may require assistance in the form of support while defecating or urinating, genital massages, catheterization, enemas, frequent changes of bedding and bathing. Many aged animals build up tartar on their teeth at an accelerated rate and may also require frequent claw or hoof trimming.

The result of nursing care can vary from prolonging the life of a terminally ill animal to complete rehabilitation and a return to normal health. The expectations for each animal must be realistic. Success may depend upon the quality of care given and the communication between the veterinarian and owner or attendant. Often the owner is in a better position to provide intensive nursing for a debilitated animal than is a technician. Also, the curative power of the bond of trust and affection between the owner and animal cannot be underrated. Cats particularly respond well to nursing care in their own home.

Death and Dying

Death is the final equalizer for all things. Rarely does one body system dictate an animal's life span. Rather, there seems to be a "concerto of decline" in which all systems play a part. Theories of aging hypothesize a gradual accumulation of toxins (free radicals, dimers, autoantibodies) or mutations, or a depletion of essential substances (hormones, etc) that causes the body to decline. Each body system has limits beyond which it cannot compensate and begins to fail.

Death must be dealt with on a clinical and personal level. There are times when euthanasia is the most loving and responsible decision. In food animal production, death is a prerequisite to human consumption. We have a humane obligation to see that the animal dies quickly, with a minimum of pain. Methods that destroy the brain or its communication with the environment have maintained their "popularity" in capital punishment of criminals and should be the yardstick used to judge the "relative experience" of dying. The method used to kill food animals depends on what product the animal's body will produce (*eg,* meat), as food products cannot be contaminated with toxins. Pets should have a quiet, dignified death.

Euthanasia is the painless, merciful killing of terminally ill, injured or unwanted animals, usually with lethal injections. Since there is no use for the body of an animal killed by injection (except where a rendering plant can make fertilizer or meat and bone meal), the bodies of most euthanized animals are buried or cremated.

Food animals are usually slaughtered, after stunning, by shooting (often with a captive-bolt device), CO_2 gas, electrocution, or with a blunt instrument (hammer, etc). Killing after stunning involves exsanguination (bleeding out) by cutting the major vessels in the throat. The animals are often blinded with bright lights so they cannot see the hand of the stunner. In certain religious communities (Jewish, Islamic), unstunned animals must be exsanguinated and the kill must be supervised or carried out by a designated person. The carcass is then inspected for wholesomeness.

Grief

In companion animal practice, the technician may be required to deal with the client's grief and bereavement after loss of a pet. The overt expression of the love, fear, anger and suspicion that accompany a pet's death or terminal illness is often embarrassing to all concerned. The technician should take steps to legitimize the client's feelings, as they are a healthy expression of the emotional bond with a pet.

Client response to a pet's death may vary from, "It's only a cat" to threats of suicide. Denial of death (or impending death) is the first step and may be a protective mechanism for the owner. The client may insist that there has been some error and that the animal is not dying or dead. In some cases, the animal may have to be discharged from the hospital to give the owner time to accept the situation. Going along with the idea that an error might have been made regarding the severity of the pet's condition may give the client time to accept the situation.

Anger often replaces denial and may be expressed toward himself/herself, the doctor, the technician or other members of the client's family. This anger is often unjustified and is frequently followed (sometimes much later) by an apology, "I just lost my head for a time."

The third stage of grief is the verbal or physical expression of the loss or impending loss. This process may be smoothed by enlisting the owner's help in caring for the pet or with explanations of the animal's condition.

Resolution is the final stage, a kind of "positive submission" to the fact of death in which an inner peace and serenity complete the pattern of loss and allow healing of the emotional scars. Condolence notes and calls can do much to further the resolution of grief so that the client is free to love another pet.

QUARANTINE

Controlling contagious disease by enforced isolation (quarantine) of animals, goods, supplies, property or people is part of state and federal law. Enforcement is charged to the sheriff or militia (National Guard). This is the only time, other than during a war or other major disturbance, when personal and civil rights can be suspended in America. The state veterinarian acts as judge, jury and executor to limit the freedom and disposition (condemnation, etc) of animals. The purpose of quarantine is to reduce exposure to disease, eliminate certain infections and preserve public health and safety. Providing quality animal products (meat, milk, fertilizer), preserving profits for food producers and reducing animal suffering and stress are additional goals.

Prevention of disease and the spread of disease (prophylaxis) can be greatly assisted by the technician. Places where animals congregate, such as race tracks, shows, parks and veterinary hospitals, tend to become sources of infectious diseases. Veterinary hospitals and many producers use large amounts of antibiotics that may encourage the growth of resistant pathogens. Vaccination, isolation of new or sick animals, and good hygiene practices are the foundations of animal health and husbandry.

Quarantine Procedures

Animals and people can be protected from infection by a variety of methods, depending upon the disease(s) and the species involved. Many diseases are species specific, so moving animals of a different species into an area of microbial contamination may be acceptable. Most animal diseases are no risk to people, but some are common to people and animals (zoonotic), such as salmonellosis, rabies and ringworm.

Some infections require only standard medical nursing to control, as they are not contagious. Diseases that are difficult to transfer (*eg*, botulism, histoplasmosis) can be treated without isolation of infected animals. Some conditions diagnosed by response to therapy must be treated as suspect infections until the final diagnosis is made.

When a potentially contagious disease occurs, isolation is an effective means of control. The period of quarantine may be defined legally, as in rabies, or established by the veterinarian through testing or experience with the disease. Sometimes animals may safely be returned to the group when clinical signs are no longer seen. Most veterinary hospitals are excellent quarantine areas as they are equipped to deal with disinfection. Moving healthy animals to a clean area and keeping infected ones confined in the area of the outbreak helps control disease spread, assuming that none of the currently healthy animals are harboring or just developing infection.

Test and slaughter is a more radical form of preventing spread of some very serious diseases. In this method, all animals in a suspect area are tested. Infected animals are slaughtered so healthy individuals cannot be exposed. Test and slaughter is effective and is practiced routinely with brucellosis, tuberculosis, feline leukemia virus infection and other diseases. It has been responsible for elimination or near elimination of several serious diseases. Owners of economically important animals are compensated for the loss of animals (market price).

Control of highly infectious diseases necessitates drastic measures, such as the destruction of any animal that has potentially been exposed. Eradication campaigns have been waged successfully in this country against foot and mouth disease and hog cholera. Though thousands of animals in a given area may be killed, protection of millions more justifies the method.

Meat Inspection

Meat inspection is also a form of disease control, as it maintains the wholesomeness of the food supply by preventing the spread of zoonoses and residues of harmful substances. Veterinary inspectors control the use of animal parts by condemning, diverting for nonfood use (rendering), or passing for alternate food use any part or all of a carcass.

The inspection starts with preslaughter observation of live animals. Any showing signs of disease may be held for observation or rejected. After slaughter, the internal organs are palpated or sectioned and visually inspected for abnormalities.

Carcass Disposal

Disposing of hazardous materials, such as contaminated bedding, bandages and carcasses, is of utmost importance in control of infectious diseases.

Toxic materials (heavy metals, pollutants, radioactive material) must be handled by toxic waste management authorities. Infectious wastes may be cremated, buried where the animal died (if this does not pollute water or soil) or turned over to a licensed rendering agent. If the dead animal must be moved, the carcass must be elevated from the ground during carcass removal to prevent a trail of contamination. Any contaminated bedding or soil should be saturated with oil and burned or turned under deeply. In some diseases (anthrax, vesicular stomatitis, exanthema), bodies must be buried with lime (though there is little evidence that this controls infection) or handled in specific ways (Fig 25).

Disinfection of Contaminated Premises

Contaminated barns, buildings, pastures and equipment used on infected animals must be made safe for susceptible animals. All litter, feces and other debris are removed. Then, the area is thoroughly swept, controlling dust with moisture. After all surfaces are cleaned with steam, detergents and scrubbing, disinfectant solutions (2% lye, formalin, etc) are applied. Drainage of wash water must be considered. New bedding or soil (placed over plastic sheeting) is brought in to replace what is removed. All utensils, tools and feed or watering apparatus must be scrubbed and disinfected.

In-Hospital Isolation

Hospitalized animals with, or suspected of having, a contagious disease should be isolated from other animals within the hospital to prevent spread of the disease. The isolation unit should be completely separate from areas where other animals are housed and the air supply should not mix with that of the rest of the hospital.

Technicians should care for the isolated animals after other patients. A separate set of coveralls or change of clothing should be available in each isolation unit. Clothing should be laundered regularly and not allowed to contact other animals. Rubber boots must be worn in stalls or kennels and thoroughly scrubbed and disinfected between uses. Boots must be clean before most disinfectants are effective. Disposable or sterilizable bedding, litter boxes, feeding supplies, and food and water containers should be used. Paper towels for handwashing and cleaning are helpful.

No visitors should be allowed into the isolation unit. Disease vectors, such as flies and mice, should be eliminated from the isolation unit. All cleaning must be done with a wet mop, cloth or sponge to prevent spread of disease through contaminated dust. Cages should

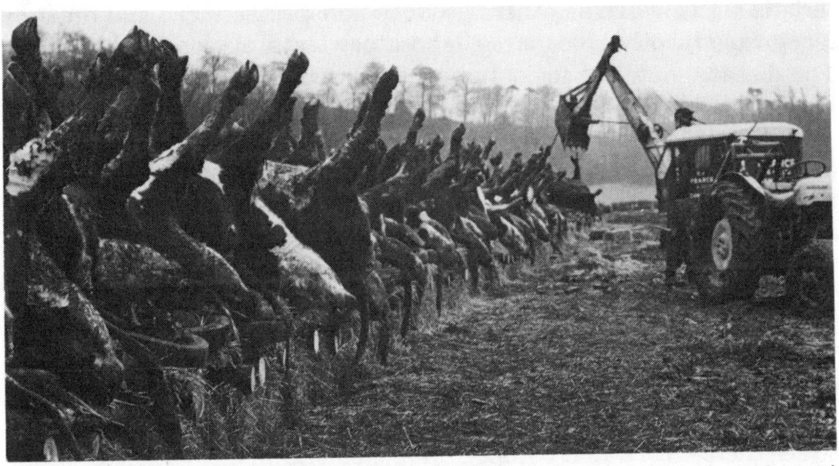

Fig 25. Cattle exposed to foot and mouth disease where slaughtered and burned during an outbreak in England in 1967-68.

be carefully disinfected regularly and all bedding and disposable equipment burned or tightly bagged. Reusable equipment must be autoclaved or otherwise sterilized before other animals come into contact with it.

Technicians should wash their hands, arms and other contaminated body surfaces before and after entry to the isolation unit. Between occupants, all surfaces in the isolation unit must be cleaned and sprayed with an appropriate disinfectant (not all organisms are killed by a single disinfectant).

INFECTIOUS DISEASES

An infectious disease is one that can be transmitted from one animal to another. Contagious diseases are infectious diseases spread by direct contact between animals. Additional means of disease transmission include fomites (inanimate objects that carry microorganisms), food, water soil, air, etc. Infectious diseases may be caused by bacteria, viruses, protozoa, rickettsiae, mycoplasmids, molds, yeast, helminths (worms) or arthropods.

Whether an animal becomes sick or not depends upon its resistance to disease, the virulence (potency) of the microorganism, number of invading organisms, route of infection, ability of the pathogen (disease-causing agent) to propagate in tissues, and the formation of toxins. The animal's response to the pathogen is manifested as fever, anorexia and various other clinical signs. Some diseases have characteristic signs, whereas others produce nonspecific signs and must be recognized by other means (*eg,* laboratory tests, exploratory surgery). The disease may last for only hours (peracute), through days (acute) to years (chronic).

Animals may clear their bodies of a pathogen and become immune or susceptible to reinfection, harbor the disease at low levels and reactivate the infection at a later date (latent infection), or appear recovered but shed the organism and infect other animals (carrier infection).

Bacterial Infections

Bacteria are very small (the oil-immersion objective must be used to see them with a microscope), one-celled organisms with a less complex cellular structure than either plants or animals. They can be motile (capable of movement) or nonmotile, and require either O_2 (aerobic) or lack of O_2 (anaerobic) for growth. Because they multiply by cell division, signs of infection usually take some time to appear, unless a toxin is present. The virulence of bacteria varies greatly; most do not cause disease.

Living organisms have good defenses against bacterial invasion, including antibody production (large molecules that enhance or activate internal defenses) and phagocytosis by WBC (engulfing and destroying the organism). However, some bacteria can circumvent these mechanisms. Good vaccines are available to protect against many bacterial pathogens (bacterins) and toxins (toxoids). Many effective antibacterial drugs (antibiotics, disinfectants) are now in common use.

Bacterial infections may be spread through the blood (bacteremia or septicemia), or may be localized to a tissue or organ. Bacterial diseases are not as specific regarding host and target tissue (area of the body primarily affected) as viral infections.

A classification scheme has been developed to separate one type of bacterium from another as an aid in recognition of pathogens and their association with specific diseases.

Bacteria are grouped by shape (rod, spiral, sphere) and by Gram-staining reaction (blue = +, pink = −). Many bacteria growing in a clump make a visible spot (colony) on culture media and may be classified by colony morphology (appearance) and reactions with various types of media, stains, chemicals, etc. Because many bacteria are similar, multiple tests are usually required to distinguish them.

Gram-Negative Bacteria

Pseudomonas: This motile, rod-shaped organism (bacillus) is usually involved in suppurative (pus-forming) processes. It is an opportunist that invades after other processes have impaired body defenses. Diseases caused by *Pseudomonas* include green wool, rhinitis and pneumonia in swine, organ abscesses, bovine mastitis, genital infections, otitis in dogs, respiratory disease in horses, and cystitis in small animals.

Supportive care involves debridement (excision of dead tissue) of infected areas and use of topical or systemic antibiotics. Because *Pseudomonas* can cause endocarditis, meningitis, pneumonia and otitis in people, especially if they are immunosuppressed or on antibiotics to which the organism is resistant, latex gloves should be worn when handling infected tissue or debris.

Escherichia coli: This organism is a normal inhabitant of the large intestine of all warm-blooded animals. It varies from a short, plump rod to filamentous in form. Certain strains are enteropathogenic (capable of causing intestinal disease) due to a toxin found in them (enterotoxin). These strains are usually species specific and cause disease in young animals. Signs of *E coli* infection include anorexia, diarrhea, fever and depression. The organism causes edema and death in pigs, mastitis in cattle, abortions in horses and septicemia in neonatal (newborn) animals. Supportive care includes good hygiene to reduce the number of organisms to which the animal is exposed (fecal contamination), and antibiotic and fluid therapy. Some vaccines are available.

Salmonella: This organism is a short rod with a variety of serotypes (subspecies classification based on surface structure of the organism) that may or may not be species specific. Young and stressed animals are more prone to infection than others. Disease usually occurs due to fecal contamination and is often an enteric (intestinal) infection but may become generalized with septicemia and internal abscesses. Salmonellosis is a highly contagious disease that is hard to eliminate once animal quarters are contaminated. Supportive care includes quarantine of infected animals and use of scrupulous hygiene and antibiotic and fluid therapy. In some cases, a vaccine may be available.

Hemophilus: This bacterium is a small or medium-sized, filamentous or pleomorphic (variable shapes in one microscopic field) bacillus (rod). It is a parasite of the mucous membranes and usually only causes disease when the animal's resistance to infection is decreased, resulting in genital (horses), respiratory (swine), and CNS (cattle) diseases. Vaccination and antibiotic therapy are used in prevention and treatment, respectively.

Pasteurella: This small, ovoid rod often stains lighter in the center than at each end. The organisms are carried as normal flora of the mouth and throat and can cause disease when the animal is stressed. General signs may include fever, respiratory distress, edema, hemorrhages on membranes, and fluid in body cavities. *Pasteurella* is a common cause of abscesses in cats and severe mastitis in sheep. Many cases in people result from animal bites. Such bite wounds are slow to heal and have a watery discharge. Bacteremia and CNS and respiratory infections may also occur in people. Treatment includes use of antibiotics, such as penicillin, and vaccination with a bacterin.

Bordetella: This organism is a motile rod that is an important contributor to bronchopneumonia after viral infection (*eg,* kennel cough, canine distemper) and atrophic rhinitis in pigs. Culling of carrier animals in swine herds, vaccination, administration of serum from immune animals, and antibiotic therapy are all involved in treatment.

Moraxella bovis: This organism is a short, curved rod found in pairs. It causes pinkeye in cattle and starts as simple conjunctivitis that may progress to blindness. Supportive care involves vaccination, use of ophthalmic preparations, and minimizing such predisposing causes as dust and bright sunlight.

Actinobacillus: These pleomorphic organisms are found in small granules in pus from infected areas. They are part of the normal mouth flora of sheep and cattle but can form large abscesses in soft tissue when introduced into deep oral tissue (foreign body penetration often introduces them). These masses often occur in the tongue (wooden tongue) but can form in the limbs and internal organs. The bacteria also cause bacteremia in foals and young pigs. Treatment involves use of a systemic iodine compound and antibiotics.

Fusobacterium and *Bacteroides:* These bacteria are anaerobes and are differentiated by gas chromatographic analysis. *Fusobacterium* normally occurs as long rods, invades damaged tissue and causes necrosis, abscesses and a foul odor. It invades the liver, mouth and throat of young calves (calf diphtheria), as well as the udder, rumen wall and hooves of adults. Sulfonamides are an effective treatment.

Bacteroides is also involved in "foot rot" (paronychia) in cattle and sheep, and may be the primary disease agent. Supportive care includes paring the hoof to expose diseased tissues to O_2, use of a topical antibiotic or disinfectant foot dip (*eg,* formalin), and vaccination.

Gram-Positive Bacteria

Staphylococcus: These cocci (spherical shape) are found arranged in grape-like clusters (in a fluid culture they may be single, in short chains or small groups). They are very resistant to drying, heat and disinfectants, and thus are often responsible for infections acquired in hospitals (nosocomial). They can be carried as normal flora of skin and mucous membranes of people and animals.

Staphylococci produce many extracellular toxins (exotoxins) and enzymes damaging to cells. Infections caused by *Staphylococcus* include many suppurative diseases, such as mastitis, equine botryomycosis, eye infections, canine pyoderma, urinary tract infections and greasy pig disease. Supportive care involves flushing of lesions if possible and antibiotic therapy based upon sensitivity test results, as many of these organisms are resistant to common antibiotics and disinfectants.

Streptococcus: These bacteria arrange themselves in chains of various lengths. They are found on mucous membranes and are opportunistic invaders. Frequently appearing in milk and milk products, they cause suppurative diseases of the udder, umbilicus, CNS, respiratory tract, uterus and joints. *Streptococcus* causes equine and porcine "strangles," when it invades lymph nodes and the upper respiratory tract. Abscesses and bacteremia often result from infection. Some diseases caused by *Streptococcus* are prevented by herd vaccination and isolation of infected animals. Antibiotics and symptomatic therapy are also given.

Erysipelothrix rhusiopathiae: This organism is a short, slender rod that causes swine erysipelas (diamond skin disease) and polyarthritis in calves and lambs. Healthy animals carry the organism in their tonsils and stress activates the disease. It is spread in urine, feces, saliva and vomitus and lives for long periods in the environment, so good hygiene is an important part of supportive care. People with small wounds have been infected by handling infected animals and tissues; therefore, latex gloves should be worn in such situations. Vaccination, immune serum (serum from recovered animals) and antibiotic therapy are used as disease control.

Clostridium: These organisms are anaerobic, spore-forming rods (spores are like plant seeds that allow the organism to resist adverse environmental conditions for long periods and germinate when conditions are right). Two organisms produce powerful endotoxins and cause tetanus (*C tetani*) (Fig 26) and botulism (*C botulinum*). Other species of the organism invade tissue and produce toxins of less po-

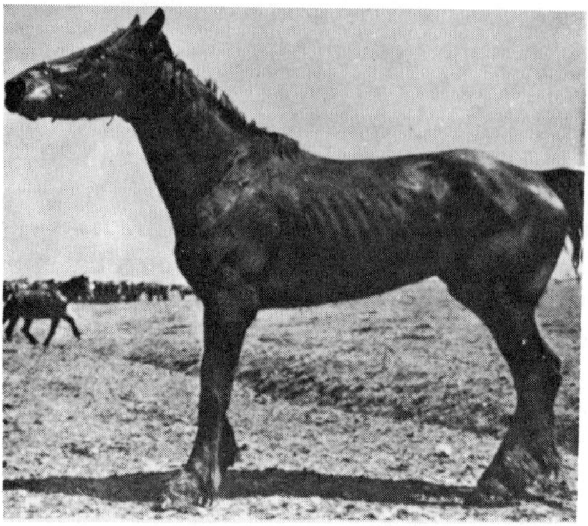

Fig 26. A horse with tetanus.

tency, causing yellow lamb disease, lamb enteritis and enterotoxemia in sheep (*C perfringens*), red water in cattle (*C hemolyticum*), black disease in sheep (*C novyi*), and black leg (*C chauvoei*) and malignant edema (*C septicum*) in ruminants. Due to the seriousness of most of these diseases, vaccination with bacterins and toxoids is widely used.

Supportive care involves use of antitoxins, transfusions, fluids, antibiotics and purgatives, reducing feed (enterotoxemia) and wound care. Spores in the environment are difficult to eradicate.

Listeria monocytogenes: This bacterium is a small rod with slight clubbing at one end. Coccoid (spherical) forms can be seen. Low pH favors its survival, especially in high-moisture silage feeds. It causes meningoencephalitis (circling disease) and septicemia in horses, ruminants and people. Treatment involves antibiotic therapy.

Corynebacterium (Rhodococcus): These organisms are pleomorphic, straight to slightly curved rods with frequent clubbing and irregular staining. They produce pus and are found in abscesses, especially of the lymph nodes, in ruminants, swine and occasionally other animals. Diseases caused include summer mastitis, pneumonia, arthritis, pseudotuberculosis, endocarditis, and genital and urinary tract infections.

Supportive care includes draining abscesses, isolation of infected animals, prevention of wounds, and good hygiene to prevent spread. Antibiotics have been useful in some cases.

Actinomyces: These bacteria produce a mycelium (mass of thread-like processes) that may branch and fragment into rods. It is the cause of lumpy jaw in cattle and abscesses in cats and dogs, and may invade the bone. Treatment includes use of antimicrobial agents, such as Lugol's iodine and penicillin. Treatment may be extended over many weeks.

Nocardia: This organism also produces a long, filamentous, branching mycelium that breaks up into coccoid or rod forms. It causes bovine mastitis and granulomatous (proliferative, tissue-like) lesions of the skin and thoracic organs of dogs and cats. Abscesses may drain pus to the bodies' surface and contain granules. Thoracic fluid from affected animals resembles tomato soup. Antimicrobial agents are used to treat nocardiosis. Needles used for intramammary infusion may be a source of spread unless disinfected between uses.

Dermatophilus congolensis: Narrow, tapering filaments, with branching at right angles to the main stem, characterize this organism. It causes streptothricosis, strawberry foot rot and greasy heel disease. Supportive care involves use of antimicrobials.

Mycoplasmas

These organisms are the smallest and simplest cells capable of self-replication. Pleomorphic (variably shaped) in form, they may appear coccoid, filamentous, spiral, or as rings, granules or globules. They cause contagious bovine and caprine pleuropneumonia, mastitis, vulvovaginitis, arthritis, conjunctivitis, bronchopneumonia, and polyserositis and enzootic pneumonia of swine. Some forms are sensitive to antibiotics; however, in others, growth may be enhanced by these drugs. Vaccination is practiced in some areas as a control measure.

Rickettsiae

These are a group of small rod-shaped coccoid or pleomorphic organisms that must live inside host cells. They are true bacteria and are usually associated with reticuloendothelial (macrophage-like), vascular or blood cells.

Arthropods (*eg,* fleas, ticks) often act as vectors, transmitting the rickettsiae with their bite. Some diseases are species specific, but many are not, and a few are zoonotic. Diseases caused by rickettsiae include tick-borne fever, benign bovine and ovine rickettsiosis, bovine petechial fever and contagious ophthalmia in ruminants, equine ehrlichiosis, canine ehrlichiosis, feline hemobartonellosis, and salmon poisoning in dogs.

Supportive care involves elimination of arthropod vectors and use of antimicrobials, transfusions and fluid therapy. Infected animals may be carriers for long periods and in some cases should not be used as blood donors.

Anaplasmas

These organisms are found on or within RBC and are transmitted by blood-sucking arthropods, transfusion or contaminated instruments. The course of the disease depends upon the number of organisms present and the health of the animal. Ruminants are tested and animals with anaplasmosis are slaughtered. In pets, hemobartonellosis and eperythrozoonosis may respond to antimicrobial therapy. Supportive care involves use of transfusions and reduction of stress.

Chlamydia

These organisms are probably bacteria that lack the machinery for extracellular existence. Included in this group are agents that cause psittacosis and ornithosis in birds, pneumonitis and conjunctivitis in cats, encephalomyelitis, polyarthritis, placental disease and enteritis in cattle, and enzootic abortion in sheep and cattle. Antibiotics are useful but most are unable to clear the infection; carrier animals should be culled. Vaccines are available for protection against some disease caused by chlamydia. Some of the infections in this group are transmissible to humans.

Fungal Infections

Fungi are filamentous or unicellular organisms with chitinous cell walls. The major pathogenic groups are molds and yeasts. Molds are composed of mycelia and reproduce by spores. Yeasts are single-celled fungi that reproduce by budding. Identification is based on morphology (physical appearance).

Two yeasts that cause superficial infections of animals are *Candida* and *Pityrosporum*. *Candida* invades mucosal surfaces, especially when the animal is stressed or on prolonged antimicrobial therapy. The superficial disease causes caseous (cheese-like), round lesions and is called thrush; however, the organisms may also produce mastitis, genital tract infections and systemic disease.

Pityrosporum can invade the ears of dogs and cats, causing inflammation (otitis) and a thick, brown exudate.

Treatment includes thorough cleaning of involved areas and long-term chemotherapy.

Mold-like organisms, including *Sporothrix*, *Aspergillus* and *Rhinosporidium*, cause granulomatous, necrotic and suppurative reactions (Fig 27). Therapy includes use of antifungal medications and surgical removal of infected tissues. Unfortunately, long-term treatment is required and often is not successful in eliminating the organism. Chronic debilitation is the frequent result of systemic mycoses.

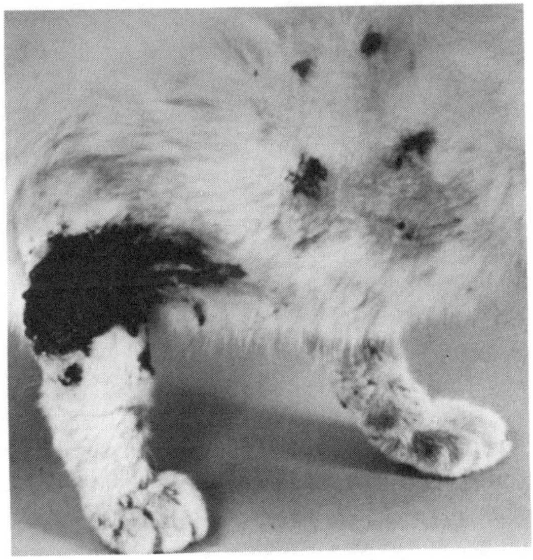

Fig 27. Cat with sporotrichosis, showing scattered skin lesions and large necrotic area on foreleg.

Protozoal Infections

Only a few of the numerous types of protozoa cause disease. These one-celled-animals are larger than bacteria, frequently motile and often have complex life cycles.

Trypanosomiases and babesiases are transmitted by arthropods and are found in the blood stream. Signs vary and may include chronic wasting, posterior paralysis, jaundice and infertility. Many effective systemic drugs are available for treatment but decreasing the numbers of the arthropod vector is essential to controlling the protozoa.

Trichomoniasis is a contagious venereal disease, principally of cattle, that causes sterility, pyometra and abortion. Slaughter of bulls and artificial insemination of cows are recommended for control.

Sarcosporidiosis occurs when the muscle of an animal is invaded by the protozoan, *Sarcocystis.* Unless animals are heavily infected, no clinical signs are seen and affected areas are trimmed after slaughter.

Coccidiosis is an acute infection caused by the invasion of intestinal mucosa by *Eimeria* or *Isospora*, resulting in bloody diarrhea. It is an important disease of all domestic animals except the horse. Because animals acquire the disease through contact with infected feces, good hygiene is important in control of the disease. Sick animals should have minimum stress, clean quarters and adequate supportive care. Use of coccidiostatic or coccidiocidal drugs and symptomatic therapy for diarrhea are indicated. Immunity to infection usually develops as animals mature.

Parasitic Infections

A parasite is an organism that lives in or upon and at the expense of another organism, called the host. Internal parasites are found inside the host and external parasites inhabit the surface of the host. They are typically multicelled, except protozoa, and usually visible to the naked eye.

Internal Parasites

Internal parasites, except protozoa, are helminths (worms) and are divided into 3 groups: flatworms (trematodes), roundworms (nematodes) and ribbon-like worms (cestodes). Internal parasitism is diagnosed by seeing the worms grossly or the eggs microscopically (in feces, vomit or tissue).

Trematodes: Trematodes are leaf-shaped flatworms of various sizes. They usually have a complex life cycle involving one or more intermediate hosts (a host, other than the primary, that is necessary for completion of the life cycle); often a snail is involved. Trematodes ma-

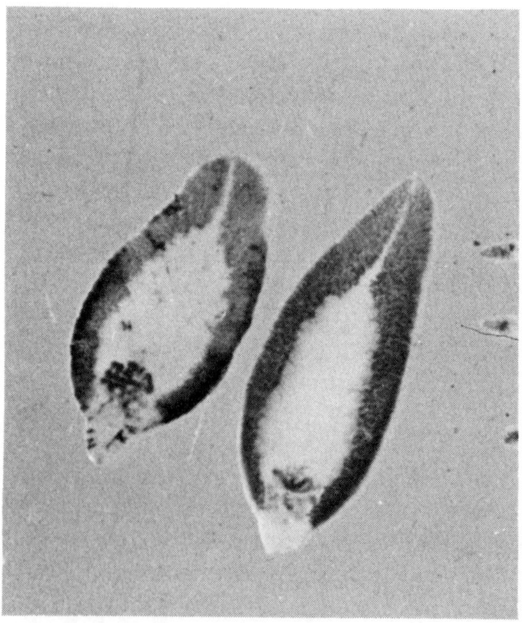

Fig 28. *Fasciola hepatica*, the common liver fluke of cattle.

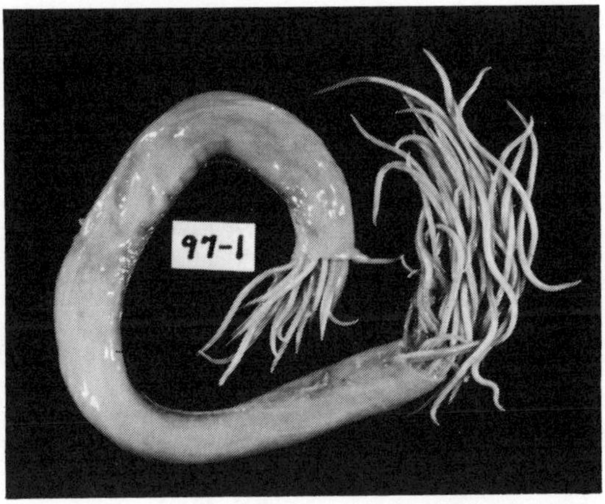

Fig 29. Impaction of the small intestine of a foal by roundworms (*Parascaris equorum*).

ture in body tissues (liver, lung), cause necrosis and inflammation, and interfere with body function.

In large animals, *Fasciola* is an important species that lives in the bile ducts (Fig 28). In small animals, *Nanophyetus salmincola* causes salmon poisoning and *Paragonimus* encysts in the lungs.

Supportive care includes use of anthelmintics, therapy to aid the animal while affected tissues heal, and protection from reinfection by elimination of contact with the intermediate hosts (snails, fish, etc).

Nematodes: Nematodes are spaghetti-like roundworms, often pointed on the ends, and may be microscopic to many inches in length. Typically, they have a direct life cycle (only a primary host is involved) and migrate within body tissues before completing their life cycles in the digestive, vascular or respiratory system. Eggs from fecal contamination are the usual source of infection but penetration of the skin and transplacental transfer may also occur in some species.

Ascarids are roundworms that occur in most nonruminants and look like large, white, rubbery earthworms. Their life cycle involves migration throughout the body (especially the liver and lungs) before adults develop in the intestine. Disease occurs by physical blockage of the intestine, competition for nutrients with the host, tissue destruction during migration, and interference with digestion (Fig 29). Affected animals are usually thin, with a rough haircoat and a pot belly. The diarrhea and vomitus of affected animals may contain worms. Because young animals are often infected before birth or from the dam's milk, mature worms may occur in animals as young as 4 weeks of age. Treatment involves deworming with an anthelmintic, followed by provision of a good diet to return the animal to good con-

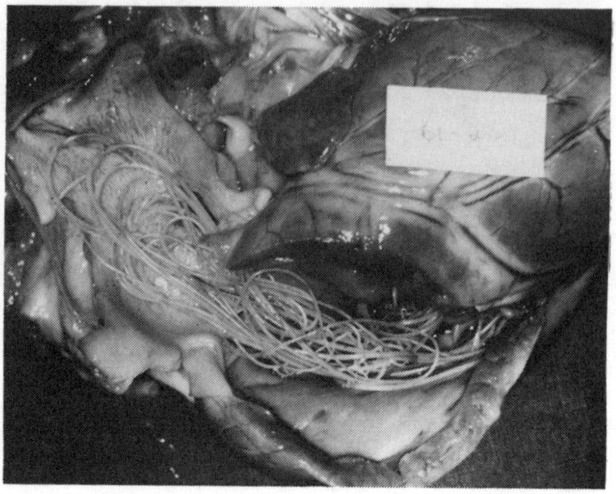

Fig 30. Adult heartworms in the heart of a dog.

dition. To avoid impaction of the intestine with dead worms in a heavy infestation, a series of dewormings may be used. Because ascarids pose a public health hazard, puppies should be checked for worms at an early age.

Large strongyles (bloodworms) in horses and *Dirofilaria* (heartworms) in dogs live in the vascular system (Fig 30). Large strongyles invade artery walls and are a common cause of colic when they compromise the blood supply to the intestinal tract. Horses should be dewormed about every 6-8 weeks. *Dirofilaria* interferes with the blood supply to the lungs and may cause dyspnea. Heartworms are transmitted by mosquitoes. Treatment involves use of drugs to kill the adults and microfilariae (larvae). People bitten by infected mosquitoes may develop granulomatous lesions in their lungs.

Hookworms (*eg, Ancylostoma*) attach to the intestinal lining and suck large quantities of blood. Infection causes melena (blood in the stool), anemia and weight loss. Heavy infections may require transfusions after deworming. Larvae may be ingested or penetrate the skin to gain entrance to the host, so good hygiene is essential to prevent transmission. Larvae that penetrate human skin do not complete their life cycle but travel subcutaneously, causing a rash and itching (creeping eruption or cutaneous larva migrans).

Whipworms (*Trichuris*) live in the large intestine and, in heavy infections, cause loss of weight, diarrhea and fresh blood in the stool. Affected animals should be treated with an anthelmintic. Because eggs are susceptible to drying, cleanliness and elimination of damp areas in the animal's environment are helpful control measures.

Pinworms (*Oxyuris*) occur only in horses and are not transmissible to people. Females lay their eggs around the horse's anus, causing intense itching. Inspecting the anal folds, cleaning the perineal area and routine anthelmintic therapy constitute a good control program.

Ruminants have a variety of small roundworm parasites (*Hemonchus, Ostertagia*, etc) that live in various portions of their digestive tracts. Depending on the number of parasites and the species, signs vary from none to weight loss, anemia and diarrhea. Good hygiene (pasture rotation, use of feed bunks, providing good drainage, manure removal) and regular deworming are necessary for control.

Lungworm infections occur in cattle and horses (*Dictyocaulus*), swine (*Metastrongylus*) and cats (*Aelurostrongylus*). The eggs are coughed up and swallowed by the host. Signs include coughing, weight loss and dyspnea. Use of anthelmintics, moving dewormed animals to a clean pasture or stall, and providing a high level of nutrition are important.

Cestodes: Tapeworms are composed of a series of identical reproductive segments (proglottids) in a chain extending from a head (scolex) that is anchored in the intestinal wall. Their life cycle always involves an intermediate host. They are usually well adapted to their host and cause little damage other than competition for nutrients. The passing of tapeworm segments can be distressing to the client and several types are transmissible to people. Weight loss may be seen. Elimination of the intermediate host to break the life cycle or regular deworming is essential to clear this parasite. Some types of anthelmintics may require hospital supervision when administered.

External Parasites

External parasites include fleas, flies, ticks, mosquitoes, lice and mites. The first 4 of these parasites spend at least part of their life cycle off the host and the last 2 remain continuously on the animal. Damage to the host includes blood loss, skin irritation, spoiling of the haircoat, transmission of disease and destruction of tissues. External parasites are often a seasonal problem and require diligence to eliminate an infestation.

Ticks: Ticks are arachnids (8-legged arthropods) and come in a variety of sizes, shapes and colors (some look like beetles, others like spiders). The female requires a blood meal for egg development and some species need a blood meal before every molting cycle (2-3 times). They are a particular problem in rural areas and may transmit a variety of diseases to animals and people (*eg,* Rocky Mountain spotted fever, tick fever).

Ticks attach themselves to the host and engorge themselves by burying their heads in the host's skin with their biting-sucking mouthparts. A variety of compounds can be applied to kill them. Wear gloves when removing ticks to prevent disease transmission. Ticks prefer to attach themselves where the skin is thin and moist. Infestation may be prevented with collars, dips, powders and sprays, though many species of ticks have built up resistance to them.

Heavy infestations may cause anemia due to blood loss. Ticks that attach near the spinal cord may cause an ascending paralysis (tick paralysis) than can kill the animal when the respiratory muscles are paralyzed. Removal of the tick causes a rapid return to normal. A neurotoxin in the tick's saliva is the apparent cause; only certain ticks cause the disease.

Flies: Flies have 3 parts to their life cycle. Adults lay eggs that hatch into larvae (maggots), which pupate (usually on the ground) and hatch into adults. Adult flies are pests that irritate animals and may spread disease, but most damage is caused by the larvae. Larvae developing in wounds produce an enzyme that liquefies tissue so they can consume it. Because the enzyme dissolves both dead and healthy tissue, maggots enlarge existent wounds or create new ones when eggs are laid on matted hair contaminated with feces or wet wool.

Some types of flies (bots in horses, warbles in cows) have modified life cycles. The larvae live inside the animal's body, protected from environmental conditions, and are released when the environmental temperature is right for pupation. Such flies destroy tissue (meat), spoil hides and, in large numbers, interfere with normal body functions.

Treatment is aimed at preventing contact between the host and fly (stabling, clipping matted hair, etc), killing adult flies with insecticides, removing fly eggs by flushing wounds or scraping eggs off the hair, removing maggots from wounds, and using internal insecticides. Good hygiene, especially proper manure disposal and protecting of open wounds in the summer, are important control measures.

Mosquitoes: Mosquitoes are flying pests that must breed in standing water. Females require a blood meal before egg production (males generally do not suck blood). The female may visit several hosts in search of blood and her proboscis (mouthparts) often transmits disease.

Control measures include draining, treating (such as adding a layer of oil to the surface) or screening standing water, using mosquito repellents to prevent bites, and using medication to prevent disease once a bite has occurred.

Fleas: These small insects are the bane of mammals in humid, temperate areas, especially in late summer and fall. Their life cycle is similar to that of flies, but adults live most of their life on the host and cause irritation with their bites. Eggs are very resistant to insecticides. The larvae eat organic debris and pupate in rugs and crevices.

In animals that develop an allergy to flea saliva, one bite is enough to cause rashes, hair loss and extreme discomfort. Adult fleas can live for months without a blood meal.

Successful control involves killing the adults and larvae on the animal, in the house (or animal's sleeping quarters), and outdoors around the yard or other premises with insecticides. The process must be repeated at intervals to kill newly hatched larvae and immature fleas until all the eggs are hatched. Eggs hatch 3-14 days after being laid, depending on the environmental temperature and humidity (increasing both speeds up the life cycle). Poor control results are obtained if any facet of environmental control is missed (only killing fleas on the animal is not enough), if newly hatched fleas mature and lay fresh eggs, or if the animal contacts fleas on another animal or area. In addition, fleas have become resistant to many insecticides on the market.

Some insecticides have residual activity or interfere with adult development to prevent reinfestation between applications. Ultrasound generators have been used to drive fleas away with some success. Internal insecticides may be useful in some cases but they may cause side effects.

There are a variety of products for flea control on the animal. The following methods of application are listed in decreasing order of residual flea-killing activity (and hence effectiveness): dips, powders, sprays, collars and baths. Heavy flea infestations can kill an animal through blood loss. Debilitated, young or old animals are especially prone to this problem as they have difficulty grooming themselves and a limited ability to respond to blood loss.

Animals allergic to flea bites (flea-bite dermatitis) should be kept as free of fleas as possible, as one bite is enough to set off a violently pruritic (itchy) reaction. If it is impossible to eliminate flea contact, the allergic reaction can be reduced with corticosteroids, but there can be undesirable side effects. Killing the flea after it has bitten the animal does not prevent the allergic reaction.

One type of tapeworm (*Dipylidium*) is carried by fleas and may infect both animals and people if fleas are consumed.

Lice: Lice are small insects, visible to the naked eye, that cement their eggs (nits) to the host's hair. The adults produce irritation by biting and sucking out tissue fluids. Heavy infestations result in loss of condition and anemia.

Control measures include periodically dusting the animal with an insecticide. Because they spend all of their lives on the animal, lice are fairly easy to control. They can be transmitted directly by close contact between animals or indirectly from grooming brushes, blankets, etc.

Mites: There are a variety of sizes and shapes of mites, but most are microscopic. They may live on normal animals without producing disease (*Demodex*) or they may burrow into the skin, consuming tissue and fluids, and causing intense irritation (Fig 31). A mite infestation is called mange.

Control measures include use of acaricides (baths, dips or pour-ons that kill mites), worked well into the skin, with use continued until all eggs hatch. In cases of otodectic mange (ear mite infestation), scabs or ear wax should be removed before instilling an acaricide in the ear to allow the medication to contact the mites. Some types of mange may not respond to treatment if the disease has manifested itself because of concurrent disease or immunosuppression.

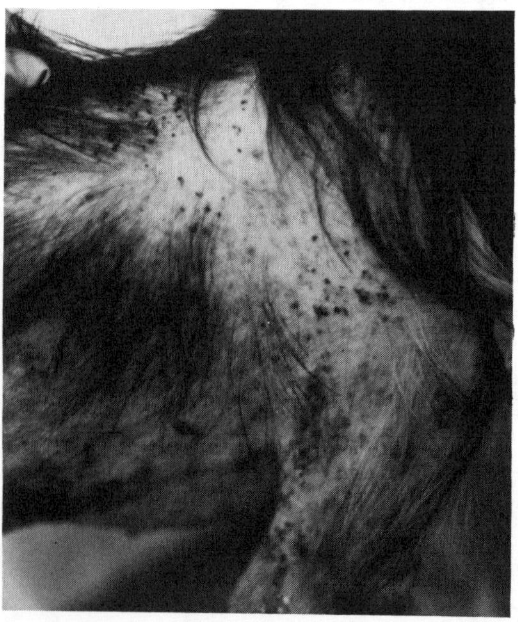

Fig 31. Severe sarcoptic mange in a dog.

Viral Infections

Viruses are composed of genetic material that may be encased in a protective coat. They reproduce by inserting their genetic material into the host cell and commanding the cell's reproductive machinery to make virus particles instead of cells. Infected cells usually die when their nutrients are exhausted, waste products build up, or the virus particles rupture the cell membrane.

Viruses are extremely small (with few exceptions) and the light microscope can only be used to visualize cell death caused by infection. Most can be seen with the electron microscope. Because they can only be cultured in living cells (eggs, tissue culture), viral diseases are often diagnosed by their effect (signs, antibody titer rise, etc) rather than finding and culturing the organism, as in bacteriologic procedures.

Viruses are classified as either DNA or RNA viruses, depending on the nucleic acids (genetic material) they contain, similar to the classification of bacteria into 2 groups by their Gram stain reaction. No virus contains both DNA and RNA. Further classification is based upon the protein coat (capsid), which protects the virus particle from enzyme degradation. The coats are described by their symmetry (icosahedral, helical, etc), size, number of units making up the protein coat (capsomeres) and sedimentation rate.

Control of Viral Infections

Most viruses are inactivated by heating at 56 C (132.8 F) for 30 minutes, and so are inactivated by boiling water. Enveloped viruses are less stable than unenveloped as the envelope is very susceptible to degradation, especially by lipolytic agents.

Many viruses are preserved by drying or cooling on dry ice. Practically all viruses are inactivated at a pH above 9 and below 5, so acids and bases are good disinfecting agents. Enveloped viruses are inactivated by most disinfectants including phenol, detergents and formaldehyde. Certain unenveloped viruses (*eg,* parvoviruses, caliciviruses) are resistant to all common disinfectants except a 1:20 bleach solution (*eg,* Clorox).

With few exceptions, antibiotics have no effect on viruses as they are protected inside living cells for most of their existence. Drugs powerful enough to kill viruses often kill host cells too.

Interferon is a natural substance produced by a virus-infected cell that prevents infection of surrounding cells by other viruses. It is species specific but not virus specific.

Disease Production

Most viruses are specific for a species (with some notable exceptions) and may even require a specific cell type for replication (reproduction).

Viruses generally first attack body surfaces, especially mucous membranes, and replicate locally. They may remain local or spread to other tissues, often via the blood or lymph. In other cases, viruses may enter mobile body cells (*eg,* WBC) and be distributed throughout the body. Some viruses cross the blood-brain barrier and many infect the fetus *in utero.* The same virus may produce different clinical signs in animals of varying ages.

The course and manifestation of disease are determined by the number of viruses involved, the type and number of host cells infected, and the nature of viral replication within the cell. The infection may cause no clinical signs, serious disease or sudden death. In some cases, clinical signs do not appear until late in the infection. Secondary bacterial (and fungal) infections often complicate viral diseases, as the virus reduces the body's resistance to bacterial invasion. This is especially true of respiratory and skin infections.

Some viruses can also change the genetic make-up of normal body cells, resulting in tumor production. Certain viruses cause chronic disease or persist in the host and are reactivated when body defenses are reduced due to stress (latent infection).

Usually the mechanisms that lead to signs of disease and death are unknown; however, vascular shock, toxicity (viral toxins or cellular metabolites) and failure of organ systems may account for disease.

Certain diseases have a seasonal prevalence and may cause explosive outbreaks in a susceptible population. Reduction of the number of susceptible animals below a certain level may terminate an outbreak of a viral disease. Many viral diseases are transmitted by vectors, such as arthropods, or contaminated material or instruments (fomites).

Immunity in most natural viral infections is absolute and relatively long lasting (as opposed to that in bacterial diseases). Serum from immune animals can be given to susceptible animals before infection occurs or before the virus is widely disseminated to produce effective but short-lived (1 to 2 weeks) immunity. The dam (mother) usually passes immunity to its offspring across the placenta and/or in the colostrum (first milk), so it is very important that neonatal animals nurse within the first 24 hours of life. Maternal antibody protection usually wanes at about 6-12 weeks of life.

Vaccination with an altered live virus (modified or attenuated so it cannot produce disease) or a killed virus confers variable immunity, depending on the virus type and immunocompetence of the host. Modified-live-virus vaccines usually give better protection as the virus actually multiplies within the host tissue. Regular boosters are usually recommended to keep immunity at a protective level.

DNA Viruses

Parvoviridae: This group contains viruses that cause feline panleukopenia, canine, porcine and bovine parvovirus infections, and hemorrhagic encephalopathy. They are very small viruses with a protein coat arranged in a many-sided geometric figure. The viruses do not have envelopes and so are resistant to disinfectants, heat and lipid solvents.

Papovaviridae: This group of viruses contains 2 genera, *Polyomavirus* and *Papillomavirus.* They are icosahedral in shape (20-sided), more than twice as big as parvoviruses and do not have an envelope. Some can cause growths (warts or papillomas) but most cause inapparent infections (Fig 32).

Adenoviridae: The genus *Adenovirus* contains a number of pathogenic organisms, including those causing infectious canine hepatitis and respiratory disease in dogs, conjunctivitis, pneumonia, diarrhea and polyarthritis in calves (weak calf syndrome), pneumonia in foals, and diarrhea and/or meningoencephalitis in swine. Adenoviruses are larger than papovaviruses but have the same geometric shape; however, they have fine, filamentous projections on some corners. They do not have an envelope.

Iridoviridae: African swine fever is caused by a virus from this group. Iridoviridae are enveloped and large, and their protein coat is composed of complex particles.

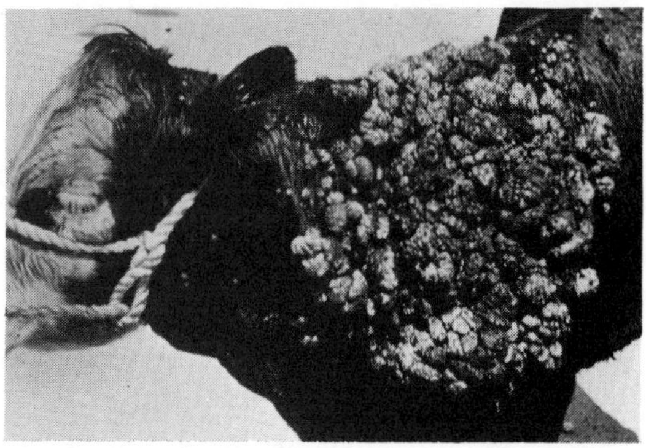

Fig 32. Severe papillomatosis in a heifer.

Herpesviridae: This family contains many viruses causing a variety of catarrhal (weepy), chronic and even neoplastic conditions. Diseases they may cause include pseudorabies, infectious bovine rhinopneumonitis (IBR), equine rhinopneumonitis, malignant catarrhal fever of cattle, bovine ulcerative mammillitis, feline rhinotracheitis, canine herpesvirus infection, and porcine inclusion-body rhinitis. Almost every animal species is plagued by one or more herpesvirus infections.

A herpesvirus is larger than an adenovirus but has the same icosahedral symmetry. Because is has a lipid envelope, it is quite sensitive to disinfectants and environmental conditions.

Poxviridae: Viruses in this group cause cowpox, swinepox, horsepox, lumpy skin disease, bovine papular stomatitis and pseudocowpox. There are no pox virus infections of dogs or cats but livestock pox viruses cause fatal and economically serious losses.

Pox viruses are very large (just visible with the light microscope) and have a complex structure composed of ovoid or brick-like components. Some have an envelope.

RNA Viruses

Picornaviridae: Diseases caused by the genus *Enterovirus* are various forms of intestinal disturbances ranging in severity. The rhinoviruses are the agents of bovine and equine upper respiratory disease; aphthoviruses cause foot and mouth disease. All picornaviruses have an icosahedral shape and are not enveloped.

Caliciviridae: Viruses in this group cause vesicular exanthema of swine and feline calicivirus infection. They are icosahedral and unenveloped.

Reoviridae: Three serotypes of this group have been associated with respiratory and enteric diseases of animals, but most infections are inapparent. They are icosahedral and unenveloped, and the only group with double-stranded RNA. An important genus, *Orbivirus,* causes African horse sickness, bluetongue and Colorado tick fever.

Togaviridae: These viruses are isometric and enveloped. They cause Western, Eastern and Venezuelan equine encephalomyelitis and louping ill. The genus *Pestivirus* causes bovine virus diarrhea and hog cholera.

Orthomyxoviridae: Viruses in this group are spherical, elongated or filamentous and have an envelope. They cause hemagglutination (cause RBC to stick together) and are sensitive to dactinomycin. Diseases caused include porcine and equine influenza.

Paramyxoviridae: These viruses are spherical or pleomorphic and enveloped, and cause hemagglutination but are resistant to dactinomycin. Diseases caused include Newcastle disease, parainfluenza, canine distemper and rinderpest.

Rhabdoviridae: Rhabdoviruses are "bullet shaped" and have an envelope. Some types can cause hemagglutination. Rabies and vesicular stomatitis are caused by viruses in this group.

Retroviridae: Retroviruses are complex and enveloped. Members of the subfamily Oncovirinae cause feline leukemia and sarcoma, mammary carcinomas, and many other types of neoplastic diseases.

Bunyaviridae: This virus particle is spherical and enveloped, and causes Rift Valley fever.

Coronaviridae: These viruses are spherical or pleomorphic and enveloped, with bulbous projections forming a crown (corona). They cause GI disease in cattle, pigs, dogs and possibly horses, infectious peritonitis in cats, and encephalitis in pigs.

Arboviruses: "Arbovirus" is a term for viruses carried by arthropods. Most have been reclassified into RNA virus groups.

Unclassified Viruses: Scrapie, ulcerative stomatitis, bovine papular stomatitis, contagious pneumonia of calves, proliferative stomatitis, ocular squamous carcinoma of cattle, and transmissible venereal tumor and mastocytoma of dogs are caused by various unclassified viruses.

Zoonoses and Public Health

Zoonotic diseases (zoonoses) are the relatively few infections transmitted from animals to people, under natural conditions. They are of particular concern in veterinary medicine because animal handlers are a high-risk group for such diseases. Veterinarians and their coworkers must educate the general public on zoonoses.

In most cases, people are accidental hosts of zoonoses, as outbreaks are usually propagated by animal-to-animal spread; person-to-person transmission is very rare. Many zoonoses must be reported to public health authorities so that steps can be taken to contain the infection and the human medical community can be alerted.

Technicians are not qualified to advise clients regarding human health matters, but they can indicate steps necessary to reduce the risks of zoonotic disease to animal owners.

Bacterial Zoonoses

Leptospirosis: Leptospira is a slender, spiral organism that infects dogs, cattle, pigs, sheep and horses. Most infections are subclinical, but jaundice, fever, hemoglobinuria (hemoglobin in the urine), abortion and death can occur. Organisms are shed in the urine of infected animals for months or years, and so may contaminate water supplies.

The disease is contracted through contact with infected urine (enters through skin wounds), ingestion of contaminated water, or by splashing infected material onto the mucous membranes. Most outbreaks are self-limiting but may be perpetuated by rodents.

Wearing gloves when handling urine and avoiding potentially contaminated water supplies for drinking are recommended, as 5% of human cases are fatal. Serologic tests, urine cultures or tissue biopsy can be used to diagnose leptospirosis. Antimicrobials are used in control of the disease. Vaccination prevents clinical signs in animals but does not eliminate the carrier state, in which organisms are shed in the urine.

Plague: Bubonic plague is caused by *Yersinia pestis,* a Gram-negative rod. Plague is not a disease of people but a natural infection of rodents (rats, ground squirrels, etc) that is spread by the rat flea. In people, *Yersinia* infects regional lymph nodes and may become systemic. The pulmonic form of plague can be spread by aerosol (droplets in the air) and is especially serious. Veterinarians have developed plague after treating cats with abscesses or respiratory infections (cats can carry plague, as diseased rats are easy to catch).

Diagnosis is by culture or inoculation of rodents. People may be vaccinated against plague and antimicrobial therapy is useful; however, the main method of control involves reducing rat populations.

Tularemia: Tularemia is an infectious disease of rodents, especially rabbits, caused by *Francisella tularensis,* a Gram-negative, pleomorphic organism. Transmission to domestic herbivores is by blood-sucking arthropods. In lambs, calves, piglets and foals, tularemia causes weakness, depression, coughing and diarrhea. The infection may remain latent for long periods.

Transmission to people occurs through contact with tissues or blood from infected animals, inhalation of aerosol, through bites of blood-sucking insects, or the bite of animals (cats, dogs, skunks, nonpoisonous snakes) that have fed on infected carcasses. Cats do not usually display signs of illness.

Infected rabbits caught by dogs and cats should be burned or buried. People should avoid sick, wild rabbits and rubber gloves should be worn when such animals are necropsied.

The disease can be diagnosed by blood culture or serologic analysis. Supportive care is based on therapy with streptomycin.

Brucellosis: Brucellosis affects cattle, swine, goats, dogs and people. The *Brucella* organism is a small, Gram-negative rod. Brucellosis is characterized by infertility, abortion and testicular infection. In horses, it is associated with fistulous withers and poll evil. In people, brucellosis causes a protracted, debilitating disease called undulant fever (fever waxes and wanes).

The organism is transmitted venereally in dogs and is contained in infected fetuses, placentas and birth fluids of all affected species. Raw milk or milk products and aborted material from infected animals are the primary sources of infection in people.

Milk and cattle are tested for brucellosis in an effort to trace infected herds. Adult cattle that test positive are slaughtered, as there is no effective treatment in animals. Antibiotic therapy is used to treat infections in people, but relapses are common. Diagnosis is based on serologic examination and culture of the organism.

Technicians can reduce their chance of infection by not drinking raw milk, wearing gloves when handling dead fetuses, placentas or birth fluids, and careful handling of the strain-19 brucellosis vaccine (this vaccine is not attenuated for people and splashing it in the eyes or injection into the skin can cause the disease).

Vibriosis: Campylobacter (formerly called *Vibrio*) is a short, curved Gram-negative rod. *Campylobacter fetus jejuni* causes hemorrhagic enteritis in dogs and people, and winter dysentery (black scours) in cattle.

The diarrhea of infected dogs may infect people. Contaminated pork and chicken is a source of disease for people and dogs.

A stool culture is needed for diagnosis. Most strains are sensitive to antibiotics. Washing the hands after handling dogs with diarrhea or raw meat is recommended to help prevent infections.

Anthrax: Bacillus anthracis, a Gram-positive, nonmotile, spore-forming rod, causes anthrax, an acute, febrile disease that can affect all species. The most common disease form consists of septicemia, with a rapidly fatal course; local and pulmonary forms are also seen.

The carcasses of infected animals often have blood oozing from the anus and nostrils and become bloated. Such carcasses should not be opened as the organism forms spores when exposed to the air; these spores can remain viable in soil for 20-30 years. People become infected by inhaling spores, especially from raw wool, hides or horse hair (wool sorter's disease), ingestion of poorly cooked meat or contact with infected tissues.

Diagnosis is based on culture, microscopic examination of tissues and blood, clinical signs and rodent inoculation. Sick animals may be treated with antimicrobials and contact animals vaccinated, but infected premises are quarantined and disinfected by state authorities.

Botulism, Tetanus: Botulism and tetanus are both caused by powerful neurotoxins elaborated by the anaerobic bacterium, *Clostridium.* All animals are susceptible to the diseases caused by this spore-forming rod.

Tetanus occurs when the organism is introduced into a wound, especially puncture wounds, and causes prolonged contraction of muscles (lockjaw). The organism is naturally found in soil, especially where horse manure is present. Toxoids, antibiotics and antitoxins are used as therapy. Puncture wounds should be made to bleed freely to help eliminate an anaerobic environment. When large numbers of animals are castrated or docked, instruments should be sterilized frequently. Iodine or chlorine application to wounds kills spores.

Botulism occurs when spoiled food (meat, bones), containing the toxin, is ingested. Paralysis progresses until death is caused by respiratory collapse. Antitoxin has been used with variable success. Control involves avoiding spoiled feed and elimination of old carcasses.

Tuberculosis: Tuberculosis, caused by a mycobacterium, is a chronic disease affecting almost all vetebrates. There are 3 main types: human, avian and bovine tuberculosis. The bovine form is responsible for human disease caused by ingestion of infected raw milk or milk products and inhalation of infectious aerosol. Wherever the organism becomes localized (usually the lungs), large masses form. Animals can also contract infections from infected people.

An intradermal skin test is used to detect the infection, along with radiographs and cultures (Fig 33). The usual control measures involve test and slaughter, but chemotherapy has also been used; however, infected animals are a health hazard to people and other animals. Infected animals shed organisms in their feces, and dust particles, food and water may become contaminated.

Salmonellosis: Salmonella organisms inhabit the intestinal tract of many birds and mammals, and quite a few species can cause GI disease in people. Infection occurs through ingestion of contaminated food. Direct infection from animals is uncommon. Cats are seldom involved in this zoonotic disease.

Ornithosis-Psittacosis (Chlamydiosis): This is an acute or chronic disease of birds caused by *Chlamydia psittaci* (in people and psittacine birds, it is called psittacosis, in other birds ornithosis). In birds, it causes weight loss, nasal discharge and diarrhea, and in people, flu-like symptoms.

Pet birds should come from an aviary free of disease, as an inapparent carrier state can occur. Screening aviaries against wild birds is

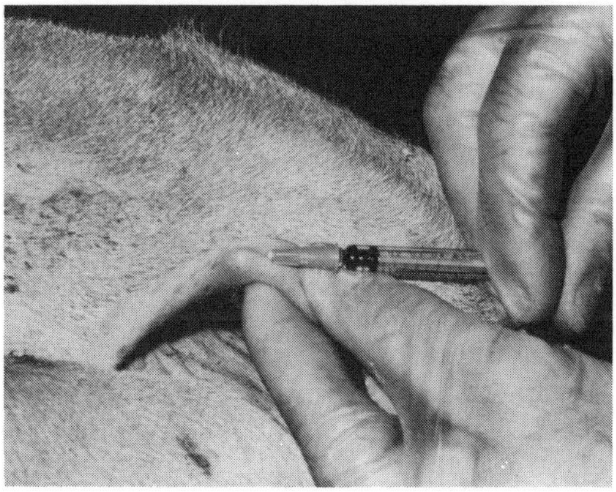

Fig 33. Intradermal injection of tuberculin in the caudal tail fold of a cow.

necessary. Tetracycline-coated seeds may be fed; however, some resistance is developing to this drug.

In people, the disease occurs after exposure to infected aerosol or dust. When necropsying birds, the feathers should be moistened with a disinfectant to prevent spread of the disease. Live birds can be examined using a surgical mask or transparent container (glove box).

Outbreaks of the disease must be reported to public health authorities.

Cat-Scratch Fever: The causitive agent of cat-scratch fever has not been isolated. The disease occurs about 4 weeks after a cat scratch has healed. The lymph node draining that region becomes inflamed and may develop an abscess. Fever, weakness and headache may accompany lymph node enlargement. It is a self-limiting disease.

Rickettsial Zoonoses

Rocky Mountain Spotted Fever: Rickettsia rickettsii causes Rocky Mountain spotted fever in people and inapparent infections in animals. The disease consists of fever, severe chills, headache, muscle pain and a rash in people and is transmitted by the wood tick (*Dermacentor andersoni*) or the dog tick (*D variabilis*). The tick must be attached to the skin for several hours for transmission of the disease.

The disease is diagnosed by symptoms, isolation of the organism, serologic examination or inoculation of rodents. It is treated with antimicrobials, though 5-10% of affected people die. Rocky Mountain spotted fever can be prevented by avoiding ticks (protective clothing), vaccination, and frequent inspection of the body. Ticks on people should be removed with forceps or with fingers protected by paper or gloves. Care should be taken not to damage ticks during removal, to prevent spread of the disease.

Q Fever: Q fever is caused by *Coxiella burnetii* and causes abortion in sheep and goats, and an influenza-like disease and chronic endocarditis in people. It is carried by a variety of ticks that must feed for several hours for transmission of the disease. Contamination of the mucosae or wounds with crushed ticks or tick feces may also cause the disease. Diagnosis is based on isolation of the organism or serologic examination.

Vaccination of people reduces the severity of clinical signs but does not eliminate infection. Killing ticks with insecticides and clearing of brush that can house ticks are recommended.

Viral Zoonoses

Rabies: Rabies is a viral disease that affects all warm-blooded animals, though some are more resistant than others. It is usually transmitted by the bite of an infected animal, but it has been transmitted by inhalation of aerosol in bat-infested caves. The disease is propagated in nature by wild animals, especially skunks, bats and foxes.

The virus travels up nerve trunks to the brain and then enters the salivary glands where it can be transmitted by biting. Therefore, clinical signs occur before the virus is present in the saliva.

The furious form presents a picture of the typical "mad" animal and the dumb form is characterized by progressive paralysis. Pharyngeal paralysis may cause the animal to act as if it has a bone in its throat.

Domestic animals that have bitten people should be quarantined for 10-12 days and watched for clinical signs. If signs of rabies appear within that time, there is a possibility the virus was in the saliva at the time of the bite and treatment of the bitten person should begin. If no signs are observed, the virus was not transmitted at the time of the bite, though the animal could still be incubating rabies. Wild animals that, without provocation, have bitten people are killed and their brains are examined microscopically for the disease. Animals that have bitten other animals must be quarantined for longer periods, as the incubation time is variable. If the biting animal has a current rabies vaccination, it is revaccinated and confined for 90 days. If the biting animal was not vaccinated, it must be placed in strict isolation for 6 months and revaccinated one month before release. Suspect livestock should be slaughtered or observed closely for 6 months.

Control measures include vaccination of pet animals, stray animal control and education of the public.

Rabies vaccination is recommended for all technicians.

Encephalitis: A number of viral zoonoses cause encephalitis (inflammation of the brain), including Eastern, Western and Venezuelan equine encephalitis, Rift Valley fever, Ross River disease, Japanese encephalitis, St. Louis encephalitis, West Nile disease, louping ill and California encephalitis. All are transmitted by mosquitoes or ticks.

The equine encephalitides are a similar group of diseases characterized by CNS disturbances. They are propagated in nature by birds or rodents and transmitted by mosquitoes. The diagnosis is based on clinical signs, geographic area and season (fall and summer) of infections, and serologic examination. Fever, convulsions, cyanosis, drowsiness and increased intracranial pressure occur in infected people. Eastern encephalomyelitis is fatal in 50% of affected horses and Western encephalomyelitis in 5-15%, as there is no effective treatment. Diagnosis is by serologic examination.

Vaccination of horses and mosquito control are used to combat spread of the disease.

Mycotic Zoonoses

Superficial Dermatomycoses: Infections by *Microsporum* and *Trichophyton*, both superficial dermatophytes, are commonly known as "ringworm." The organisms feed on keratin found in the skin, hair and nails. The lesions grow centrifugally (in a circle) and result in hair breakage and thickened, scaly patches of skin. Long-haired cats may carry dermatophytes without demonstrating clinical signs. Lesions in people may occur on exposed areas, such as the arms, and appear as red, circular or blotchy patches that slowly enlarge.

Therapy includes topical or systemic antifungals (*eg,* griseofulvin). Because fungal spores remain viable in the environment for several months, infected animals should be confined to an area where thorough cleaning is possible. Contaminated brushes, collars, bedding and other items should be sanitized or replaced.

Systemic Mycoses: Such diseases as histoplasmosis, blastomycosis, coccidioidomycosis and cryptococcosis are not directly transmissible from animals to people. However, infected animals contaminate the environment and may increase the likelihood that people, especially very young, old or immunosuppressed people, will contract these potentially serious infections.

Parasitic Zoonoses

Cestodes: A variety of tapeworms are transmissible to people, including *Taenia saginatta* in undercooked beef, *Taenia solium* in undercooked pork and *Diphyllobothrium latum* in raw fish. *Hymenolepis nana* does not require an intermediate host and infects people through food contaminated by infected rodents. *Dipylidium caninum* infects people when fleas are accidentally consumed. These parasites mature into adult tapeworms in the human intestinal tract, where they cause mild enteritis, compete with the host for nutrients and produce proglottids (tapeworm segments), but no serious disease.

Echinococcus, on the other hand, may follow a similar pattern when undercooked meat is eaten; however, if an egg is consumed (from fecal contamination), a hydatid cyst develops in the liver, lungs, kidneys, spleen, heart, skeletal muscles, brain or bone marrow. The cyst is filled with fluid and scoleces (worm heads) and can grow very large.

Control is by fecal examination for animals, elimination of intermediate hosts and careful food preparation (well-cooked meat).

Trematodes: Fasciola hepatica, a fluke that inhabits the liver and bile ducts, is transmitted to people when contaminated raw greens (*eg,* watercress) are eaten. It is found where snails, moisture and herbivorous animals are combined. Cooking of wild greens and treating infected animals are recommended control measures.

Nematodes: The roundworm of swine (*Ascaris suum*) can infect people through ingestion of food or water contaminated with the feces of infected swine. The roundworm then completes its life cycle as in the natural host.

Toxocara (roundworm of dogs and cats) also infects people in a similar fashion but does not complete its life cycle (humans are an aberrant host). Instead, it wanders throughout the tissue (especially damaging to the brain or eye), causing damage until the worm dies (larva migrans).

Hookworms (*eg, Ancylostoma*) and *Strongyloides* penetrate the skin and migrate subcutaneously, causing itching, inflammation and a rash (cutaneous larva migrans or creeping eruption). *Strongyloides* has a free-living cycle and can heavily contaminate the environment. It may cause clinical enteric disease in people and, if the infective stage is activated internally, can penetrate the colon or skin around the anus with fatal results in a person with an immunodeficiency.

Domestic animals, especially young puppies, should have a fecal sample examined routinely to reduce the public health hazard of these parasites.

Trichinella spiralis encysts in the muscle of pigs and may be consumed in undercooked pork. In people, the parasite prefers highly active muscles, such as the tongue and diaphragm, where the cysts cause pain and even death.

Table 1. Zoonotic Parasites

Parasites of Food and Water
Taenia solium (pork tapeworm)
Taenia saginatta (beef tapeworm)
Diphyllobothrium latum (broad fish tapeworm)
Trichinella spiralis
Entamoeba histolytica
Toxoplasma
Parasites of Dogs
Enchinococcus granulosus
Toxocara canis (dog roundworm)
Dipylidium caninum (flea-transmitted tapeworm)
Ancylostoma braziliense (hookworm)
Dirofilaria immitis (heartworm)
Strongyloides canis
Trypanosoma cruzi
Ctenocephalides canis (dog flea)
Parasites of Cats
Toxocara cati (cat roundworm)
Toxoplasma gondii
Ctenocephalides felis (cat flea)
Sarcoptes (sarcoptic mange mite)
Notoedres (notoedric mange mite)
Miscellaneous Parasites
Strongyloides
Cryptosporidium
Giardia
Sarcocystis
Ascaris suum (swine roundworm)
Fasciola hepatica (liver fluke)
Hymenolepis nana
Balantidium coli
Echinococcus multilocularis
Cheyletiella

Heartworms (*Dirofilaria*) cause granulomatous lung lesions in people bitten by infected mosquitoes.

Protozoa: Consumption of water contaminated by *Entamoeba* and *Giardia* can lead to enteritis (diarrhea) and weight loss.

Toxoplasmosis (*Toxoplasma gondii*) is a protozoal infection of domestic animals and many birds. The sexual phase of its life cycle takes place only in the intestinal tract of cats. Ingestion of oocysts in cat feces leads to cyst formation in other species (eating cysts in undercooked meat causes cyst formation in the new host). Cyst formation is of particular concern to pregnant women, as it can cause serious deformities in the fetus. Clinical disease in people resembles influenza or infectious mononucleosis; chronic disease can result in ocular abnormalities.

Precautions involve completely cooking meat, washing hands after handling raw meat, avoiding cat litter pans when pregnant, and covering children's sandboxes when not in use.

Cats usually pick up the infection through hunting and may be tested for toxoplasmosis. People with prior exposure may have protective antibody levels.

Ectoparasites: Flies, fleas, ticks and mosquitoes may transmit a variety of diseases through their bites. *Sarcoptes, Notoedres* and *Cheyletiella* are burrowing mites that can cause rashes in people. Direct contact with infected animals is necessary for transmission. Bright-red, itchy papules are formed, especially in areas where clothing fits tightly. Elimination of infection on animals often clears the rash on people, but topical insecticides may be required.

Recommendations

Prevention of zoonotic disease involves some very simple measures. Do not eat, drink or smoke unless your hands have been thoroughly washed. Do not eat undercooked meat or drink contaminated water. Protect open wounds from animal waste, saliva, pus and other contaminants. Wear rubber gloves when handling dead animals, aborted fetuses, placentas or birth fluids and wash hands well after cleaning up animal waste or vomit. Get vaccinated for tetanus and rabies. Educate clients regarding the value of fecal examinations and vaccinations in preventing zoonotic diseases. Finally, encourage owners to obey leash laws, control stray animals and clean up after their pets in public areas.

Recommended Reading

1. Siegmund: *The Merck Veterinary Manual.* 5th ed. Merck and Co, Rahway, NJ, 1979.
2. Blood *et al: Veterinary Medicine.* 5th ed. Lea & Febiger, Philadelphia, 1983.
3. Robinson: *Current Therapy in Equine Medicine.* WB Saunders, Philadelphia, 1983.
4. Howard: *Current Therapy in Food Animal Practice.* WB Saunders, Philadelphia, 1981.
5. Kirk: *Current Veterinary Therapy VIII.* WB Saunders, Philadelphia, 1983.
6. Pratt: *Feline Medicine.* 1st ed. American Veterinary Publications, Santa Barbara, 1983.
7. Mansmann and McAllister: *Equine Medicine and Surgery.* 3rd ed. American Veterinary Publications, Santa Barbara, 1982.
8. Amstutz: *Bovine Medicine and Surgery.* 2nd ed. American Veterinary Publications, Santa Barbara, 1980.
9. Kirk and Bistner: *Handbook of Veterinary Procedures and Emergency Treatment.* WB Saunders, Philadelphia, 1981.

4

treatment technics for small animals

R.B. FORD, J. RASMUSSEN, C.S. INTRAVARTOLO & K. KAZMIERCZAK

ROUTES OF DRUG ADMINISTRATION
by R.B. Ford

Any discussion of technics as routine as administering drugs, fluids and vaccines may seem unnecessary in a textbook for experienced veterinary technicians. However, the frequency with which drugs and vaccines are given to small animal patients mandates that technicians not only be familiar with the various routes of administration but that they also be aware of specific contraindications, potential complications and alternative routes of administration.

In veterinary medicine, drugs are given parenterally, orally or topically. Parenteral administration of drugs involves injection of medication into the patient. Parenteral routes include intravenous (IV), subcutaneous (SC) and intramuscular (IM) routes when systemic distribution of a drug is desired. The term parenteral applies even to those drugs that, when injected, are intended to have local or regional effects only, *eg,* infiltration of the skin with a local anesthetic. Since the parenteral administration of any drug or vaccine is not without some risk of complication, products that must be injected are generally given within the veterinary hospital by trained personnel. Injection of insulin to diabetic dogs or cats is one notable exception.

Oral administration of medication involves giving a drug by way of the mouth. While there are numerous technics for giving a drug by the oral route (*per os,* PO), the discussion that follows emphasizes methods of avoiding personal injury while giving drugs PO and alternative strategies for animals that resist this route of administration.

Topical application of medication to small animals, particularly dogs, is quite common. However, improper application of topical medication often complicates the response to therapy. In addition, improper application of topical medication can become extremely expensive. The discussion in this section emphasizes skin preparation and proper technic with respect to maximizing the efficacy of topically applied drugs.

Parenteral Routes

Parenteral administration of drugs, fluids or vaccines is never without some risk of complication. Though infection subsequent to parenteral administration of drugs is rare, most such infections can be easily avoided through use of routine aseptic procedures. With the exception of placing indwelling IV catheters, it is more customary than it is necessary to "cleanse" the patient's skin at the site of injection immediately before inserting the needle. Skin preparation with alcohol or other disinfectant solutions does not sterilize the skin. In fact, alcohol may be an additional source of irritation and pain as the needle penetrates the skin. However, most clients expect their pet to receive some form of skin preparation before injection. In contrast to single-dose injections, skin preparation is of utmost importance before inserting an indwelling IV catheter.

Subcutaneous Route

The subcutaneous (SC) route involves injection beneath the skin but not into muscle underlying the skin. It is probably the most common parenteral route used in small animals. In dogs and cats, SC injection may be at any convenient site. However, preferred sites are body regions where the skin is loosely attached to the subcutis and muscle and where pain sensation is minimal. In dogs and cats, the skin between the scapulae (shoulder blades) and on the dorsal midline best fits these criteria.

Subcutaneous injection is relatively simple. However, occasionally the technician must instruct the owners of an animal to give SC injections to their pets, such as diabetic pets. Adherence to proper technic is important.

Technic: A common and convenient technic used for SC injections entails lifting the skin between the scapulae with the thumb and first 2 fingers of one hand, forming a "tent" of skin (Fig 1). With needle and syringe in the opposite hand, the needle is thrust through the pa-

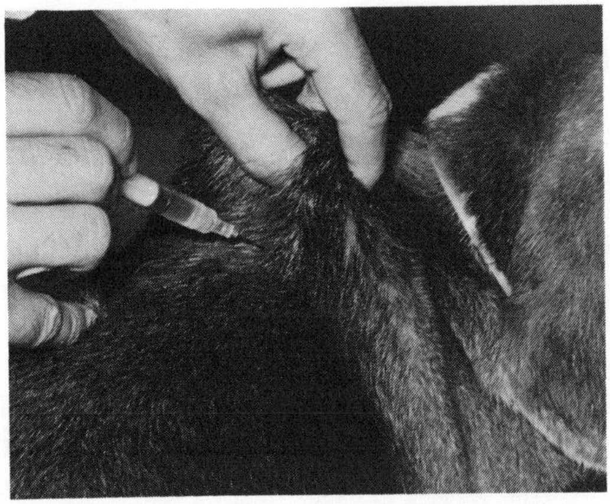

Fig 1. Needle placement for SC injection.

tient's skin at the base of the "tent." In small dogs and kittens, it may be easier and less painful to the patient to pull the skin over the needle.

Use of disposable 22- through 25-ga needles is recommended. Smaller-diameter (25-ga) needles are reserved for young and small animals. When the tip of the needle is properly positioned in the SC tissue, it is not necessary to aspirate (briefly withdraw the syringe barrel to apply suction) before injection.

Subcutaneous injection of large volumes of fluid is a common means of treating dehydrated patients. A single needle should be inserted SC to give the total fluid volume. Generally, redistribution of the fluid deposited in SC tissues is rapid enough that the patient can accept large volumes over several minutes. The disadvantage of SC fluid therapy using multiple sites of needle insertion is the increased risk of infection associated with multiple skin punctures.

Indications: The SC route is used *only* with drugs approved by the Food and Drug Administration and recommended by the manufacturer for SC injection. *Do not* assume that any drug intended for IV or IM use may also be given SC.

Complications: The most common complications associated with SC injections include pain, infection and improper needle placement.

Some pain is to be expected, particularly in puppies and kittens, as the needle penetrates the skin. An intense painful response can be associated with inadvertent intradermal (within the skin) injection or injection of an irritating material (*eg,* chloramphenicol succinate).

Infection and abscessation at the injection site are attributed to use of a contaminated needle or injection of contaminated drugs. Some drugs intended for IM or IV use are particularly irritating when given SC, resulting in a sterile abscess and sloughing of skin around the injection site.

Inserting the needle through the skin, into the subcutis, and through the skin a second time occasionally occurs, even with experienced individuals. The drug is injected onto the haircoat rather than into the patient. This problem is best corrected by collecting one's pride and reattempting the injection. This problem is most likely to occur in severely dehydrated animals or in those that are difficult to restrain during needle insertion.

Intramuscular Route

With the intramuscular (IM) route, the drug is injected into one of the large skeletal muscle groups in the body. The most common site for injection in dogs and cats is into the lateral thigh. However, IM injections may be given at other sites as well. In larger dogs, for example, the lumbar muscles and shoulder muscles may be used.

Technic: Once the appropriate site is selected, the needle, with syringe attached, is inserted deeply and rapidly in the muscle. Since the needle could be inadvertently inserted into a vein or artery, one must gently withdraw the syringe barrel before completing the injection. If blood is not withdrawn into the syringe upon aspiration, the drug is then injected. If, however, blood appears in the syringe during aspiration, the needle should be withdrawn and discarded and the injection reattempted at another site.

Disposable 21- through 25-ga needles are routinely used for IM injections. The 25-ga, 5/8-inch needle should be reserved for cats and small dogs. In large or overweight animals, the 5/8-inch-long needle may not be of sufficient length to penetrate down to muscle.

Complications: Pain associated with IM injections can be attributed to tissue injuries stemming from deposition of material into the muscle. Injection of large volumes (2 ml or more in cats and small dogs, 5 ml in larger animals) by the IM route is discouraged. Irritating solutions, particularly acidic (low pH) solutions, may elicit a painful response regardless of the volume injected.

Deposition of a drug into or, more likely, around a major nerve (perineural) may cause serious and permanent nerve damage. Paralysis and muscle atrophy in the affected leg may become evident within a week after injection. There is no way to determine when a perineural injection is about to be made. Extreme pain is not necessarily evident.

Nerve injury associated with IM injection is not usually treatable. It is, however, preventable. Cats and small dogs are at greater risk of complication following IM injection because of their smaller muscle mass as compared to that of larger animals. Furthermore, most nerve complications are associated with IM injections in the thigh.

Intravenous Route

Intravenous (IV) injection involves positioning the needle tip in the lumen of a vein. Intravenous catheters and needles are generally inserted into a vein in the same direction as the flow of blood, *ie,* toward the heart. Though any vein will suffice, the large, superficial veins should be used. These include the jugular, cephalic, femoral, saphenous (cats) and lateral saphenous (dogs) veins. In emergency situations, the lingual vein may be used for IV injections in anesthetized or unconscious animals.

Technic: Successful placement of a needle or catheter into a vein is one of the most demanding skills required of technicians and veterinarians. With experience, IV injections become routine. However, even the most experienced individual occasionally encounters an animal in which IV injection is particularly difficult.

The probability of unsuccessful venipuncture increases in direct proportion to the urgency of the situation. Stated another way, when needed the most, successful IV catheterization is quite likely to be most difficult to accomplish. There are, in fact, some logical reasons for this axiom. The most demanding situations in which IV catheterization is required are typically emergency situations. Not only does an atmosphere of tension exist among those tending to the patient's vital needs, but there is a very natural tendency to work rapidly. Too often, this translates into decreased efficiency. The unconscious patient that is becoming cyanotic may be thrust onto a makeshift examination table, or even onto the floor, where inadequate light, improper vein preparation and poor positioning seriously complicate attempts to resuscitate the patient.

The first and most important goal in successful IV catheterization is adequate visualization of the vein. This includes at least the following steps:

Patient Position: The patient should be elevated to a height that is comfortable for the technician. Inserting a needle into a vein while kneeling, squatting or sitting on the floor with a patient is difficult. Though it is possible to give IV injections or withdraw blood while working alone, additional assistance not only decreases the time involved but also decreases the risk of injury to the technician and patient.

Vein Preparation: It is not always necessary to clip hair from the skin overlying a vein before IV injection or catheterization. Wetting the hair with alcohol, using a cottonball or sponge swept in the direction of the hair, enhances visualization of the vein, even in long-haired breeds. Overweight animals and certain breeds (*eg,* Collies) tend to have veins that are difficult to visualize. In these cases, clipping the hair *and* wetting the skin with alcohol are often necessary. The alcohol not only cleans the skin of hair, oil and superficial debris but, by virtue of its irritant properties, also makes the vein more prominent beneath the skin.

Adequate Light: A properly prepared vein in a well-positioned patient can be difficult or impossible to visualize in poorly lit areas. Use of a focal, moveable light source is important when attempting IV injection and catheterization.

Use of a Tourniquet: Veins carry blood from peripheral tissues back to the heart under low pressure (systemic venous pressure may be less than 5 mm Hg, vs 110 mm Hg in systemic arteries). Adequate visualization of a vein, therefore, necessitates occluding the vein at some convenient point between the site of intended venipuncture and the heart. As the segment of vein distal to the point of obstruction fills with blood, the diameter of the vein lumen increases. In turn, the enlarging vein causes a prominent bulge in the overlying skin.

Routine insertion of a needle or catheter into a vein requires practice. While inserting a needle into a vein, particularly when using large needles such as those used with IV catheters, it may be helpful to use a 2-step technic. First, insert the needle through the skin into the SC tissue, parallel and adjacent to the vein. The needle should be completely through the skin before entering the vein. Second, direct the tip of the needle toward the vein and thrust the needle into, not through, the vein. The needle should be threaded into the vein until the needle hub contacts the skin surface (Fig 2). The vein should be stabilized by *extending* the animal's limb before attempting venipuncture (Fig 3).

To ensure proper positioning of the needle within the vein, a small quantity of blood should be aspirated into the syringe *before* removing the tourniquet. Only when blood flow into the syringe is confirmed by aspiration may the tourniquet be released and the injection completed. Any attempt to inject into an obstructed vein results in leakage around the venipuncture site, which could cause serious complications if caustic solutions are being injected.

A needle tip that has passed through the vein and is positioned within SC tissues contains a small amount of blood. In such cases, at-

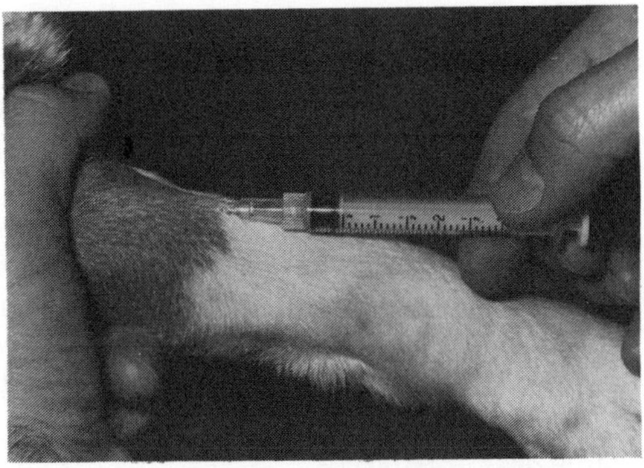

Fig 2. Proper placement of needle and syringe for IV injection or withdrawal of blood.

tempts to aspirate frequently yield a small quantity, but not a flow, of blood. Injection should not be made under these circumstances.

The correct technic for withdrawing a needle or catheter is too often overlooked, even by experienced individuals. If blood flow has been obstructed during venipuncture, it is important to restore the flow of blood before withdrawing the needle. Even when using a tourniquet, release the tourniquet completely before taking the needle out of the vein. If an assistant is holding the animal and occluding the vein, the assistant should be told when to release pressure on the vein. Blood flow must be restored before removing the needle. This technic of needle withdrawal is intended to prevent hematoma (a SC blood "bubble") formation. Some blood leaks out of the veins even though blood flow has been restored before needle withdrawal. Such leakage is minimized by compressing the skin over the venipuncture site for 15-30 seconds after needle withdrawal. In some cases, particularly when a large needle has been inserted into a limb vein, it may be

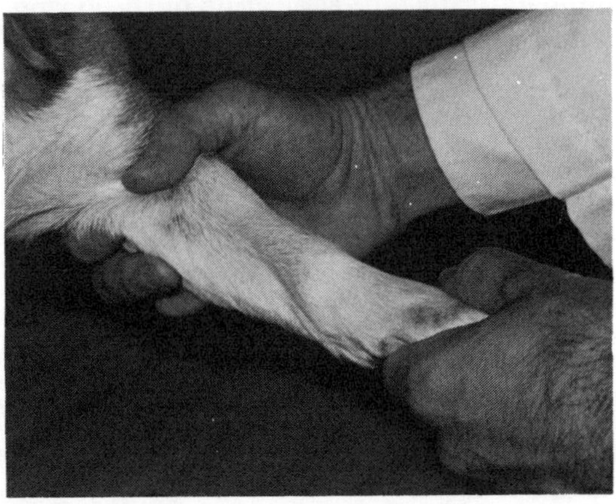

Fig 3. Extending the leg before attempting an IV injection stabilizes the vein beneath the skin.

necessary to place a compression bandage over the venipuncture site for several minutes.

Complications: Problems associated with IV injections include hematoma formation, collapse of the vein, needle occlusion and infection.

The swelling caused by extravasation (leakage) of blood through the venipuncture site into SC tissues is called a hematoma. Inadvertently passing a needle *through* the vein or making multiple attempts to insert the needle into the vein commonly results in hematoma formation. Also, withdrawal of a needle from a vein in which blood flow has been restricted (as with a tourniquet) invariably results in hematoma formation.

Once a hematoma develops, IV injection should not be attempted at the level of the hematoma or at any point distal to (farther from the heart) the hematoma. If IV injection is necessary after a hematoma has formed, another vein should be selected. However, if another vein is not available, the injection must be proximal to (closer to the heart) the site of hematoma formation. For this reason, the most distal site available should be used for the initial venipuncture attempt.

Use of excessive pressure to impede blood flow may be counterproductive. Veins are thin-walled structures that collapse easily under pressure; only the minimal amount of pressure necessary to collapse the vein at one point is necessary. Inordinately tight tourniquets or excessive manual pressure can preclude venous filling by restricting arterial circulation and causing excessive skin tension over the vein.

In small dogs and cats, blood can be withdrawn from a vein faster than the vein can fill. This causes the walls of the veins to collapse around the needle tip. Gentle and intermittent squeezing of the distal limb, intermittent aspiration of the syringe and loosening of the tourniquet are often helpful.

Formation of a small blood clot in the lumen of a needle can prevent blood return into the syringe during aspiration. This is most likely to occur during repeated attempts at venipuncture using the same needle. During its excursions through the SC tissue, enough blood and tissue thromboplastin may enter the tip of the needle to activate extrinsic clotting mechanisms and effectively occlude the needle.

Before inserting an IV catheter, the hair should be clipped from the skin over the vein and the skin prepared with a surgical scrub. Failure to do this can result in serious infection at the site of venipuncture, particularly when the catheter will be in place for several hours or days.

Intraperitoneal Route

Injection of medication directly into the peritoneal cavity of an animal can achieve high drug concentrations in the blood. Fluids may also be given by intraperitoneal (IP) injection in dehydrated animals that do not have veins suitable for catheterization.

The IP route, however, does carry a significant risk of infection and must not be used indiscriminately.

Technic: In dogs and cats, regardless of age or size, IP injections are given at the level of the umbilicus, to the right or left of the midline on the ventral aspect of the abdomen. A 1-inch disposable needle is sufficient for most animals; in large dogs or overweight animals, a 1½- to 2-inch-long needle may be necessary.

The hair is clipped from the injection site and the skin prepared with a surgical scrub. Injection of local anesthetic into the skin at the site of penetration can be quite irritating to the patient and, furthermore, is rarely necessary. The patient is restrained in lateral recumbency and the needle is inserted perpendicular to the skin, into the peritoneal cavity. The hub of the needle should touch the skin's surface.

Once inserted, the injection is completed without aspirating and without excess movement of the needle. Aspiration may plug the needle tip with abdominal fat or mesentery. Movement of the needle hub causes wide excursions of the sharp needle tip within the abdomen. The risk of damaging tissue with the needle tip is increased as either patient or needle moves during IP injection. The needle is quickly withdrawn after injection.

Due to the inherent risks associated with IP injection, the decision to use this route should be made by the clinician responsible for the case.

Complications: Infection is the most significant complication associated with IP injection. Introduction of bacteria into the abdominal cavity during IP injection may cause death from septic peritonitis (bacterial infection within the abdomen). Since the risk of serious bacterial infection following IP injection is significantly greater than the risk in IV injection, strict aseptic technic should be used when giving drugs or fluids by the IP route.

Intralesional Route

Injection of a drug directly into a lesion is common in small animal practice. With few exceptions, intralesional injections involve injection of small amounts of a drug into small, discrete lesions of the skin, such as small cutaneous tumors or "hot spot" lesions. Intralesional injections are not to be used when the objective of treatment is to obtain significant systemic drug levels.

Skin lesions are typically contaminated with bacteria, particularly when the patient has been licking or chewing the lesion. Therefore, skin preparation is important before intralesional injection. Preparation can entail only an abbreviated surgical scrub or may involve clipping of hair, thorough surgical scrubbing of the lesion, rinsing and drying.

Though chronic skin lesions are frequently devoid of sensory nerve endings and may be anesthetic, the patient should be restrained by an assistant during intralesional injection. Injection of any drug into normal skin adjacent to a lesion can be quite painful.

Topical Route

The topical route of drug use involves application of a drug directly to a particular body area, such as the skin, eye or ear. Of all drug administration routes, topical application is among the most common for treating the skin, haircoat, eyes and ears. The technic of instilling topical eye and ear medication is discussed later in this chapter.

Numerous prescription and over-the-counter products, such as creams, ointments, powders and soaps, are available for use in treatment of skin and haircoat disorders. Correct use of the appropriate product can provide relief from clinical signs and may even treat the primary cause of disease. However, if used inappropriately, many of these same products can intensify clinical signs and worsen the disease. Some topical drugs may be absorbed through normal skin, ultimately reaching toxic levels in the blood. Fatalities stemming from excessive topical use of flea and tick products have been reported.

Problems associated with use of topical skin care products center more around preparation of the patient and frequency of drug administration than on the actual method of taking the product from the bottle, jar or tube and placing it onto the patient's skin. The cost and efficacy of topical drugs are dramatically increased when medication is applied to a skin lesion that is dirty, greasy or covered with hair. Before treatment, hair around the skin lesion should be clipped to permit thorough cleansing. Because clipping the hair from large lesions is disturbing to some owners, the client should be advised that it may be necessary to remove hair to effectively treat the lesion. Avoid any unnecessary clipping.

Oral Route

Numerous technics have been used to give oral medication to dogs and cats. Unfortunately, most have never been described. The most familiar and probably the most often used technic entails opening the patient's mouth with one hand and depositing a tablet or capsule on the caudal aspect (base) of the tongue with the opposite hand. After releasing the medication into the oral cavity and removing one's hand, the mouth is held closed until the patient swallows. However, the patient may not swallow and if it does, the medication may not be swallowed. Individual pecularities among certain animals may warrant use of varying strategies to successfully treat a dog or cat *per os* (PO).

Giving liquid medication PO is not difficult, at least until the patient tires of being treated. Use of a small bulb syringe or eye dropper facilitates drug administration. The liquid is dispensed directly over the tongue or into the space between the upper dental arcade and upper lip. Note that liquids should only be given to animals that do not have swallowing disorders. Liquids must never be given PO to heavily sedated or anesthetized animals, since they may aspirate the medication and develop pneumonia.

Though giving oral medication presents little risk to the patient, the person giving it may be injured if the patient resists treatment, particularly with cats. Their sharp teeth, agility and numerous pathogenic bacteria in the oral cavity warrant extreme caution when medicating a cat PO.

Client Education

Since most oral medication is dispensed to the client at the time the patient is examined, it is unlikely the technician will be involved with giving oral medication on a daily basis to one patient. The patient's response to therapy hinges on 2 critical factors: the client's willingness to comply with the medication instructions, and the client's ability to give the medication.

Though it may appear there is little the technician can do to ensure a client actually gives the medication to the patient, the technician should review the medication instructions with the client, review possible side effects, precautions and complications, if any, and reinforce the importance of giving all of the medication prescribed. Additionally, requesting the client to bring all prescribed medications when returning for a follow-up examination helps evaluate how well the owner has complied with the instructions.

Never assume a client can give a tablet, capsule or liquid to a dog or cat. Always ask the client if he or she is familiar with an appropriate and safe technic. Ideally, the technician should demonstrate or at least recommend a technic that is acceptable to the individual giving the medication. Note that the client may not necessarily be the same individual that actually treats the patient.

When giving tablets or capsules to dogs, instruct the client to facilitate opening the dog's mouth by placing the thumb of one hand on the hard palate and using the opposite hand to place the medication on the base of the tongue (Fig 4). With the head held in its normal horizontal position, the mouth is generally held closed for a few seconds to encourage the dog to swallow. Coating the tablet or capsule with a small amount of butter or salad oil may expedite swallowing.

Disguising medication in a small bolus of food (*eg,* hamburger, cheese, canned food) often facilitates medicating dogs PO. Some dogs, even when all other methods have failed, eagerly accept tablets or capsules if offered as a "food reward" for obeying a command.

While the same technics used to treat dogs can be effectively applied to cats, there is one notable exception. Passing one's finger into a cat's mouth to push or place a tablet onto the base of the tongue is not recommended. Instead, the tablet or capsule, coated with butter or another edible lubricant, should be dropped, not placed, into the vertically oriented mouth. Holding the mouth closed for several seconds, with the head in its normal horizontal position, increases the chances the medication will be swallowed. Commercial "pilling guns" are available for cats as well as dogs and may be the preferred method of treating some animals.

Note that after a tablet or capsule is placed in an animal's mouth, the head should be returned to its normal horizontal position, as

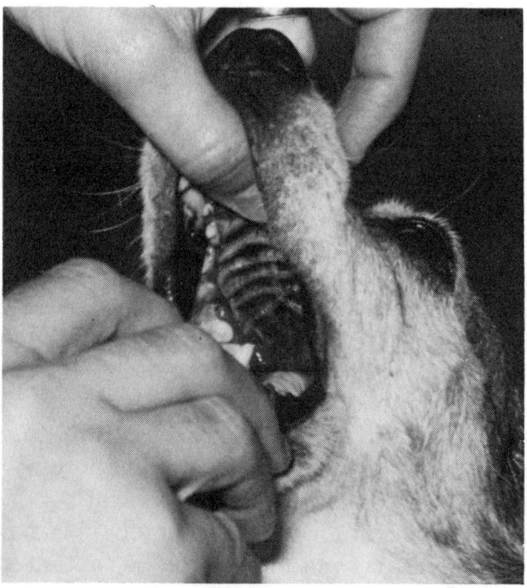

Fig 4. Technic for examining the oral cavity or giving oral medication.

swallowing is nearly impossible while the neck is extended and the head is held vertically.

TUBE FEEDING

by R. B. Ford

General Considerations

Of the many reasons for passing a tube into the stomach or esophagus of a dog or cat, delivering nutrients and/or water into the gastrointestinal (GI) tract is the most common. Several disorders may result in unwillingness or inability to grasp food (*eg,* mandibular fractures), chew food (*eg,* large oral tumors) or swallow food (*eg,* megaesophagus). In such cases, supportive therapy that includes tube feeding nutrients facilitates healing, shortens the recovery period, and maintains normal bowel function until the patient can eat on its own. Animals with severe congenital or inherited defects, such as cleft palate, may be successfully maintained if fed by stomach tube. However, the nature of this disorder, if not feasible to correct surgically, necessitates lifelong therapy.

Passing a tube through the esophagus and into the stomach (gastric intubation) can have therapeutic value. In dogs with gastric dilatation-torsion, passing a stomach tube and relieving gaseous distention of the stomach may be life saving.

Gastric intubation has diagnostic application as well. Contrast radiography of the stomach and small intestine requires accurate delivery of a specified volume of contrast material, usually barium sulfate, into the stomach. Attempts to force feed barium sulfate, particularly to cats, are likely to be resisted. Effective, efficient preparation of patients for upper GI contrast radiography is useful in a busy small animal practice.

Instruments

To be prepared for intubating patients of various sizes, tubes of varying lengths, diameters and rigidity must be on hand. Since most stomach tubes are constructed of material that can withstand repeated cleaning and sterilizing, a large inventory of similarly sized tubes is generally unnecessary.

Technic

Note that the term "stomach tube" is somewhat of a misnomer since there are relatively few situations that require the tube to actually pass into the stomach. To feed animals, it is only necessary that the feeding tube be passed well into the esophagus. From there,

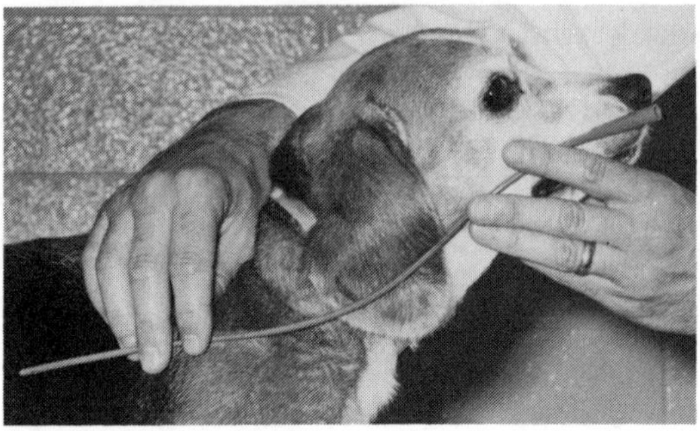

Fig 5. Feeding tubes need not be passed into the stomach but should at least reach the thoracic esophagus.

deposited nutrients enter the stomach by virtue of normal esophageal peristalsis.

Puppies and Kittens: Tube feeding young animals is best accomplished with a pediatric feeding tube or similar pliable plastic tubing that has 2 or more side holes ("eyes"). Though the tube can be lubricated with an aqueous lubricant, such as K-Y Jelly, saliva in the oral cavity is generally sufficient for passage into the esophagus. The tube should be of sufficient length to enter at least the thoracic portion of the esophagus (Fig 5).

The tube must be tested *before insertion* to ensure that the material to be infused will actually pass through the tubing, as suspensions of food pieces that are larger than the tube's inside diameter or the "eye" will plug the feeding tube. Therefore, when feeding small or very young animals, nutrient solutions or finely homogenized suspensions should be used.

In puppies and kittens, use of a speculum to prevent the animal from biting the tube during passage may occasionally be necessary. However, in most young animals, a feeding tube may be inserted at an interdental space (between the teeth) while holding the patient's mouth closed. Generally, less restraint is required with this procedure than with use of a mouth speculum.

In neonates (newborn animals), biting is not a problem since the teeth have not erupted to the extent that they can penetrate the tube. The tube can be passed into the esophagus with one hand while the animal is held with the opposite hand.

Slight resistance is encountered as the tube passes into the esophagus. If no resistance is detectable or if persistent coughing develops during the insertion, the tube may have inadvertently passed into the trachea. Occasionally, a debilitated animal shows no signs of tracheal intubation. For this reason, before introducing the nutrient solution, 1-2 ml of room air should be injected through the tube while the stomach is auscultated. The absence of air-injection sounds suggests the tube is in the trachea. The tube should then be withdrawn and the procedure attempted again.

Tube feeding is relatively safe in neonates. The small size of the glottis (laryngeal orifice) and the normal protective reflexes in neonates permit the tube to pass into the esophagus with little likelihood of tracheal intubation. Testing tube placement by air injection is rarely necessary in neonates. Because of the safety of this procedure, clients can learn tube-feeding technics for care of large litters of very young dogs and cats.

Adult Dogs: The size of the dog and composition of the material to be infused into the stomach determine the size of the tube to be used. Generally, tubes larger than 1.5 cm in diameter are not necessary. An oral speculum (guard to prevent mouth closure) should be used in any dog that is not anesthetized. Even sedated dogs may reflexly bite with sufficient strength to penetrate and even divide a plastic feeding tube.

If a tube is to be passed into an unanesthetized dog, a roll of 1- or 2-inch-wide adhesive tape often suffices as a speculum (Fig 6). The plastic case of a disposable syringe may also be used in some dogs. A hard rubber "bite block" with an appropriately sized hole can also be purchased for this purpose.

Tube lubrication is recommended in adult dogs, particularly in those that are not sedated or anesthetized during the procedure. Most lubricants have some degree of taste and, at least to some degree, may divert the patient's attention as the tube is passed. In most dogs, even anesthetized dogs, some degree of resistance can be felt as long as the tube is in the esophagus. Persistent coughing or no resistance to tube passage suggests the tube is in the trachea. Tube

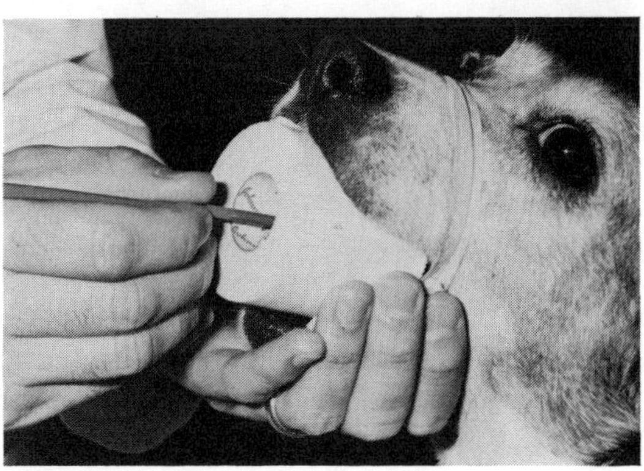

Fig 6. A roll of adhesive tape is an effective speculum when passing a tube into the esophagus.

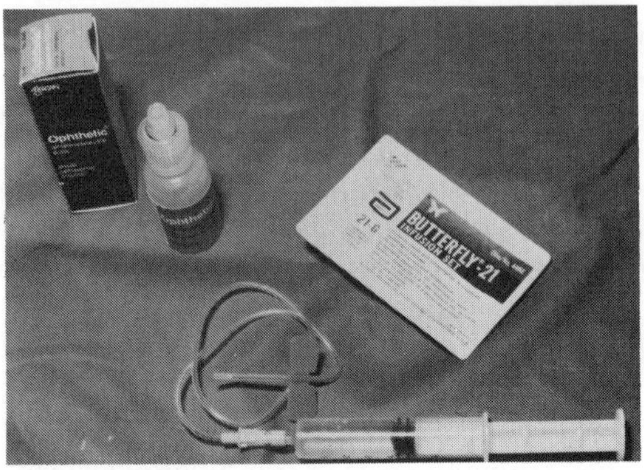

Fig 7. Materials needed for tube feeding cats.

position can easily be checked in dogs by carefully palpating the neck. If the tube is in the esophagus, 2 rigid structures can be palpated in the ventral aspect of the neck. The trachea is the more superficial rigid structure and the esophagus, in which the feeding tube should be positioned, is the deeper rigid structure. If the tube has inadvertently been passed into the trachea, only one rigid structure, the trachea, is palpable. Should there be any question as to the proper position of the feeding tube, the entire procedure should be repeated.

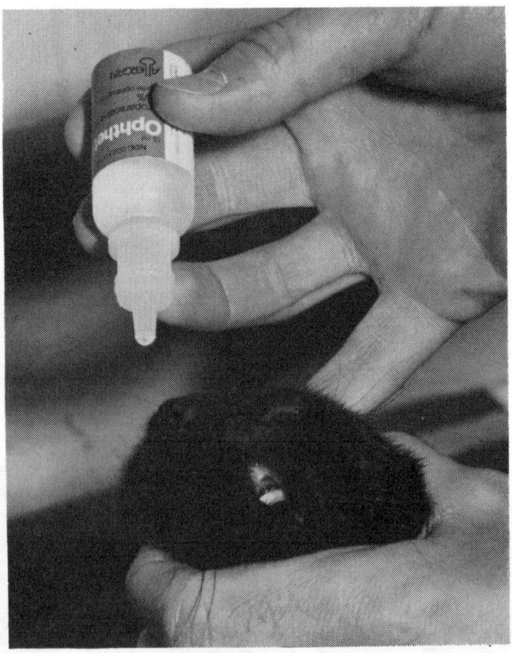

Fig 8. A topical ophthalmic anesthetic is instilled directly into one nostril before passing a flexible feeding tube.

Adult Cats: In contrast to the technic used in kittens, puppies and adult dogs, tube feeding adult cats is significantly different. Attempting to insert an oral speculum or bite block into a cat's mouth and passing a tube through the oral cavity into the esophagus can be difficult as well as dangerous. For these reasons, cats should be tube fed with a nasogastric tube. This method entails passing an appropriately sized tube through one nostril and the nasal cavity, into the oropharynx, and into the esophagus or stomach. The oral cavity is completely bypassed.

The equipment needed for tube feeding cats is simple and inexpensive (Fig 7). Since small-gauge nasogastric tubes for use in cats may be difficult to acquire, a suitable alternative involves cutting the needle off of a 19- or 21-ga Butterfly catheter (Abbott Laboratories) (Fig 7). The plastic tubing is cut at right angles, 1-1.5 inches from the point of attachment on the needle.

The following steps are used when performing nasogastric intubation in cats:

Step 1. Prepare the cat by instilling 4-5 drops of a topical ophthalmic anesthetic into one nostril (Fig 8). The cat may sneeze initially. This step is repeated 2-3 minutes later using only 2-3 drops of anesthetic. During instillation, the cat's head should be vertically oriented, permitting the anesthetic to contact the nasal mucosa (Fig 8).

Step 2. With the cat's head restrained, the lubricated tube is gently inserted into the ventral aspect of the anesthetized nostril (Fig 9). Some cats struggle as they perceive the pressure (not pain) caused by the tube in the nostril.

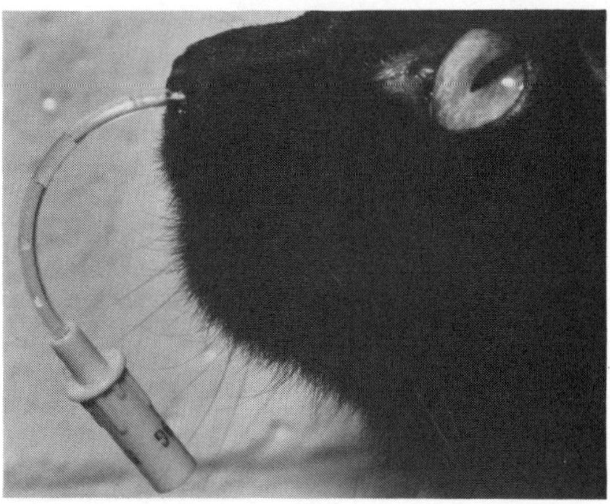

Fig 9. The feeding tube is passed ventromediad through the nasal cavity.

Step 3. About 6-8 inches of tube is advanced through the nostril. If the tube becomes abruptly lodged, gentle rotation of the tubing may permit continuation. If this fails, the tube should be removed and relubricated. A second attempt is made through the same nostril without need for additional anesthetic. Occasionally it is necessary to repeat the entire procedure using the opposite nostril.
Step 4. Slight resistance to passage of the tube can be expected as it passes through the esophagus. It is not essential that the end of the tube reach the stomach, since liquid deposited into the distal esophagus readily passes into the stomach.
Step 5. Before injecting any nutrient or contrast material into the nasogastric tube, about 1 ml sterile saline or water is infused through the tube. If the tube has inadvertently been placed into the trachea, a very rare occurrence, the cat may cough or air bubbles in the tubing move with respiration. Any sterile saline or water entering the lungs is absorbed within seconds and causes no complications. If this does occur, the tube should be withdrawn and the procedure is repeated using the opposite nostril.
Step 6. If there is no response from the cat after the 1 ml test injection of sterile water or saline, an appropriate volume of contrast material or feeding solution is given through the tube at a constant rate of infusion.
Step 7. The nasogastric tube is then removed, cleaned and stored for use at a later time. If several daily treatments are necessary, it may be feasible to maintain the tube in place by affixing it to the side of the head or neck (Fig 10). Obviously, the success of long-term placement of a nasogastric tube is largely dependent on the cat's willingness

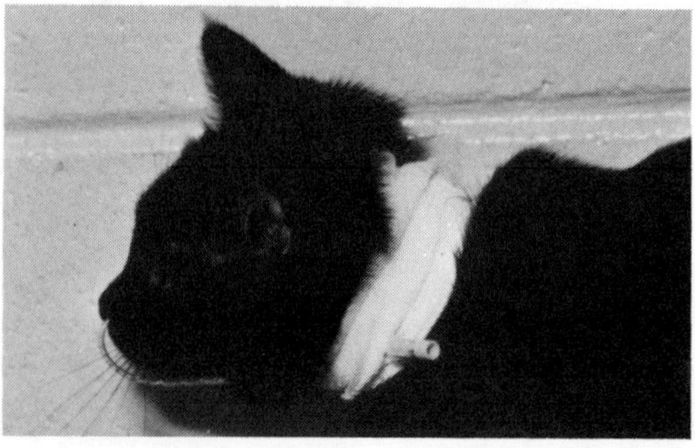

Fig 10. For long-term placement, the feeding tube may be affixed to the cat's neck.

to tolerate it. There is no contraindication to passing a nasogastric tube several times daily. However, if this is necessary, the opposite nostril should be intubated each time the technic is repeated.

Complications

The most serious risk associated with tube feeding is pneumonia. Inadvertent placement of the tube into the trachea, followed by infusion of nutrient solution or barium sulfate, may seriously compromise the patient's ability to breathe.

Relatively large volumes of liquid, including such compounds as barium sulfate, may be introduced into the lower airways with minor *initial* discomfort or stress experienced by the animal. However, other compounds, particularly fat, can predispose to severe or fatal pneumonia. On the other hand, introduction of small volumes of water or sterile electrolyte solutions into the lower airways is unlikely to cause serious complications since these liquids are absorbed from the lower portion of the lung into the vascular system within a few seconds.

DENTAL PROPHYLAXIS

by R. B. Ford

Veterinary dentistry in small animal practice offers veterinary technicians the opportunity for an active role in patient treatment and client education. It is estimated that 85% of all dogs 6 years of age or older in the US have significant dental disease. While some of these animals may have severe disease that requires specialized dental procedures, most need only routine dental prophylaxis.

The role of veterinary dentistry within small animal practice is expanding as new, more specialized technics are developed and equipment becomes available and affordable. In a sense, veterinary dentistry is rapidly becoming a subspecialty of small animal medicine and surgery. Descriptions of dental radiology, periodontal therapy, oral surgery, endodontics and dental orthopedics are appearing in the literature with increasing frequency. Additionally, the availability of dental instrumentation designed specifically for veterinary dental procedures is stimulating interest among veterinarians to offer advanced dental services. Veterinary technicians willing to learn more about dentistry and specialized dental procedures will find themselves taking on greater patient responsibility within the practice.

As routine as it may seem, the dental prophylaxis (teeth scaling) is the first step in recognizing serious, underlying dental disease. Fur-

Table 1. Dental Formulae of Dogs and Cats

Deciduous		Permanent
$2\ (I\ \frac{3}{3}\ C\ \frac{1}{1}\ PM\ \frac{3}{3}) = 28$	Dog	$2\ (I\ \frac{3}{3}\ C\ \frac{1}{1}\ PM\ \frac{4}{4}\ M\ \frac{2}{3}) = 42$
$2\ (I\ \frac{3}{3}\ C\ \frac{1}{1}\ M\ \frac{3}{2}) = 26$	Cat	$2\ (I\ \frac{3}{3}\ C\ \frac{1}{1}\ PM\ \frac{3}{2}\ M\ \frac{1}{1}) = 30$

I = incisor teeth
C = canine teeth
PM = premolars
M = molars

The numbers beside each letter represent the number of teeth ($\frac{\text{maxillary}}{\text{mandibular}}$) on *one* side of the head.

thermore, if done correctly, it involves special skills in handling tissue, examining teeth and gingivae, recognizing evidence of disease, and properly using dental instruments.

Anatomy of the Teeth and Periodontium

As in people, dogs and cats have 2 sets of teeth during life: deciduous and permanent teeth. The deciduous (temporary) teeth of young animals have very long roots that, during adolescence, are resorbed, loosen and eventually fall out. All deciduous teeth are normally shed by 6-8 months of age. Though they are only temporary, the deciduous teeth are important, since their position affects the route of eruption and resting position of the permanent teeth. The dental formulae (numbers and arrangement) for deciduous and permanent teeth in dogs and cats are listed in Table 1.

Teeth comprising the upper arcade are situated in the maxilla and are termed maxillary teeth; teeth of the lower arcade are termed mandibular teeth. The names of the teeth and their respective positions

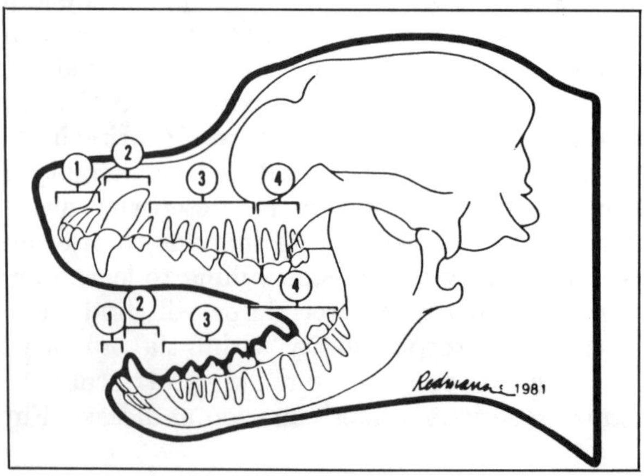

Fig 11. Dentition of the adult dog: (1) incisors; (2) canine teeth; (3) premolars; (4) molars. (Courtesy of Jane Redmann)

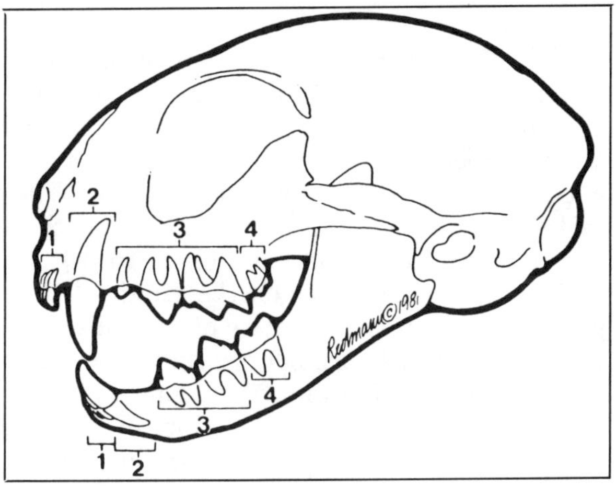

Fig 12. Dentition of the adult cat: (1) incisors; (2) canine teeth; (3) premolars; (4) molars. (Courtesy of Jane Redmann)

are depicted in Figures 11 and 12. In recording the presence of defective or diseased teeth, descriptive terminology is important, particularly when entering information into the medical record, *eg,* fractured left fourth upper premolar.

Each tooth is composed of 3 layers: enamel, the outermost layer and the hardest tissue in the body; dentin, the middle layer; and pulp,

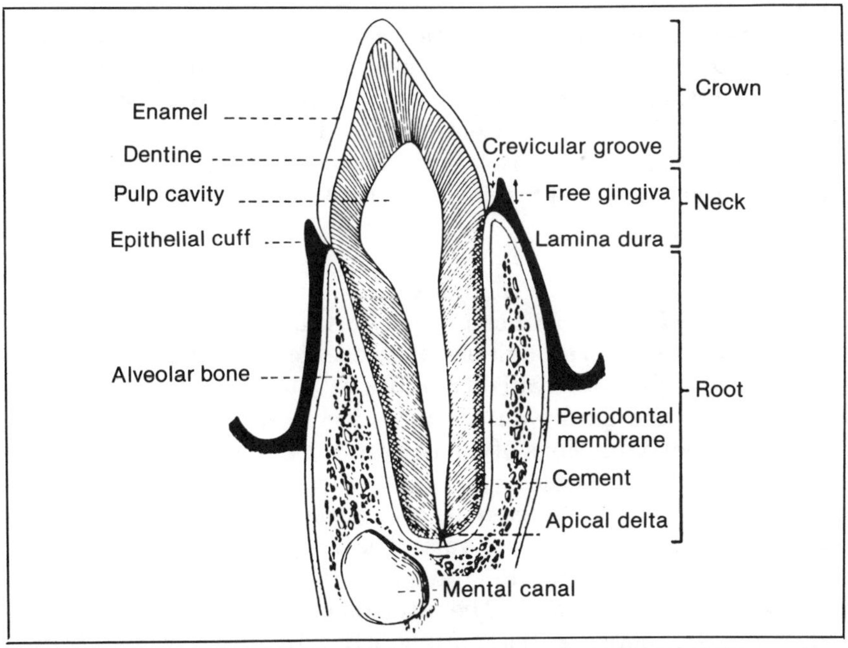

Fig 13. Anatomy of the tooth. Modified from Bell, *J Sm Anim Pract* 6 (1967), courtesy of Lea & Febiger.

the inner core of the tooth that contains the nerves and blood vessels (Fig 13). The enamel is located above the gingival (gum) line; the outermost layer of the root (below the gum line) is termed the cementum.

The periodontium consists of tissues that support and sustain the teeth (Fig 13). The free gingival margin is normally pink or pigmented and firmly affixed to the neck of the tooth. The gingival sulcus, a normal space between the free gingiva and the tooth, is the point at which dental disease is most likely to begin. The epithelial attachment is the point at which the gingiva attaches to the tooth. The periodontal ligament consists of specialized tissue that attaches the entire tooth root to the bony socket. Alveolar bone is the last component of the periodontium. Periodontitis is an inflammation, usually associated with bacterial infection, of the periodontium. The objective of dental prophylaxis is to prevent periodontitis.

Origin of Dental Disease

Plaque, not calculus, causes periodontal disease. Plaque, a slimy, white film usually concentrated at the free gingival margin, is comprised of food, debris, salivary glycoproteins and bacteria. The bacteria, though varying in type from one animal to another, can invade the gingiva and are the most common cause of periodontal disease in dogs and cats.

Untreated, plaque accumulates, resulting in progressive periodontal disease, ulcerative gingivitis, loose teeth, dental abscesses and severe infections. Animals with severe periodontitis may become septicemic from the heavy concentration of bacteria in the oral cavity and periodontium. Death from bacterial endocarditis can occur subsequent to routine dental prophylaxis in patients not pretreated with antibiotics.

Instruments for Dental Prophylaxis

Mechanical Scalers: Much of the effort involved in cleaning teeth has been eliminated through use of mechanical scalers. Two kinds of mechanical scalers are available for use in veterinary dentistry: ultrasonic scalers and air-driven turbine scalers. Mechanical scalers use high-frequency vibrations of a metal tip to remove plaque and calculus from the tooth surface.

Though effective and easy to use, ultrasonic scalers can damage the teeth, particularly the gums. The handpiece of an ultrasonic scaler is designed to vibrate at about 25,000 times a second and can generate considerable heat. The ultrasonic scaler is therefore attached to a water source; water continuously flows over the metal tip to dissipate heat. Without the cooling effect of water, an ultrasonic

Fig 14. Manual scalers used for routine dental prophylaxis.

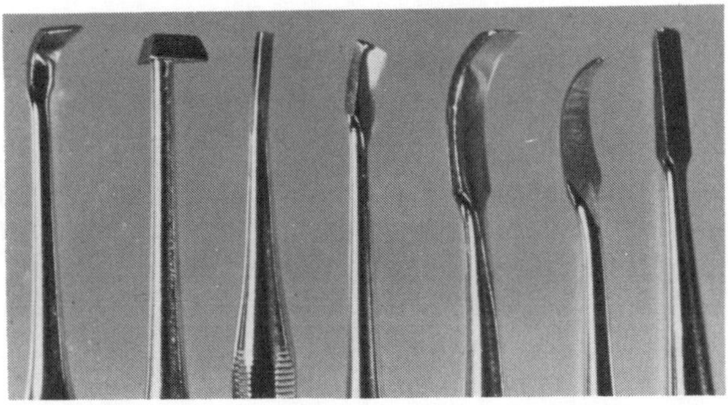

scaler can damage the enamel, pulp and gingivae. Ultrasonic scalers should never be used to clean or retract soft tissues.

Air turbine scalers operate similarly to ultrasonic units but are powered by compressed air, which causes oscillation of the metal tip. Because considerably less heat is generated on the tooth surface, the risk of injury to the teeth and gingivae is minimal. Though a water source is not required, the turbine scaler must be powered by an air compressor.

Manual Scalers: Various instruments are available for manually scaling plaque and calculus from teeth (Fig 14). Remember that these instruments are, in fact, delicate surgical instruments that if properly cared for will provide years of use. Storing instruments together without adequate separation substantially decreases their utility and may be a source of injury to the patient.

Polishing Equipment: An electrical bench engine or air-driven power source with low-speed rotary handpieces can be adapted for polishing enamel (Fig 15). The soft, rotating endpiece of the polisher is used with dental pumice to smooth the surface of enamel after scaling. Not only does this process "repair" any damage to the

Fig 15. Low-speed, rotary handpiece used to polish enamel.

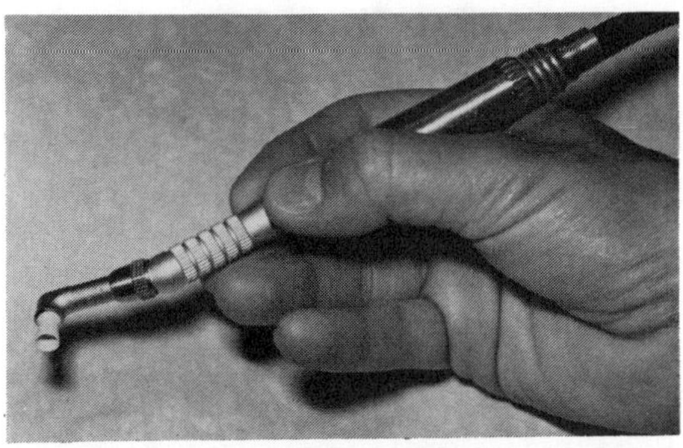

enamel subsequent to scaling, but it discourages further accumulation of plaque by eliminating surface irregularities.

Scaling Technic

Dental prophylaxis involves a 5-step procedure: examining the oral cavity, gums and teeth; removing supragingival debris (hair, food, calculus, plaque) with a mechanical (ultrasonic) scaler; removing subgingival debris with a manual scaler; polishing the enamel; and irrigating the oral cavity.

Oral Examination: A dental probe is used to test the integrity of the periodontium (Fig 16). The gingival sulcus around each tooth is gently probed in an attempt to identify deep periodontal pockets or abscesses. If present, periodontal pockets should be cleaned and flushed. Loose teeth should also be identified. Since not all loose teeth must be removed, the veterinarian should decide which teeth are to be extracted. Very loose teeth should be extracted. Other significant lesions (*eg,* tumors, ulcers) should be noted in the medical record and brought to the attention of the attending clinician.

Mechanical Scaling: Supragingival plaque and calculus are readily removed with a mechanical scaler. If using an ultrasonic scaler, the operating tip must emit water while the instrument is in operation. Water not only flushes the gingiva and tooth but also dissipates the heat generated by the vibrating metal tip.

The operating tip must be moved continuously in arcs over the enamel. Concentrating the operating tip on one tooth for 10-15 consecutive seconds can damage the pulp by overheating the tooth, resulting in devitalization.

The air turbine scaler, which is driven by compressed air as opposed to sound waves, is used in the same manner as an ultrasonic scaler. However, the heat generated by air turbine scalers is negligible and will not damage teeth.

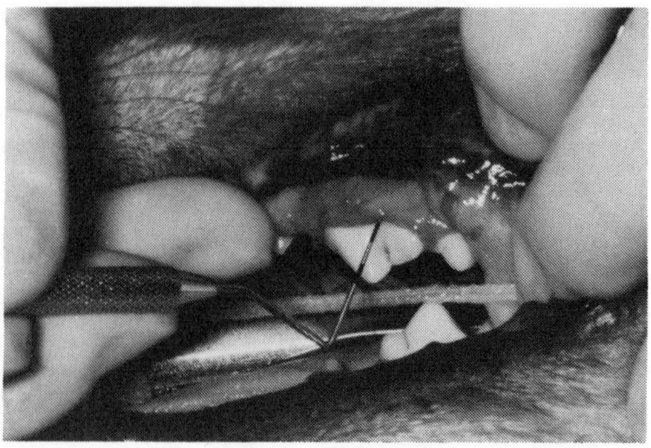

Fig 16. Periodontal probe. The depth of the gingival sulcus can be measured using the 3-mm markings on the probe.

Manual Scaling: Despite the availability of several instruments designed for scaling, root planing and extracting teeth, dental instruments are among the most improperly used instruments in veterinary practice. Technicians responsible for performing dental prophylactic procedures should be familiar with the types of instruments available and their correct use.

The 3 principal dental instruments used in scaling/root planing teeth are the simple scaler, the curet and the hoe. Table 2 lists their uses.

Manual scaling entails dislodging calculus and plaque from the enamel surface using a pull stroke. The instrument is placed on the tooth at the level of the gingival margin and is pulled forcefully with a short stroke away from the gingiva. The curet should be the only instrument used with a pulling *or* pushing stroke. When using a pushing stroke, *ie,* scaling toward the gingiva, care must be taken not to force the instrument's blade into the soft gingival tissues.

To achieve maximum control and tactile sensitivity, manual scalers should be held in the same manner as a pencil. While scaling, the hand holding the instrument should be stabilized by resting it against the opposite hand or the patient as force is exerted along the tooth surface.

Scalers, curets and hoes should be sharp. A high-quality sharpening stone can be used to maintain the cutting edge of these instruments.

Polishing: Dental pumice is applied to the enamel with a small rubber cup attached to a rotary dental handpiece. Because the friction caused by polishing can generate enough heat to damage the pulp, the polishing cup should never remain on the same tooth for more than a few seconds at a time.

Irrigation: Blood, debris, pumice, etc should be flushed from the oral cavity before the endotracheal tube is removed.

Complications

Most complications of dental prophylaxis are the result of improper use of equipment, particularly manual scalers.

Heat Injury: Ultrasonic scalers and rotary handpieces generate heat on the tooth surface. Heat may be transferred to the pulp, resulting in injury sufficient to cause death of the tooth. These instruments can also burn soft tissue and therefore should not be used on the gingiva.

Trauma: Soft tissue injury is a common sequel to improper instrument use, such as pushing toward the gingiva instead of pulling. Injury can also result from use of improper instruments, such as using a dental elevator to scale teeth.

Table 2. Description and Use of Dental Instruments for Oral Prophylaxis

Instrument	Description	Purpose	Placement/Movement
Explorer/Probe	The narrow shaft of the probe is marked in easy-to-read increments on one end. Blunted, pointed explorer tip on the opposite end. (*eg,* ST-4, Henry Schein)	Aids detection of decay and assessment of the periodontium.	Explorer is placed perpendicular to the tooth surface and lightly passed over the tooth to detect surface irregularities. Probe is placed parallel to the tooth and passed gently into the gingival sulcus.
Scaler	Curved blade with 3 cutting edges. Is the most versatile dental instrument for scaling. (*eg,* ST-2 and ST-3, Henry Schein)	Debridement of sub- and supragingival plaque/calculus.	Short, powerful strokes from the gingival margin toward the cusp tips. Blade must remain against the enamel surface.
Curet	Elongated curved blade with 2 cutting edges. Blade terminates in a round end. The outer edge is the working (scaling) edge. (*eg,* Gracey curets 11-12 and 13-14)	Subgingival scaling. 11-12 Gracey for incisors, canine premolars. 13-14 Gracey for premolars, molars.	Gentle retraction of the free gingival epithelium with the curet. Blade is placed against the tooth surface and stroked toward the cusp tip.
Hoe	Single, right-angle cutting edge. (*eg,* ST-1, Henry Schein)	Gross debridement of supragingival calculus on the flat tooth surface.	Blade is positioned perpendicular to the tooth and pulled away from the gingival margin.

URINE COLLECTION
by R. B. Ford

General Considerations

Urine is collected from dogs and cats by catheterization of the urinary bladder, cystocentesis, and manual expression of the urinary bladder. Since the patient could be injured with each of these technics, the technician must be familiar with the basic anatomy of the urinary tract, the equipment used to collect urine, and the reason urine is being collected.

Anatomy

Urine is a complex ultrafiltrate produced by the glomeruli and nephrons of the kidney. Urine is excreted into the renal collecting duct system and subsequently passes through the ureters into the urinary bladder. The urinary bladder is a reservoir in which urine is stored until it is convenient for the animal to voluntarily void. Urine collection technics are designed to overcome the bladder's physiologic ability to retain urine. Figure 17 depicts the key anatomic structures of the lower urinary tract of dogs. Reference to these anatomic structures will be used throughout this discussion.

Instruments

Various catheter types are available for collecting urine from dogs and cats. The following discussion addresses the basic types of catheters available, and their indications and contraindications.

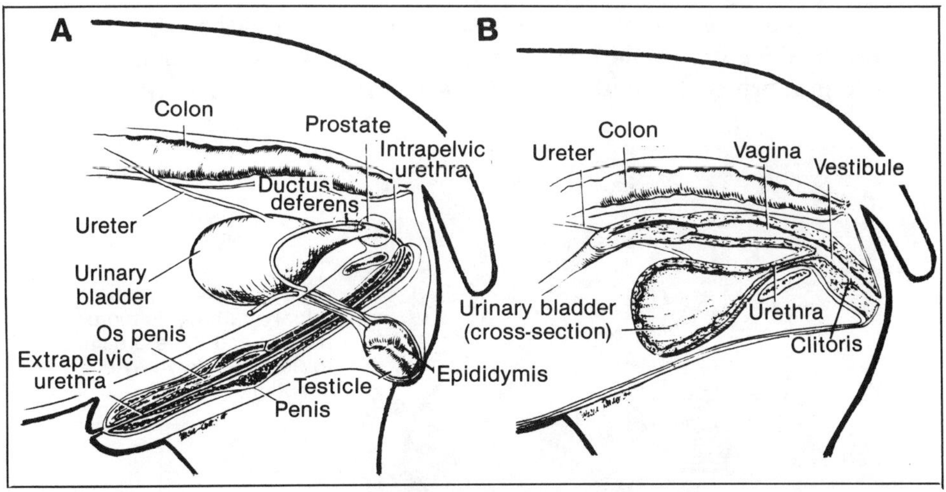

Fig 17. Lower urinary tract anatomy. A. Male dog. B. Female dog.

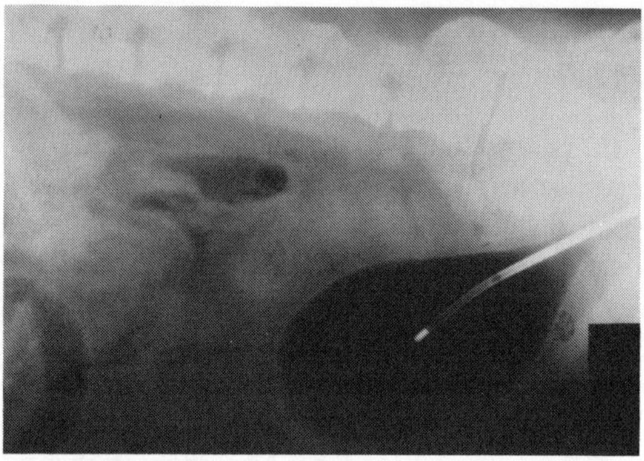

Fig 18. Rigid, metal urinary catheter in the bladder of a female dog. Air has been injected into the bladder to demonstrate proper placement.

Rigid Catheters: These are metal, reusable catheters used to collect urine from female dogs (Figs 18, 20). Because they are inflexible, rigid catheters may injure the bladder, urethra or urethral orifice if the patient is not well restrained during catheterization.

Polyethylene Catheters: These are semirigid, plastic catheters produced in several sizes and shapes appropriate for use in male dogs and male cats. The male feline urinary catheter (Tom-Cat Catheter: Sovereign) can be used to catheterize the bladder of female cats as well. Polyethylene catheters can be resterilized and reused.

Soft Catheters: Soft, rubber urinary catheters are available for use in male and female dogs (Fig 10). They are flexible and present minimal risk of injury to the patient during catheterization. Though these catheters are reusable, they may be slightly more difficult to use, particularly small-diameter catheters.

Urinary Speculum: Use of a speculum during catheterization of the bladder of female dogs and cats enhances visualization of the urethral orifice. Several types of specula are available to expand the

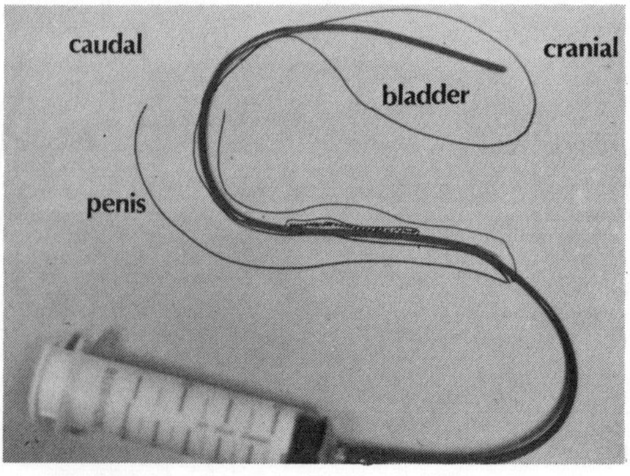

Fig 19. The soft, rubber urinary catheter is more flexible and therefore safer to use than polyethylene (plastic) catheters.

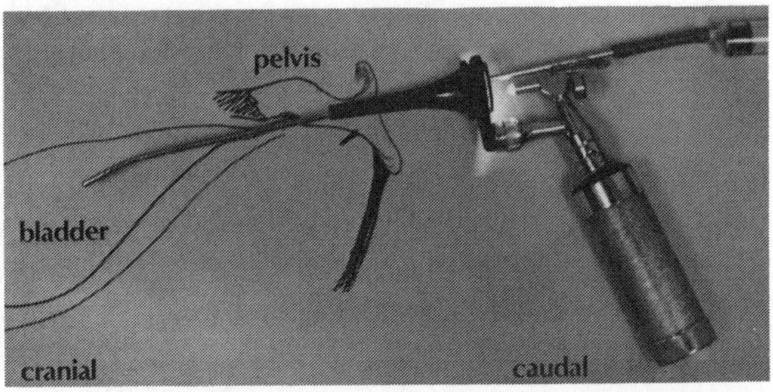

Fig 20. Use of a veterinary otoscope to facilitate urinary bladder catheterization in a female dog.

vaginal lumen. In female dogs, an otoscope speculum provides fair visualization and may be attached to a hand-held light source (Fig 20). In female cats, a small-diameter veterinary otoscope speculum may be used. Human anoscopes (Welch-Allyn), available in varying diameters, provide the best visibility of and access to the urethral orifice in female dogs.

Collection Technics

Catheterization and urine collection may be required for diagnostic studies and/or patient treatment. The specific technic used to collect urine is determined by the patient's condition. For example, repeated attempts to catheterize a male cat or dog with urethral obstruction may cause serious damage to the urethra. In such cases, cystocentesis may be indicated. On the other hand, urine collected by catheter is likely to be contaminated with bacteria from the urethra; this is taken into consideration by the clinician when interpreting urinalysis results.

The greatest risk associated with urine collection is that of bacterial infection of the urinary bladder following catheterization. This risk, however, can be minimized by using sterile technic and sterile catheters when collecting urine. Use of the following technics is recommended:

Male Dog: Selection of a flexible polyethylene or rubber catheter long enough to reach the bladder lumen is essential. The catheter diameter used is determined by the size of the dog and experience of the operator with the type of catheter being used.

The patient may be catheterized while standing or in lateral recumbency. The catheter tip is coated with sterile lubricant gel, such as K-Y Jelly, and the prepuce is retracted toward the scrotum, exposing the penis and urethral opening. The catheter tip is then introduced into the urethra.

As the catheter is advanced, resistance is typically encountered at the ischial arch and at the level of the prostate gland. Resistance can be overcome by continuing to advance the catheter using gentle pressure. Forceful thrusts and back-and-forth movements must be avoided. Urine usually does not appear in the distal catheter until the catheter tip has entered the bladder.

Male Cat: Catheterization of male cats requires a polyethylene urinary catheter designed specifically for cats. An end-hole catheter is preferred over side-hole catheters. Catheterization of cats usually requires sedation or general anesthesia to achieve adequate restraint. With the patient in dorsal recumbency, the prepuce is grasped ventral to the penis and then moved toward the anus. Properly done, this technic straightens the curved urethra, exposes the penis and urethral opening, and protects the penis against unnecessary manipulation and possible injury.

The lubricated catheter tip is introduced through the urethra and into the bladder. Minimal resistance is encountered as the catheter traverses the urethra. NEVER FORCE OR ROTATE THE URINARY CATHETER WHILE IT IS IN THE URETHRA.

Female Dog: Urinary catheterization of female dogs is most likely to be successful when the urethral orifice can be visualized. With the patient standing or in dorsal recumbency, a nasal speculum, otoscope or anoscope is inserted into the vagina (Fig 21). The lubricated catheter tip is inserted through the speculum, into the vagina and into the urethra. There should be no resistance encountered as the catheter tip is advanced.

Since a rigid, metal catheter is most commonly used to catheterize female dogs, the patient must be well restrained. Abrupt movement of the patient or urinary catheter may tear the bladder wall or seriously injure the urethra.

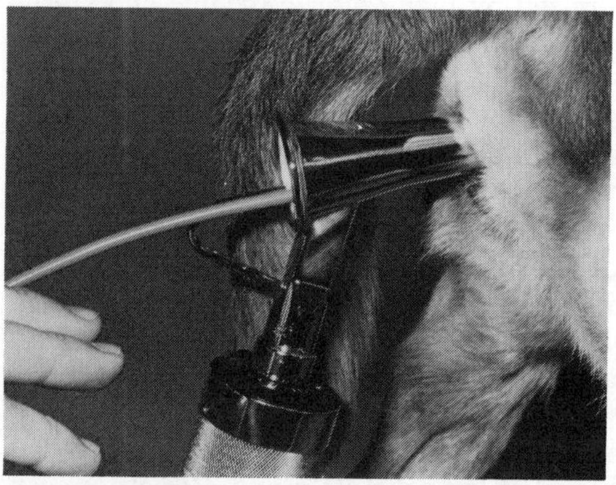

Fig 21. Use of a human anoscope (Welch-Allyn) to facilitate urinary bladder catheterization in a female dog.

Female Cat: It is possible, though seldom done in practice, to pass a male cat urinary catheter into the bladder of a female cat. This technic requires sedation or general anesthesia. With the cat in dorsal recumbency, the urethral orifice can be visualized using a small speculum and, preferably, an attached light source (*eg,* otoscope).

Cystocentesis

The urethra and urethral bacterial flora can be bypassed by collecting urine from the bladder via cystocentesis. This entails direct penetration of the bladder wall, through the abdominal wall, using a sterile, hollow needle. The procedure is safe and effective, can be repeated in the same patient, and may be performed on male and female dogs and cats.

Equipment required for cystocentesis includes a syringe (usually 10- to 12 ml) and a 20- to 22-ga, 1-inch needle. Patient preparation entails clipping hair from a small area of skin between the umbilicus and the pelvis. Female cats and dogs and male cats may be clipped on the midline; male dogs should be clipped lateral to the penis to avoid the superficial vein of the glans. The skin is cleansed, rinsed and dried before needle penetration.

Two people are required for cystocentesis. While one person holds the patient in lateral recumbency, another identifies the urinary bladder and performs cystocentesis. *Do not attempt cystocentesis unless the bladder can be clearly identified and its movement in the abdomen restricted.* The needle is thrust through the abdominal wall and into the bladder (Fig 22). It is not necessary to withdraw all of the urine from the bladder before withdrawing the needle.

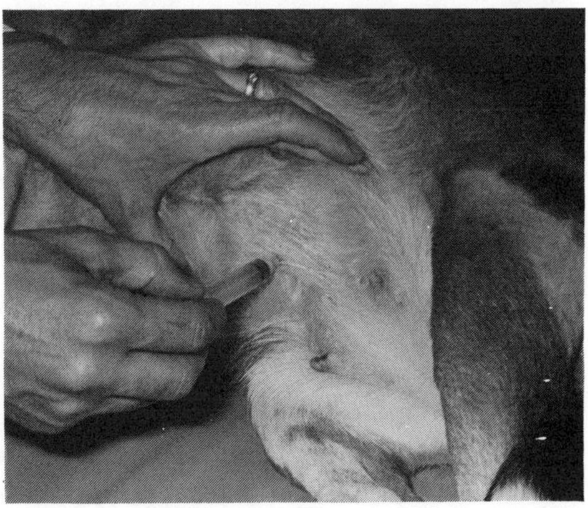

Fig 22A. Cystocentesis for urine collection.

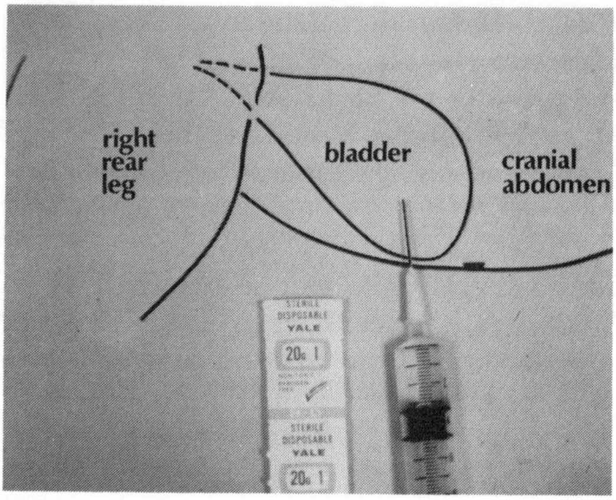

Fig 22B. Proper needle placement during cystocentesis.

Manual Expression

In some animals it is possible to force urination by physically compressing the bladder through the abdominal wall. In normal, unanesthetized animals, extreme pressure is usually required to cause urination. Generating high intravesicular (within the bladder) pressures may cause the bladder mucosa to tear and bleed. Generally, manual expression of urine from the bladder is reserved for animals with decreased muscle tone of the urethral sphincter and no obstruction to urine outflow. For example, dogs with severe intervertebral disc disease may lose the ability to void urine voluntarily (urinary incontinence). As a result, urine dribbles from the urethra continuously as the bladder fills. Manually expressing urine from incontinent patients is easy and helps prevent urine scalds in patients unable to stand.

Attempting to express urine from a patient with an obstructed urethra (*eg,* cats with feline urologic syndrome) can have disastrous consequences. Because there is no way to determine the intravesicular pressure being generated during compression nor can the integrity of a potentially diseased bladder be established, the bladder may rupture.

ENEMAS
by R. B. Ford

General Considerations

An enema involves injecting a solution into the rectum and colon to promote elimination. Enemas are not intended to flush colonic contents from the patient but to gently distend the rectum and distal colon, thereby initiating normal expulsive reflexes. In veterinary medicine, the most common reasons for giving enemas to dogs and cats is to promote defecation and to conduct diagnostic studies. Certain drugs may also be given rectally. In such instances, these drugs exert their action at the level of the rectal and large intestinal mucosa (*eg,* hydrocortisone enemas in patients with ulcerative colitis). Certain drugs, however, after being delivered into the rectum and intestine, are absorbed rapidly into the circulation (*eg,* ultrashort-acting barbiturates), where they exert a systemic effect on the patient. Though drugs are infused rectally only under special circumstances, the veterinary technician must be aware that certain constituents of enema solutions, especially phosphate-containing saline enemas, can be absorbed through the large intestinal mucosa into the systemic circulation and result in toxicity or death. It is as important to appreciate the possible consequences of giving an enema as it is to know the correct technic.

Instruments

The materials needed to give an enema are simple, inexpensive and readily obtainable. Special enema sets, intended for human use, include a large reservoir for the enema solution, attached rubber tubing, and a rigid catheter tip for rectal insertion. However, their use is somewhat limited, by virtue of the catheter tip diameter, to medium-sized and large dogs.

Depending on the size of the patient, a 5- to 60-ml syringe can be used as a reservoir for the enema solution. Polyethylene or rubber tubing, such as an infant feeding tube or stomach tube, can be attached to the syringe. The free end of the catheter is inserted rectally for administration of the solution.

Such syringe and tubing sets are easily modified for use in kittens, puppies, cats and large dogs.

Enema Solutions

Water: Warm tap water is the preferred enema solution. The action of water as an enema solution is not to flush feces from the colon but to promote defecation reflexes by distending the rectum. Not only is water inexpensive and readily available, it can be introduced into the rectum without concern for injury to the patient following absorption. In addition, patient and area clean-up is facilitated by using aqueous (water-soluble) enema solutions.

Addition of detergent soaps to water used as an enema solution is not recommended, as soaps can irritate the rectal and colonic mucosa. Furthermore, they provide no additional value in promoting defecation.

Oil: Mineral oil is the most common nonwater-soluble material used as an enema solution. Like water, it is inexpensive and easy to obtain. However, the additional time required to clean a patient's haircoat after a mineral oil enema may limit its use to patients with severe constipation (obstipation).

Mineral oil, when used as an enema solution, penetrates, softens and lubricates feces. It may also temporarily inhibit further colonic absorption of water from the feces. These actions enhance the patient's ability to pass stool from the rectum. Mineral oil enemas should not be given to patients that have had recent rectal or anal surgery since it interferes with wound healing.

Saline: Several saline cathartics, comprised of magnesium and sodium sulfates and phosphate, are available for use as enema solutions. Saline enemas promote defecation since they are osmotically active and, therefore, promote retention of water in the colon to produce a semifluid or watery evacuation. In small animals, particularly cats and very young dogs, some absorption of component ions can occur and may produce systemic toxicity. For example, absorption of phosphate salts from the colon of animals receiving sodium phosphate enemas (*eg,* Fleet Enema) may reduce the concentration of ionic calcium in the plasma, resulting in clinical signs related to hypocalcemia.

Table 3 summarizes the various types of enema solutions and their preparation and use.

Giving an Enema

Enema solutions intended to promote defecation are given by lubricating the catheter tip and inserting the catheter into the rectum and lower portion of the colon. While the enema tubing can be inserted to the cecum and higher, this is unnecessary. The most effective insertion distance appears to be at the level of the colorectal junction, located 1-3 inches cranial to the anus in most adult dogs and cats.

The rate at which the solution flows into the colon by gravity is the rate at which solution should be infused when using a syringe or commercial enema-delivery unit. Rapid infusion of enema solutions is less effective and wasteful.

The total volume of solution required to promote defecation is determined by the patient's size and degree of constipation. Though dosages for enemas have not been published, the volume of enema solution needed to promote defecation need not equal that volume required to fill the colon. In fact, use of excess amounts of enema solution may result in the solution entering the small intestine and inducing vomiting by the patient.

Table 3. Enema Solutions

	Formulation	Volume Used	Comments
To Promote Defecation			
Water	—	2-5 ml/lb body wt; may be repeated in 20-30 minutes.	Is preferred; safe, inexpensive and effective.
Soapy Water	1-2 oz liquid soap/pt water.	2-5 ml/lb body wt.	No advantage over water; may irritate bowel mucosa.
Mineral Oil	Use undiluted; commercial kits are available.	Up to 1 ml/lb body wt; may be repeated in 1-2 hours.	Softens and lubricates hard feces; indicated in obstipation; cleanup is difficult and messy.
Saline Solutions	Sodium phosphate; commercial kits are available.	0.5-1.0 ml/lb body wt.	Not recommended for use in cats and small dogs.
For Diagnostic Studies			
Barium Sulfate	10-15% suspension in water.	Total volume of 10-15 ml/lb body wt; given in increments of 5 ml/lb body wt.	*Contraindicated* in patients with severe bowel disease and within 24 hours after bowel surgery or intestinal biopsy; patient is anesthetized for infusion; cuffed catheter is required for administration; may cause dehydration.

Enemas do not stimulate immediate defecation. After infusion of enema solution, the patient should be permitted to rest, preferably in a run or outside, 20-30 minutes before repeating the enema, if necessary. This provides adequate time for the solution to promote defecation. If the patient does not have a bowel movement, the enema solution will be mostly expelled after this time, and a second enema given.

Complications

"Through-and-Through Enema": Administration of several enemas or use of inordinately large volumes of solution over a short period can cause the patient to vomit enema solution mixed with small and large bowel contents. While this is not necessarily harmful to the patient, it greatly exceeds the requirements for evacuating, or even cleansing, the large bowel.

Hypothermia: Administration of cold enema solutions to young or small animals may reduce body temperature to critically low levels. Enema solutions for adult dogs and cats should be given at no less than room temperature (70-75 F), while solutions given to young animals should be warmed to above room temperature but not in excess of body temperature.

Postenema Constipation: Because an enema can completely disrupt normal colonic physiology, the animal may be constipated for 24-48 hours following an enema.

Barium Enemas

Barium sulfate is used as an enema solution in dogs and cats when performing positive-contrast radiography of the colon. Before receiving a barium enema, the patient is prepared by giving a cleansing enema of tepid, rather than warm, water. The enema is repeated until clear water is passed after infusion. Because larger enema solution volumes are required to prepare a patient for a barium enema than are required to stimulate defecation, use of commercial hypertonic enema kits is not recommended in such situations.

A barium sulfate suspension (15-20% w/v) is given as an enema at about 10-15 ml suspension/lb body weight. The suspension is infused into the anesthetized patient through an inflated, cuffed rectal catheter at increments of 5 ml/lb body weight. Since variations in this technic are dictated by the disorder being studied and the severity of the disease, the technician should consult the attending clinician before giving a barium sulfate enema.

EYE CARE

by R. B. Ford

The eye is a highly specialized sense organ that converts visual images into electrical impulses that are transmitted to the brain by way of the optic nerve. The study of eye diseases, ophthalmology, includes not only the eye but the eyelids and the nasolacrimal system as well. Figure 23 depicts the basic ocular anatomy common to dogs and cats. An excellent review of the anatomy and physiology of the eye has recently been published (Cook, 1983) and, therefore, will not be discussed further in this section.

Restraint for Eye Care

Any animal with visual impairment of any degree should be approached and handled cautiously. Attempts to treat or otherwise han-

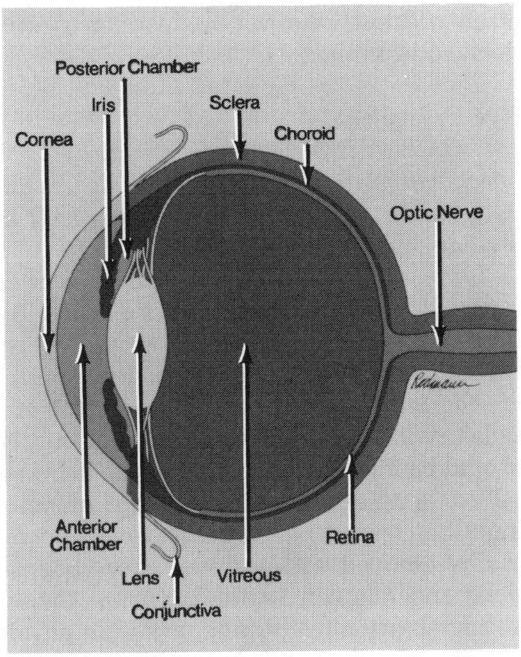

Fig 23. Basic ocular anatomy. (Courtesy of Jane Redmann)

dle a blind or visually impaired animal may startle the animal and provoke it to bite. Furthermore, ocular injuries can be quite painful, causing the patient to resist restraint. However, use of excessive restraint may further damage the eye. Visually impaired animals should be gently talked to and comforted verbally before handling. One person usually can handle and treat most small animals with ocular disease.

Since ocular diseases are often painful, the technician must protect the patient from self-inflicted injury during hospitalization and treatment. This is particularly true during the immediate postoperative period. The front dewclaws should be padded and covered with a bandage throughout the course of treatment. Animals that continue to rub the affected eye with the rear foot or on inanimate objects should wear an Elizabethan collar (see Chapter 2) until the irritation subsides.

Before medication is instilled, the eye must be free of extraneous debris. Animals with ocular diseases and those recovering from eye surgery are particularly susceptible to secondary eye infections. Large amounts of pus and mucus may accumulate around the eye within only a few hours. Medication instilled into an eye that is not clean will not be effective, leading to waste, needless expense, and delayed healing.

Eye Treatment

IMPORTANT: Never apply any drug to the eyes unless that drug is specifically intended for ophthalmic use and has been prescribed by a veterinarian. Failure to do this can result in serious complications, including loss of vision.

Two topical drug forms, ointments and solutions, are used in routine topical treatment of eye disease. Topical medication approved for use in eyes is always appropriately labeled "ophthalmic," "for intraocular use," etc. *Do not use any solution or ointment that is not appropriately labeled.* Since treatment of ocular disease usually entails frequent application of medications, the eyelids and conjunctiva should be inspected for extraneous debris each time medication is instilled. With accumulations of pus, mucus or crusty material, the eye must be cleaned before treatment. Accumulations of dry debris are easily removed with a damp gauze pad or cotton ball. Moist secretions and pus can be flushed from the eye with a commercial irrigating solution (collyrium) or sterile physiologic saline.

Ointments

Since ointments are easy to apply and generally have a longer duration of action, they are generally prescribed more often than solutions to treat eye disease.

In both cats and dogs, the ointment is instilled by pulling the lower eyelid ventrad (downward) to expose the delicate conjunctiva of the lower lid. A single ribbon of ointment, about ¼-½ inch long, is applied directly to the conjunctiva (Fig 24). The eyelid is then released, allowing dispersion of the medication over the cornea. If the ointment

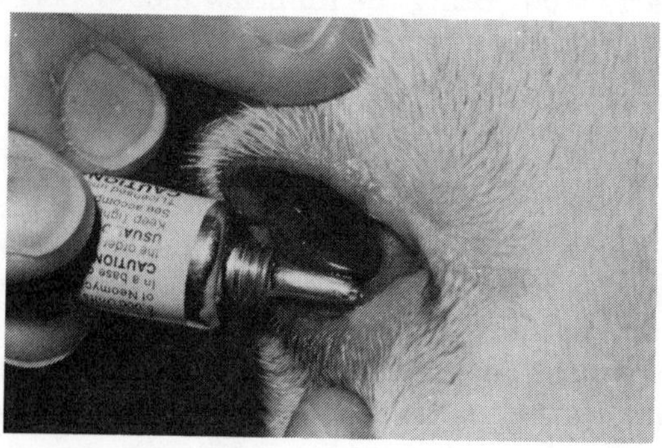

Fig 24. Medicating an eye with ophthalmic ointment.

is applied to the eyelid margin or the skin of the eyelid, an adequate amount of drug does not contact the eye.

Solutions

It may be necessary to prescribe eye medication in the form of a solution rather than an ointment despite the fact that the same concentration of drug is available in both ointment and solution forms. Depending on the disease, the veterinarian may elect to treat one eye with an ointment and the other eye with a solution.

Solutions are generally more difficult to apply than ointments. In addition, they must be applied as often as every 2-3 hours, which many dogs, cats and owners find objectionable. The technician must be familiar with the correct procedure for effective, safe application of ophthalmic solutions and ensure that the client can properly medicate the eye at home.

While several varieties of this technic may be used, the general principles of solution instillation should be strictly adhered to:

1. With one hand, the nose is lifted dorsad (upward) at about 45 °above horizontal. Since drops of solution only fall downward, the eye should be situated beneath the descending drop of solution.
2. The opposite hand is used to spread the eyelids apart and deliver the solution (Fig 25).
3. The prescribed number of drops of solution is preferably deposited on the sclera (white portion of the eye), rather than on the cornea, because the sclera is somewhat less sensitive to cold solution than is the cornea.
4. To prevent contaminating the entire bottle of solution, never allow the tip of the bottle to contact the eye or any other surface. The cap should be tightly in place when the drug is stored.

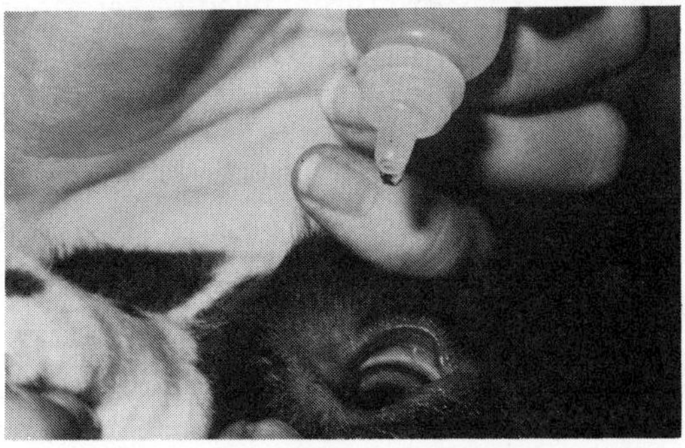

Fig 25. Instillation of an ophthalmic solution.

Concurrent Use of Ointments and Solutions

Occasionally it is necessary to prescribe both an ointment and a solution for treatment of one or both eyes. When both drugs are to be given at the same time, the solution should be given first. Wait at least 5, and preferably 10-15, minutes before applying the ointment.

EAR CARE
by R. B. Ford

Anatomy and Physiology

Anatomically, the ear is divided into 3 compartments (Fig 26). 1) The external ear includes the pinna and external ear canal. The tympanic membrane (eardrum) is the proximal limit of the external ear. 2) The middle ear is a hollow cavity in which the delicate, bony ossicles are situated. 3) The inner ear contains neuroreceptors for sound and balance (cranial nerve VIII). Each of these 3 compartments plays a critical role in hearing. The external ear collects sound waves, the middle ear transmits sound waves through vibrations on the eardrum and bony ossicles, and the inner ear converts sound wave vibrations into electrical potentials that are transmitted to the brain for interpretation.

The inner ear has a dual function. In addition to perceiving sound, the inner ear is the peripheral receptor for balance (the vestibular system). This explains why animals with unilateral (1-sided) ear disease may have a head tilt, and animals with bilateral (2-sided) ear disease may stumble, be reluctant to walk or jump, and appear incoordinated. Early recognition of ear disease and institution of proper treatment are important.

Ear-Care Instruments

Though various sophisticated otologic surgical instruments are available, they are rarely used in veterinary medicine. Because most otologic disease in small animals involves the outer ear, a few basic pieces of equipment that allow visualization and proper cleaning of the ear canal are adequate for treatment of most ear diseases. The following items constitute the basic ear treatment pack:

Two Bulb Syringes: One syringe is used to irrigate the external canal with a warm detergent solution; a second syringe is used to rinse the ear canal.

Open-End Catheter: Attached to a 6- to 12-ml syringe, an open-end catheter (Tom-Cat Catheter: Sovereign) facilitates removal of residual rinse fluid from the external ear canal by aspiration.

Forceps or Straight Hemostats: These are used to remove hair, large accumulations of debris, and foreign bodies from the external ear canal.

Wire Ear Loop: An ear loop is an otologic instrument designed for removal of foreign material from the external ear canal. Various sizes are available through many surgical supply companies.

Otoscope and Specula: Once the ear is cleaned of debris and hair, careful examination and additional fine cleansing are best done through an appropriately sized speculum attached to an otoscope.

Sterile Cotton-Tipped Applicators: These are used to obtain specimens for bacterial culture, *not* to remove debris from the ear canal.

Gauze Sponges: These facilitate cleaning of the external ear canal and pinna.

Cleaning and Medicating the Ear

Routine Cleaning: Accumulations of cerumen (ear wax) and bacterial debris are found in virtually all dogs and most cats over 1-2 years of age. These accumulations may not be harmful but, if not

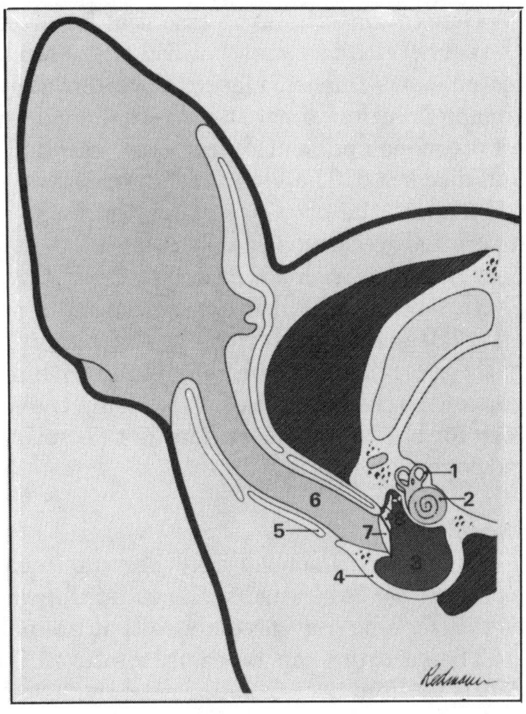

Fig 26. Anatomy of the ear: (1) semi-circular canals; (2) cochlea; (3) tympanic cavity (middle ear); (4) tympanic bulla; (5) cartilage of the external ear canal; (6) external ear; (7) tympanic membrane (eardrum). (Courtesy of Jane Redmann)

removed, can predispose to bacterial otitis (inflammation with infection). Continued neglect or improper treatment may ultimately lead to progression of the infection into the middle ear, inner ear and even the brain.

Routine cleaning does not require general anesthesia, though some fractious animals may require sedation. The procedure entails cleaning the pinna and outermost segment of the external canal with gauze sponges and cotton-tipped applicators (*eg,* Q-Tips: Johnson & Johnson). Cotton-tipped applicators should never be used to clean the proximal (deep) portion of the ear canal, since this actually forces debris deeper into the canal, predisposing to infection.

Hair normally grows in the ear canals of some dog breeds (*eg,* Poodle). The higher incidence of ear infections in these animals may be attributed to entrapment of debris and bacteria in hair within the ear canal.

Surgical Cleaning: Animals with severe otitis usually have large, visible accumulations of debris on the pinnae, malodorous and painful ears, and occasionally a head tilt or difficulty walking. Neither routine cleaning nor application of topical medication to a debris-filled ear is effective treatment. Such an ear canal must be first thoroughly irrigated and cleansed before topical drug therapy.

General anesthesia is essential for effective surgical cleansing of the ears. With the anesthetized animal in lateral recumbency, the affected ear is flushed vigorously, alternately with detergent and then rinsing solution, until the external canal and pinna are clean. Using an otoscope and suction catheter, residual rinse solution is removed and discarded. The veterinarian may then inspect the canal carefully to rule out the presence of foreign body, tumors or a ruptured eardrum. Large clumps of debris situated deep within the ear canal are best removed with a wire loop passed through the otoscope.

If a bacterial culture is indicated, a sample should be obtained after cleansing and rinsing the ear. This eliminates most nonpathogenic bacteria normally found within the ear and not considered part of the disease process. Cleansing the ear before obtaining a specimen for bacterial culture does not decrease the chances of recovering pathogenic bacteria.

Complications

Debris and bacteria may become impacted around the eardrum while the ear is cleaned with cotton-tipped applicators. Repeated use of this technic may predispose that animal to serious ear infection.

The eardrum can be easily ruptured during attempts to remove debris or fluid accumulated near the eardrum. After the eardrum is

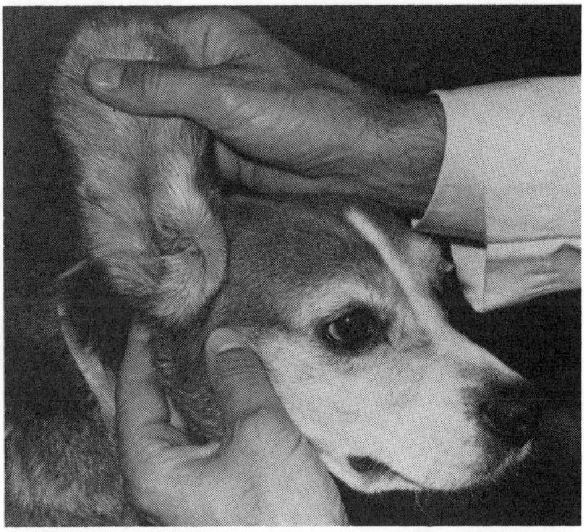

Fig 27. Dispersing otic medication throughout the external ear canal.

perforated, bacteria in the external ear canal may easily enter the inner ear, causing serious, chronic infection (otitis media).

Client Education

Topical medication is frequently prescribed to treat external ear infections. Dispensing these drugs to a client does not ensure the drug will be used, nor, if it is used, that it will be used correctly. Clients that have been properly instructed on treating the ear with topical medication are more likely to treat the patient properly.

Whether ointments or solutions are used to treat ear infections, effective distribution of the medication within a clean ear canal is the key to successful therapy. Owners unfamiliar with treating an ear infection should be instructed to gently massage the ear canal for a minute after drug instillation. The owner should massage the vertical ear canal, rather than the pinna, to properly distribute the medication (Figs 26, 27).

NAIL TRIMMING
BY R. B. Ford

Anatomy

Each weight-bearing digit of dogs and cats consists of 3 bones called phalanges: the proximal (first), middle (second), and distal (third). The 3 phalanges of the digit are comparable to bones of the human finger. The toenail (unguis) is merely extended horn-like tissue that emerges from the surface of the distal (third) phalanx. The toenail grows continuously in dogs and cats. It covers and protects the vascular bed of the ungual process.

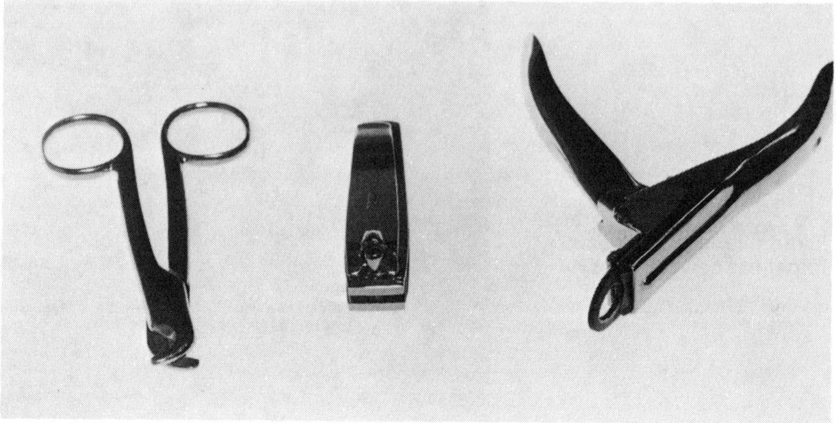

Fig 28. Toenail clippers: scissor type (left); human toenail type (center); guillotine type (right).

Instruments

Toenail clippers most commonly used on dogs are the shearing or guillotine type and the scissors type (Fig 28). Either type can be used on large and small dog breeds. All cutting edges must be sharp enough to efficiently cut through a normal nail. With continued use, the cutting edges become dull; eventually, the blade crushes more and cuts less. This is quite painful to the animal and may actually irreversibly injure the nail.

A variety of scissors-type toenail clippers can be used on cats, kittens and puppies to remove sharp toenail tips. However, a pair of toenail clippers intended for human use are just as effective and less expensive (Fig 28). A toenail clipper used on human toenails is similar to the type used on fingernails, only larger. They are easy to use and the technic of trimming a cat's toenails is generally well accepted by owners of indoor cats and kittens, as well as of puppies.

Regardless of the type of toenail clipper used, these instruments should be treated with the same care as a pair of surgical scissors. Though it is unnecessary to sterilize toenail clippers after each use, they should be thoroughly cleaned and washed if necessary. The cutting edges should be sharpened or replaced at regular intervals.

Nail Trimming

In dogs and cats, the objective of toenail trimming is to shorten the nail to a point such that the distal end, or toenail tip, does not extend ventral to (below) the level of the bottom of the digital pads.

With the animal standing on a flat, horizontal surface, the nail should not be so long as to contact the supporting surface. Neglected toenails that have been allowed to grow may seriously distort the foot and cause lameness when in contact with a hard surface. Neglected toenails, especially on dewclaws, may continue to grow in an arc; left untreated, these nails may grow into the footpads (Fig 29).

Dogs with unusually long toenails should have the nail trimmed to the appropriate length. However, as the toenail grows, the highly vascular ungual process (quick) also extends distad along the nail. When the toenail is cut to the proper length in such animals, bleeding should be anticipated. For this reason, excessively long toenails should not be trimmed in the owner's presence. Cats, on the other hand, are unlikely to have problems associated with excessively long nails since they intermittently shed the outer layer of nail. Overgrown nails are seldom encountered in cats with access to scratching posts or trees.

Bleeding from a closely trimmed toenail does not cause serious blood loss in normal dogs and cats. Any bleeding from nail trimming should be completely stopped before releasing the animal, since the

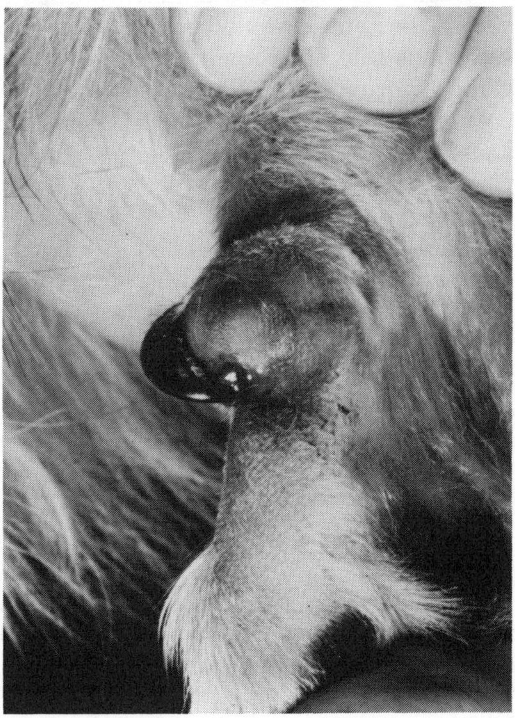

Fig 29. Neglected dewclaw nail penetrating the skin of the digit, causing painful digital infection.

blood can stain fabrics and alarm the owner. Silver nitrate applied topically to the tip of the bleeding nail stops bleeding but may cause pain. In addition, silver nitrate sticks discolor skin and stain clothing. Other topical suspensions containing aluminum sulfate and a collagen protein are available. These products are quite effective in controlling minor bleeding and do not irritate sensitive tissues.

Complications

While bleeding is often regarded as a complication of nail trimming, it is not a serious problem. Injury to the nail and underlying structures is most likely to occur when dull or damaged instruments are used. Split and broken toenails permit bacteria to invade the vascular structure beneath the toenail, which may result in an infection of the toenail bed (paronychia).

ANAL SAC CARE
by R. B. Ford

Anatomy

Dogs and cats have 2 subcutaneous anal sacs located on either side of the anus. The wall of the sac is composed of glands that expel secretions into the lumen of the sac. The secretion produced by the gland is normally liquid to pasty in consistency, is foul smelling and is normally easily expressed by applying manual pressure around the anus.

Expressing Anal Sacs

In normal dogs and cats, the anal sacs need not be routinely expressed. Generally, these sacs empty spontaneously during defecation. Occasionally, however, the anal sac may become infected or ulcerated, or the orifice may become occluded with unusually thick secretions. In such cases, the animal, particularly dogs, "scoots," *ie,* drags the anus across the ground, to relieve the irritation. Owners frequently describe this problem as being associated with "worms." Whereas tapeworms may cause an animal to "scoot," the usual cause is impaction or infection of the anal sacs.

The anal sac is best emptied by placing a gloved index finger into the rectum and then using that finger and the thumb to "milk" the secretions caudad (rearward) from the sac. Occasionally, the veterinarian will medicate the sac with an antibiotic and/or corticosteroid ointment after it has been emptied.

Complications

The most serious complication associated with expressing anal sacs is caused by emptying the anal sac at the beginning of the physical examination rather than at the end. The odor can be intolerable. Additionally, excessive manipulation of the anus may cause minor injury to the perianal tissue. This may cause sufficient pain to cause the animal to not defecate for up to 24 hours.

PHYSICAL THERAPY

by J. Rasmussen

Physical therapy is the treatment of disease or injuries by physical agents, such as light, heat, cold, water, electricity, massage and exercise. When properly applied, physical therapy can expedite healing of injured tissue, prevent disability and help restore normal function. Physical therapy can be used to rehabilitate animals with diseases of bones, muscles, joints, nerves and skin, as well as dislocations, fractures, arthritis, paresis, paralysis, infections and decubital ulcers.

The modes of physical therapy range from simple to complex. The most important factor determining the quality of the therapy is the person administering it. A good therapist must have an optimistic attitude, a general interest in the welfare of each animal, and a great deal of patience.

Massage

The simplest form of physical therapy is massage, in which the hands and fingers are used to manipulate soft tissues of the body. The primary objective of massage is to increase blood flow through the massaged tissues. Massage also enhances the flow of lymph from tissue spaces, providing quicker elimination of wastes and flow of nutrients into the site. Massage can decrease the likelihood of fibrosis, which is an abnormal formation of adhesions between connective tissue layers.

A massage medium may be used to reduce friction and soften the skin or scar tissue. Some commonly used media are mineral oil, cold cream, olive oil and petroleum jelly. Powders, such as talc or baby powder, are used more frequently in veterinary medicine in place of lubricants because they provide the same effect and are easier to remove. The medium should be placed on the hands and then massaged into the patient's skin instead of being applied directly to the skin, and never be applied to open wounds or fresh incisions. At the conclusion of therapy, the lubricant can be removed with isopropyl alcohol.

Factors that must be considered when administering massage include direction, pressure, rate and rhythm of the stroke, and duration (usually 15 minutes is enough) and frequency of massage. These factors vary, depending on the size of the area treated, and the animal's size, condition, response to and progress with treatment.

Specific conditions that massage can benefit include tight and contracted tendons, ligaments and muscles, subacute and chronic traumatic and inflammatory conditions, peripheral nerve injuries, scar tissue, and subacute and chronic edema. Specific conditions for which massage is contraindicated include acute or inflammatory processes of soft tissues, bone and joints, fractures, sprains, foreign bodies under the skin, hemorrhage or lymphangitis, and advanced skin diseases.

The 3 basic types of massage are effleurage, foulage and friction.

Effleurage

Effleurage, or stroking, is a gentle massage that accustoms the animal to the touch of the therapist, allowing it to relax before a deeper form of massage is applied. The patient is massaged from the periphery of the limb or affected area toward the center. Effleurage can be done with a light or heavy stroke, but uniform pressure is required. A light stroke, at a rate of 15 strokes/minute, should be applied for a sedative effect. A heavy stroke, at 5 strokes/minute, should be applied to enhance drainage in veins and lymph channels. A 10-minute session should generally prepare the patient for more extensive therapy.

Foulage

Foulage, also called kneading, compression or pétrissage, is used primarily on muscle groups, individual muscles or a part of a muscle to enhance circulation and stretch muscles, tendons and adhesions. The muscle should be compressed from side to side as the hands move up it, always in the direction of venous return (toward the heart). The procedure should be gentle and never forceful enough to cause reflexive withdrawal of the leg.

Friction

Friction massage is used to aid absorption of local effusions and loosen superficial scar tissue and adhesions. In friction massage, the skin is moved over underlying tissue in small, circular, rhythmic motions, with the greatest pressure applied at the lowest part of the circle. The frequency and duration of friction massage varies with the animal's condition and size.

Exercise

Another simple form of physical therapy is exercise. Therapeutic exercise is used to strengthen, improve or maintain musculoskeletal function. Exercise can improve a debilitated animal's balance, stability, coordination, and cardiovascular and respiratory function. Two important effects of exercise are increased endurance and increased range of motion of the limbs. The 2 types of exercise used in physical therapy of small animals are passive and active.

Passive Exercise

Passive exercise is used on patients that are paralyzed or very weak, or with fractures. Passive exercise is accomplished by a therapist, with no activity on the part of the patient. Each affected joint is put through its normal range of motion 5-10 times per treatment without any muscle contraction by the animal. This type of exercise helps prevent joint ankylosis ("freezing") and disuse atrophy. Passive exercise can also be used after certain types of surgery, such as that

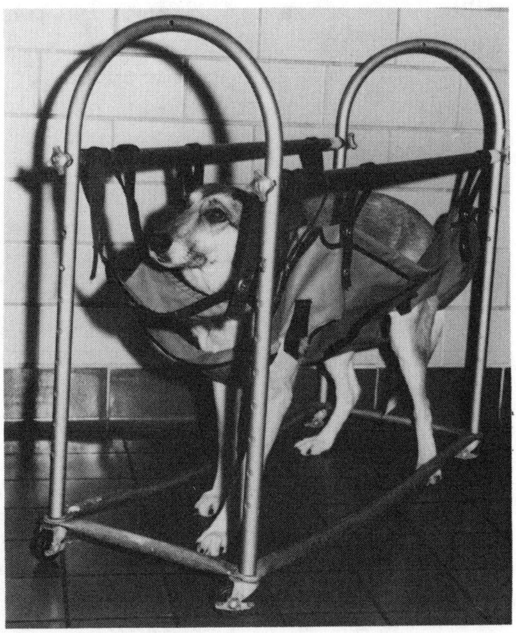

Fig 30. Full-support exercise cart.

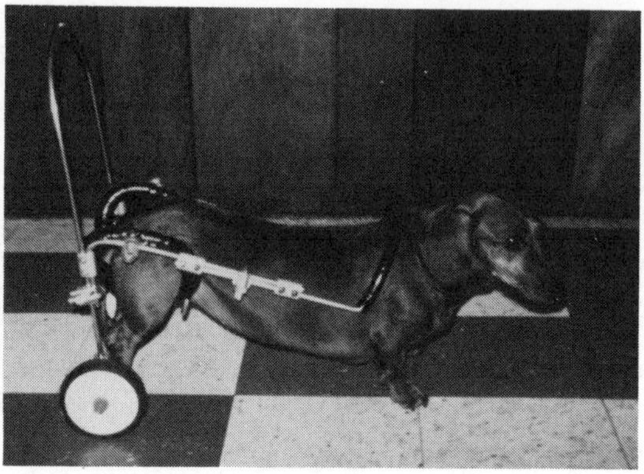

Fig 31. Exercise cart for a dog with posterior paresis.

for intervertebral disc disease. These patients should have their hindlimbs flexed and extended for 10-minute sessions several times daily. A limb should never be forced beyond its normal range of motion during passive exercise.

Active Exercise

The most beneficial form of exercise is active exercise, which entails voluntary muscle contraction by the patient and includes many types of exercise, from walking to swimming. Some patients may be willing to exercise on their own, but reluctant patients may require some stimulation and support.

Many devices can provide added support and assistance for nonambulatory (unable to walk) animals. One such device is an exercise

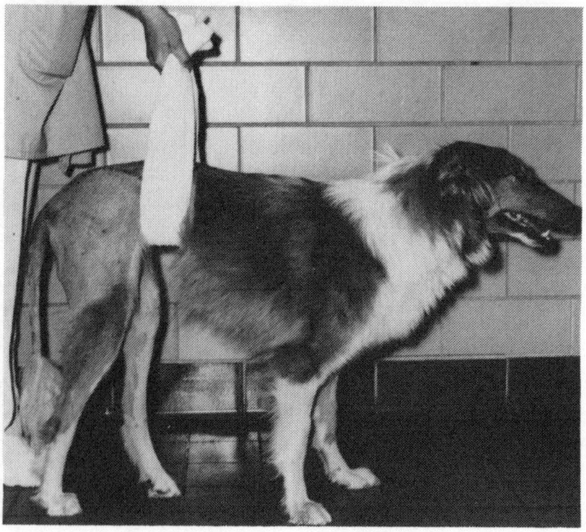

Fig 32. Use of a towel to provide active exercise therapy to a dog with posterior paresis.

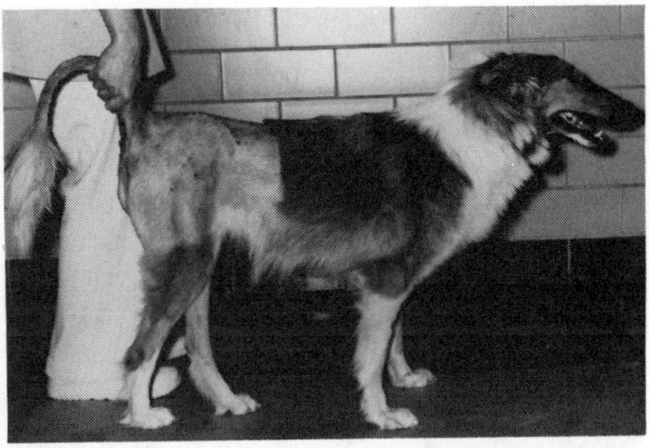

Fig 33. "Tailing" a dog to provide rear-end support during active exercise therapy.

cart, which is available commercially or can be constructed from inexpensive aluminum rods and lawn mower wheels (Figs 30, 31). The cart supports the animal's torso, allowing limb movement and exercise for patients unable to support their own weight. Carts are especially useful in rehabilitation of patients with posterior paralysis.

If an exercise cart is not available or is not well tolerated by the patient, a sling can be made with a bath towel (Fig 32). The towel should not be allowed to pull against the top of the thigh because this impedes leg motion. "Tailing" exercise, which includes using the tail to support the rear quarters of the animal, can also be used intermittently with the exercise cart to prevent dependency of the animal on the cart (Fig 33). Care must be taken to grasp the tail at its base to prevent injury.

Hydrotherapy

Underwater exercise is another method of providing support for an animal with locomotor difficulties. The physical properties of water provide the animal with support. Water movement or turbulence, as in a whirlpool bath, can be added to create a massage effect. Buoyancy provides a lifting effect, allowing voluntary exercise that would otherwise be impossible in animals unable to stand or walk.

The temperature of the water should be 65-75 F for active exercise and 96-104 F for inactive patients. With warm-water therapy, the animal gains and produces heat during exercise. These 2 combined factors increase the peripheral blood supply due to dilation of superficial blood vessels, which causes increased heart and metabolic rates.

Animals undergoing underwater therapy must never be left unattended; the possibility of drowning should always be kept in mind. If the patient has a disorder of the neck or an extremity, a sling arrangement should be used for support.

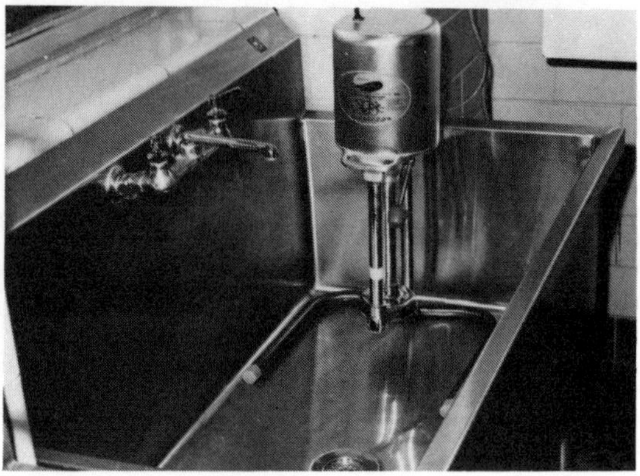

Fig 34. Portable water agitator used in hydrotherapy.

Another patient safety consideration is fear. If the patient is afraid of water, the first few therapy sessions should concentrate on acclimating it to the water.

Febrile patients should not be treated with warm-water therapy until their rectal temperature has been normal for at least 72 hours.

A povidone-iodine concentrate can be added to the water (¼ oz povidone-iodine for each 1 gal water) to decrease the possibility of transmitting infections from one patient to another. The concentration can also help prevent urine scald, infection of decubital ulcers, and superficial pyodermas.

Whirlpool Baths

The whirlpool bath, an important mode of hydrotherapy, achieves its therapeutic effects through turbulence or movement of water, accomplished with an electric turbine ejector and aerator that circulates an air-water mixture. Portable agitators are adaptable for use in almost any tank, bathtub or pool (Fig 34).

A non-skid surface should be placed on the bottom of the tub for weight-bearing patients to aid traction. The water temperature should be 105-110 F. The turbine must be electrically grounded and not started until the water is in the tank and the patient is safely positioned in the tub. Contrary to belief, the turbine should be directed so the water is emitted *away* from the affected body part. Treatments should be given after the animal has urinated and defecated to avoid contaminating the whirlpool bath. The length of whirlpool treatment should be about 20 minutes and should not exceed 30 minutes.

The effects of whirlpool baths are the same as those of underwater exercise. In addition, whirlpools combine the effects of gentle massage and superficial heat. The swirling action of the water helps clean and debride damaged tissues, thereby combating infection.

Scar tissue is softened and metabolism, respiration and mobility of extremities are increased.

Whirlpool baths are indicated for patients with fractures in the late stage of healing, arthritis, stiff joints, adhesions, dislocations, amputations, subacute and chronic inflammatory disease, diseases associated with decubital ulcers, and skin diseases.

In treating animals with dermatologic disorders, the water aids healing by removing exudates, crusts, scales, bacteria and debris from lesions, wounds and fistulas. The whirlpool also helps alleviate pain and pruritus associated with skin disorders. The water softens the keratin of the skin and promotes epithelialization.

Whirlpool therapy is contraindicated for animals with peripheral vascular disease, acute injuries, acute inflammation, recent surgery, acute edema, fever and cardiac or respiratory disorders.

Swimming

Swimming is good exercise for animals that require more extensive exercise for rehabilitation or that are in the last phase of rehabilitation. Swimming animals are forced to move continuously, while the water's buoyancy allows an increased range of motion of their limbs.

Small patients can swim in a bathtub at the veterinary hospital and continue therapy at home under owner supervision. Children's wading pools offer an inexpensive alternative for larger patients.

Thermotherapy

Thermotherapy (heat therapy) involves use of radiant, conductive or converted heat to treat disease. The purpose of thermotherapy generally is to increase tissue temperature, causing analgesia (pain relief) in affected tissues and some sedation. The resulting vasodilation and increased circulation in the injured site enhance movement of phagocytes, oxygen, antibiotics and nutrients to the area. Heat relieves pain, relaxes muscle spasms and promotes wound healing. It usually relaxes the patient, increasing its sense of well-being.

Animals with contusions and sprains benefit from heat applied 48-72 hours after the causative injury. Animals with bursitis, tendinitis, impaired circulation or noninflammatory edema have a decreased tolerance to heat and should not be subjected to thermotherapy.

Radiant Heat

Radiant heat transmits energy to the skin and superficial tissues, which absorb the rays and convert them to heat.

Long-wave rays are emitted by all heated bodies and by such items as heating pads and hot-water bottles. Because long-wave rays only penetrate about 2 mm into tissue, being absorbed mostly in the upper skin layers, they are not recommended for therapy.

Short-wave rays, emitted by generators or lamps, are the most effective rays used in physical therapy. These rays can penetrate up to 5-10 mm into tissues, influencing blood vessels, lymph flow, nerve endings and subcutaneous tissues.

Infrared radiation is a powerful form of radiant heat therapy. Animals receiving heat therapy can be severely burned by ultraviolet light (sunlamps). Infrared radiation should be used cautiously, particularly over healing skin and scar tissue and on animals with impaired circulation. It should not be used in very old or very young patients.

Conductive Heat

Conductive heat is heat transferred from an object with a higher temperature to one with a lower temperature. Hot packs are the most common method of applying conductive heat.

A protective layer of toweling should be placed between any hot pack and the skin surface. The skin should be checked every few minutes. If it feels hot or appears red, an additional layer of toweling should be added. Hot packs should never be applied over newly healed skin or scar tissue.

Hot packs are commercially available. One type is a reusable pack filled with silica gel. When heated to 170 F, the pack retains heat for 20-30 minutes, which is the usual maximum application time. The pack should be covered with a towel to delay cooling and must be kept constantly wet or it becomes unusable. Units are available for heating the water and storing the packs. These packs last for years if used with care.

Instant, nonreusable packs are also available. These are activated by breaking an inner bag and shaking the pack to mix the contents. A chemical reaction of the enclosed chemicals generates moderate heat.

Warm (about 100 F) whirlpool baths are another form of conductive heat therapy. The moist heat is more effective in relieving pain and muscle spasms than is dry heat.

Converted Heat

Converted heat results from conversion of one energy form to heat in the body tissues. Ultrasound, a mode of converted or deep-heat therapy that provides deeper heat than radiation therapy, consists of mechanical vibrations that are identical to acoustic or sound vibrations except in their frequency and mode of emission. The frequency of ultrasound waves, which is over 20,000 cycles per second, makes them inaudible to the human ear.

Ultrasound waves are transferred from the machine producing them to the affected body area through a hand-held transducer. To eliminate air pockets between the transducer and skin, a coupling medium, such as mineral oil or lubricating gel, is used. For best results, the animal's hair should be clipped from the area to be treated.

Ultrasound therapy is applied in 3 ways. The most common is the contact technic, which is used on smooth, muscular surfaces and involves a coupling medium. The weight of the transducer or the light pressure applied usually does not cause pain.

A second method is underwater ultrasound therapy. This technic is used to treat very uneven surfaces, such as the olecranon (elbow) or stifle (knee), where good transducer-body contact is impossible. Only the area of treatment need be immersed in water.

The cushion technic, the third method of ultrasound administration, is used over bony prominences or curvatures that prevent good transducer contact yet cannot be submerged in water. For this type of ultrasound treatment, a plastic bag filled with tepid water is placed between the transducer and the gel-coated skin.

Ultrasound is used for a variety of neuromuscular and musculoskeletal conditions to soften scar tissue, reduce pain of neuromas and degenerative joint disease, and treat arthritis and bursitis. The chief danger in using ultrasound is a burn. The patient should never feel any pain or discomfort during the treatment; excessive movement or other signs of pain during treatment indicate inappropriate application of ultrasound. Ultrasound should not be used over the eyes, spinal cord, brain, growing bones, heart, anesthetized areas, ischemic areas, tumors, reproductive organs, acutely infected areas, or areas previously exposed to radiation.

Cryotherapy

Cryotherapy (cold therapy), administered with cold packs, cold water or ice, is indicated within the first 48-72 hours following an injury. It decreases tissue temperature, reducing pain and muscle spasms. Cold is also thought to decrease nerve conduction and create mild analgesia at the application site. Cryotherapy also causes local vasoconstriction and decreased capillary blood flow, thereby decreasing edema. Applied within the first 24 hours after an injury, cryotherapy can greatly reduce hemorrhage into tissue spaces.

Cold Packs

Commercial cold packs are manufactured for use in human medicine but can also be used in veterinary medicine. They are available in various sizes and forms (Fig 35). A disposable instant cold pack is activated by squeezing, which breaks an inner bag, mixing the contents and causing an immediate drop in temperature. The pack provides a temperature of 20 F for about 45 minutes.

Reusable cold packs contain a liquid that does not harden even when frozen (Fig 35). This type of pack can be bulky and heavy, so it should not be applied to a fracture site. Both instant and reusable packs should be covered with a towel when applied so as to prevent frostbite. Application time is generally 5-20 minutes.

The most commonly used cold packs are those used by drug companies for shipping drugs. These packs stay frozen longer than ice and are reusable. If commercial packs are not available, apply ice to the affected site. The ice should be in a plastic, leak-proof bag wrapped in a towel. A washcloth or towel soaked in ice water can be used on injuries in body areas to which ice cannot conform, such as joints and bony prominences.

Cold-Water Immersion

Immersion of an injured limb in cold water (60 F) is another effective cryotherapeutic method. Only the affected areas should be immersed. Open wounds should not be immersed unless a disinfectant is added to the water.

A limb should not be immersed in cold water for longer than 20 minutes at a time. Large wounds should not be immersed, as this can delay healing.

Cold-water immersion is used specifically to rehabilitate muscles, ligaments, tendons and joints, combat high fevers, and treat burns

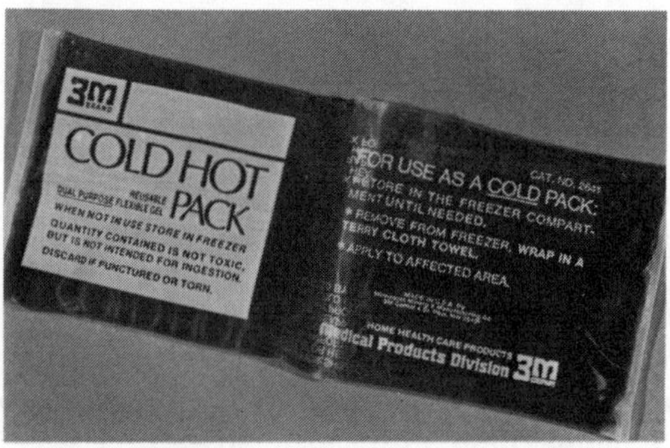

Fig 35. A reusable hot and cold pack.

and traumatic inflammatory conditions. Cold-water immersion is also indicated in cases in which thermotherapy has been unsuccessful.

Rehabilitation or recovery of a patient depends on the care it receives. The importance of conscientious nursing care, with generous amounts of affection, cannot be overemphasized. Many patients have special needs for rehabilitation. It is the technician's responsibility to recognize and attend to these needs. It is also vital that the patient have a desire to recover. The technician should interact with the patient as a friend by talking in a pleasant tone and addressing the patient by name.

Hospitalized animals should be discharged as soon as possible because their familiar surroundings at home tend to improve the animal's sense of security and speed recovery. Most clients are willing to participate in the rehabilitation program at home. Physical therapy methods should be demonstrated to the client so they are applied properly at home. The importance of maintaining the prescribed treatment schedule should be stressed, as failure to treat the animal properly may result in a relapse. Complete, written home-care instructions concerning diet, medication, exercise and treatment should be provided. Frequent communication with the client is necessary to monitor the patient's condition at home. Many animals must be returned to the hospital for additional checkups and treatment.

BLOOD COLLECTION AND TRANSFUSION

by C. S. Intravartolo

Blood Groups

Eight different dog erythrocyte antigens (DEA), also called blood groups, have been identified in dogs.[1] The canine blood groups are DEA-1, DEA-2, DEA-3, DEA-4, DEA-5, DEA-6, DEA-7 and DEA-8. Because DEA-1 and DEA-2 are the most reactive antigens within the blood groups, they are most often associated with transfusion reactions.[2] Blood incompatibility is caused by antigens on the donor's red blood cells (RBC) that react with antibodies in the recipient's plasma. More than half of the dog population has DEA-1 and DEA-2 on their RBC. These dogs should not be used as blood donors.

Little information is available about blood groups in cats. Few transfusion reactions have been noted, especially if repeat transfusions are not given.[3]

Blood typing is not a routine procedure in veterinary practices because sera required for testing are difficult to obtain; however, some commercial laboratories have facilities for typing blood in donor dogs (Dr W. Jean Dodds, N.Y. State Dept. of Health, Albany, NY 12237; Dr A. Hurvitz, Animal Medical Center, New York City, NY 10021; Dr R. Bull, Michigan State University, East Lansing, MI 48824).[4] Heparinized blood is collected from the potential donor, mixed with an equal volume of Alsever's solution and sent to the laboratory. Samples should be shipped on ice by air freight or air mail. The laboratory should be notified before shipment. To ensure faster transport, samples should be mailed at the beginning of the week.

Cross Matching

Cross matching is performed to determine donor and recipient compatibility before transfusion. It is not a substitute for blood typing. However, it is the best alternative when typing has not been done or when a suitable donor is not available.[4]

Both major and minor cross matches can be performed. A major cross match involves mixing the recipient's serum with the donor's RBC. A minor cross match combines the donor's serum with the recipient's RBC. Significant resultant hemolysis or agglutination indicates incompatibility between donor and recipient.[5] Transfusion with cross-matched blood decreases the possibility of a transfusion reaction; however, it does not eliminate the possibility of sensitizing a patient, which may result in a reaction to future transfusions.[4]

Donor Compatibility

Recipients should never be transfused with blood from an incompatible donor. However, transfusion of incompatible blood into a patient that has never been transfused is unlikely to cause a transfusion reaction, due to the lack of naturally occurring canine anti-DEA-1 or -2 isoantibodies.[2,6] Instead, the patient develops antibodies that may destroy the constituents of the transfused blood within 7-10 days. Such antibody formation does not cause illness but sensitizes the patient to future transfusions. If the patient were to receive a second transfusion with incompatible blood, RBC destruction could begin within one hour. Subsequent transfusions with incompatible blood increase the likelihood of a serious or fatal transfusion reaction.

Never give canine blood to cats. Studies have shown that about 95% of canine RBC transfused to cats are destroyed within the first 24 hours. These cells provide no benefit to the patient and, in fact, further stress the patient by increasing the work load of the kidney and liver in excreting the breakdown products.[7] Cross-species transfusions are always contraindicated.

Blood Donor Selection

Animals selected as resident hospital blood donors should be healthy, young adults, 1-5 years old, that have never received a transfusion. Dogs selected should weigh at least 40 lb and should not be obese. The animals should be free from parasites and blood disorders.[5] Dogs should be negative for *Dirofilaria immitis* and *Brucella canis.*[8] Cats should be tested for feline leukemia virus (FeLV), feline infectious peritonitis (FIP) and *Hemobartonella felis.*[8]

Advantages of maintaining resident blood donors in a veterinary practice are several:[7] (1) The animal is maintained in good physical condition and can be fed a diet known to support blood production. (2) Blood counts can be performed routinely to ensure adequate levels in the donor. (3) The animals are of adequate size and disposition to allow blood collection with minimal difficulty. (4) Blood-typed donors reduce the possibility of giving incompatible blood and (5) The veterinarian has a readily available source of whole blood.

Name ______________________ Species ______________________

Breed ______________________ Birth ______________________ Sex ____

Blood type ______________________

Vaccination History

Date												
Rabies												
DHLP												
Parvovirus												
FVRC-P												

Preventive Care Checklist

Date												
Fecal												
CBC												
Platelets												
Heartworm												
Weight												
Other												

Donation Record

Date	Amount	Next Use	Date	Amount	Next Use

Fig 36. This type of record sheet for blood donors provides a convenient record of vaccinations, diagnostic test results and blood donations. [From *Comp Cont Ed Anim Health Tech* 2 (1981) 302, courtesy of Veterinary Learning Systems]

The technician should maintain accurate records for each donor animal. Records must be kept of every donation and of routine preventive care for donors, such as immunizations and fecal and heartworm examinations. The technician may wish to develop a record sheet for records of all donors (Fig 36).

Blood Collection

The number and frequency of transfusions given in a practice determine how often blood is collected. Blood may be collected and stored for future use or collected at the time it is used. Because most transfusions are given as part of emergency treatment, fresh blood is usually collected when it is needed.

Collection Materials

Drugs for Sedation or Anesthesia: Blood can usually be collected from most hospital donor dogs without chemical restraint. Cats often require mild sedation or anesthesia for ease of collection. Tranquilizers and anesthetics should be available when needed.

Clippers and Preparation Materials: Strict asepsis must be maintained during collection, storage and administration of blood. The blood collection site should be clipped with a #40 blade and surgically prepared with a suitable antiseptic, such as providone-iodine (*eg,* Betadine: Purdue Frederick), to prevent infection in the donor animal.

Blood Collection and Administration Equipment: Blood collected for transfusion in dogs is collected in commercially available vacuum bottles or plastic bags. The most commonly used anticoagulants are acid citrate dextrose (ACD), citrate phosphate dextrose (CPD) and heparin.

Vacuum bottles contain ACD and are available in 250-ml and 500-ml sizes (Fig 37). The bottles require a separate blood collection set, also called a donor set, when the blood is withdrawn.

Plastic collection bags (Fenwal Labs, Deerfield, IL 60015) are available with ACD or CPD (Fig 37). The blood collection set is incorporated into the bag, eliminating the need for a separate donor set. The bags are available in a variety of styles for human use. Two styles that are practical for use in most veterinary hospitals are the CPD Single Blood-Pack Unit (Fenwal) with a 15- or 16-ga needle for collection of whole blood and the CPD Double Blood-Pack Unit (Fenwal) with an attached 300-ml Transfer Pack (Fenwal) suitable for harvesting plasma.

In many instances plastic bags are preferred over bottles for blood collection. Collection in glass bottles is usually quicker because of the built-in vacuum. A disadvantage of using bottles is the difficulty in

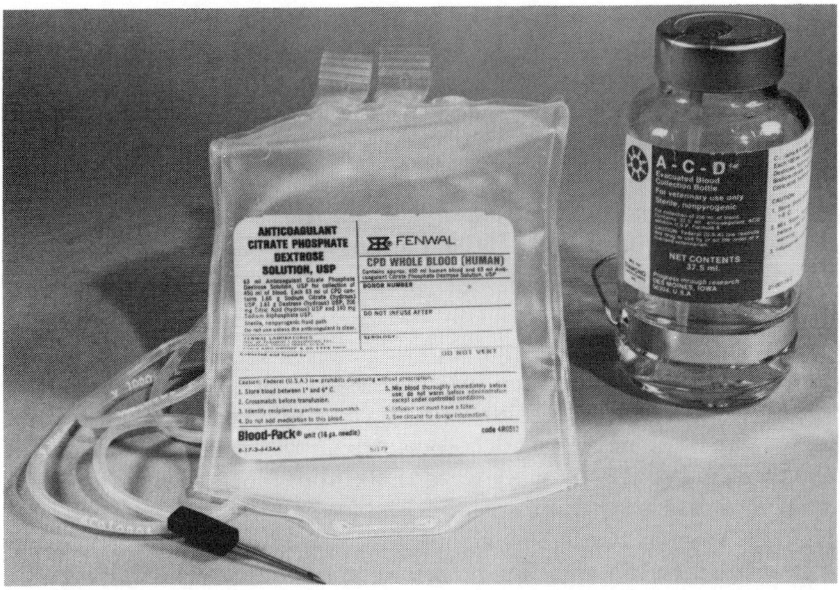

Fig 37. The CPD Single Blood-Pack Unit (Fenwal Labs) (left) and the ACD collection bottle (Diamond Labs) (right) are suitable for blood collection and short-term storage of whole blood. [From *Comp Cont Ed Anim Health Tech* 2 (1981) 302, courtesy of Veterinary Learning Systems]

maintaining sterility because the bottles must be vented during administration.[8] The advantages of using plastic bags include: minimal loss of platelets; collection tubing and needle are conveniently attached; bags are unbreakable; bags require less space for storage before and after use; the gravity flow of the bag eliminates the foaming and

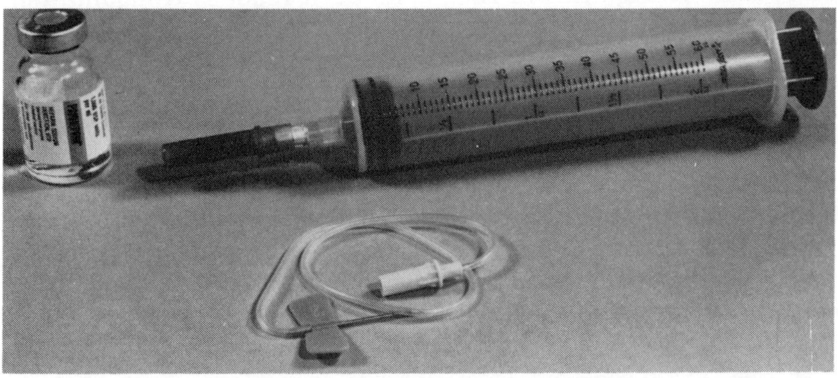

Fig 38. Blood can be collected from donor cats with a 21-ga Butterfly catheter (Abbott Labs) attached to a 60-ml syringe [From *Comp Cont Ed Anim Health Tech* 2 (1981) 302, courtesy of Veterinary Learning Systems]

mechanical trauma caused by vacuum-bottle collection;[9] and plasma can be harvested from outdated blood units.

To collect blood from donor cats, a heparinized 60-ml syringe and 21-ga Butterfly catheter (Abbott Laboratories, North Chicago, IL 60064) work well (Fig 38). The syringe is rinsed with heparin before venipuncture, using about 0.25 ml of sodium heparin for every 50 ml of blood collected.[2] Avoid using too much heparin, since this may result in heparinization of the patient, with subsequent clotting disorders.

Blood Collection from Donor Cats

The most common sites for collection from cats are the jugular vein and heart. The jugular vein is the preferred site, since most technicians are not trained to perform intracardiac puncture. The average adult cat can safely donate 40 ml of blood every 3 weeks.[5]

Donor cats are usually anesthetized for blood collection. Ketamine HCl (*eg,* Vetalar: Parke Davis), given IM at 5-10 mg/kg, works well for this procedure. The jugular area is clipped and surgically prepared with povidone-iodine scrub. The Butterfly catheter is inserted into the vein craniad (against the flow of blood) and the required amount of blood is withdrawn into the heparinized syringe. Once the cat is anesthetized, the entire procedure can be completed in 10 minutes with relative safety and minimal stress to the cat.

Blood Collection from Donor Dogs

The most common sites for collection from dogs are the jugular vein, femoral artery and heart. Collection from the femoral artery causes less trauma to RBC and platelets than collection from any other site.[6] Though this method is quick, it requires tranquilization and sometimes general anesthesia. Donor dogs can safely give 5-10 ml blood/lb body weight every 3 weeks.[4]

Sedation or anesthesia is rarely necessary when collecting blood from donor dogs, unless the femoral artery is used. Most resident blood donor dogs are quite familiar with the procedure and easily handled. The jugular area is prepared as with cats, the collecting needle is inserted into the vein craniad, and blood is collected in the appropriate container. Because the collection bottle or bag contains a specific amount of anticoagulant, it is important to completely fill the container with blood.

Donor Care After Collection

Following blood collection, the technician should place a bandage over the venipuncture site to prevent infection and hematoma formation. If the donor was anesthetized, the animal should be monitored during recovery. If the veterinary practice has the equipment available to harvest plasma, RBC may be given back to the donor if they are not immediately used.

Blood Storage

Whole Blood

The dextrose in the anticoagulant helps preserve RBC. Citrate phosphate dextrose is a better anticoagulant for blood storage since CPD-stored blood more efficiently delivers oxygen to body tissues than ACD-stored blood.[10]

All whole blood and plasma should be labeled, dated and stored at 32-43 F.[2] It can be safely stored in a refrigerator for 21 days.

Heparinized blood contains no preservative and should be used immediately or stored in the refrigerator and used within 48 hours.[2]

Plasma

Plasma is the liquid portion of blood. It differs from serum in that serum is plasma from which fibrinogen has been separated during clotting. Plasma may be harvested from blood simply by allowing the RBC to settle for 24 hours and then aspirating the plasma from the top of the blood container. Use a 3-inch, 20-ga needle attached to a 50 -or 100-ml syringe to collect the plasma. It may be stored in a refrigerator up to 26 days after collection or kept frozen for as long as 2 years.[7] Plasma from various donors may be pooled and stored in large containers or packaged in smaller containers.[7]

Preparing Stored Blood and Plasma for Use

Stored blood should not be warmed unless it is given faster than 50 ml/kg/hour.[2] Before it is transfused, the bottle or bag should be inverted gently several times until the RBC are in suspension. Discard any previously stored blood that is not used; avoid rechilling it. Bacteria are found in blood that has been warmed, not used and rechilled[8] A dark-brown to black color of the plasma indicates bacterial growth.[6]

Blood Administration

Handling the Recipient

The technician must remember that patients in need of transfusion are usually in poor condition. Most such animals are depressed and weak; some may be toxemic and even hypoxemic, depending on the underlying disorder. Stress of any kind may result in sudden collapse, even death. For these reasons, the technician must handle recipients as gently as possible.

Routes of Administration

Whole blood may be given IV, IP (intraperitoneally), or directly into the intramedullary canal of a long bone. Blood should not be given SC because nearly 97% of the RBC are destroyed in the SC tissue, resulting in no benefit to the patient.[7]

Whole blood is most effective when given IV. The most common sites are the jugular, cephalic and lateral saphenous veins. One method combines use of commercially available blood administration sets (Fenwal) and indwelling IV catheters (Sovereign Catheter: Sherwood Medical, St. Louis, MO 63103). Never use standard fluid administration sets for blood transfusion. Blood administration sets differ from fluid administration sets in that they contain a special filter chamber that prevents large blood clots from entering the patient. Improperly filtered blood may cause pulmonary microembolization and respiratory distress.[8] The blood should be given through a 20-ga or larger indwelling catheter placed aseptically into the vein. Using a smaller needle or catheter may cause hemolysis of the transfused blood.[3]

No other drugs should be mixed with blood or plasma during transfusions, as incompatibility between the drug and blood or anticoagulant may cause complications. Certain drugs and fluids (*eg*, Ringer's solution) can cause recalcification and coagulation of the blood. Saline is the only safe fluid for diluting blood for transfusion.[8]

Sometimes IV administration of blood is difficult. Occasionally an animal's blood pressure is so low that a vein cannot be catheterized. An alternative method is to give the blood IP. The blood is dripped in by gravity through a 20-ga needle inserted through the aseptically prepared abdominal wall. Though this method is considered safe, the RBC are not as effectively used as when the blood is given IV. With IP transfusion nearly 65% of the RBC are absorbed into the blood within 48 hours.[5,7] This is an acceptable method for animals that do not require an immediate increase in blood volume or RBC numbers.

In small puppies and kittens, it is sometimes difficult to catheterize a vein. Blood and other fluids can be given directly through a needle placed in the intramedullary canal of the femur. A standard 18- or 20-ga needle usually can be placed in the bone without problems. If the needle plugs with medullary bone particles, a 20-ga needle with a stylet may be used. When the needle is securely placed, blood or other fluids may be dripped in by gravity or injected through a syringe. Care should be taken to inject slowly to minimize the endosteal pain often associated with this method.[2] One disadvantage of this method is the risk of possible osteomyelitis.[2]

	Recipient's weight	10 lb
	Recipient's PCV	8%
	PCV of donor blood	40%
	Desired post-transfusion PCV	18%
	Approximate blood volume of cats	35 ml/lb
10 lb	Recipient's weight	
× 35 ml/lb	Blood volume of cats	
350 ml	Recipient's approximate total blood volume	
350 ml	Recipient's total blood volume	
× 8%	Recipient's PCV before transfusion	
28 ml	Recipient's total RBC before transfusion	
350 ml	Recipient's total blood volume	
× 18%	Desired post-transfusion PCV	
63 ml	Total required RBC volume	
63 ml	Total required RBC volume	
− 28 ml	Recipient's total RBC volume before transfusion	
35 ml	Total RBC volume required from transfusion	

$$\text{Volume of donor blood required} = \frac{\text{Total RBC volume required (ml)}}{\text{PCV of donor blood (\%) (including anticoagulant)}} = \frac{35\text{ ml}}{40\%} = 87.5\text{ ml}$$

Fig 39. Equation to determine volume of blood required for transfusion in cats.[3] The same equation may be used for dogs, using an approximate total blood volume of 40 ml/lb and desired post-transfusion PCV of 28-30%. (Courtesy of Veterinary Practice Publishing Co)

Amount and Rate of Administration

The amount of blood transfused depends upon the indication for the transfusion. Blood may be given to effect, in amounts to replace known losses, or generally on the basis of 5-10 ml/lb body weight.[5-7]

The average cat can usually accept about 40 ml of blood over a 30-minute period. An equation has been developed to determine blood replacement requirements, based on the recipient's weight and PCV, the PCV of donated blood, the desired post-transfusion PCV in the recipient, and the blood volume of dogs and cats (Fig 39).[3]

The usual rate for IV administration of blood is less than 10 ml/kg/hour.[2] Most blood administration sets are designed to deliver 10 drops/ml (always refer to package inserts for exact directions); therefore, the administration rate in drops per minute can be calculated. A slow IV drip is safer and more desirable for the recipient than a large, rapidly administered IV dose.[5] Dogs with heart failure cannot tolerate transfusion rates above 2 ml/lb/hour.[8] Cats may vomit during rapid administration of blood.[7] Single IP injections may be given with relative safety and few harmful side effects.[3] When possible, the entire required volume of whole blood should be given within an 8-hour period, particularly if the patient needs platelets more than RBC.

During transfusion, the technician should closely monitor the recipient for signs of a reaction to the transfusion. Specific clinical signs include dyspnea (difficult breathing), shivering, vomiting and urticaria (hives). If these signs occur, transfusion should be immediately discontinued and the patient reevaluated by the veterinarian.

References

1. Bull, in: *Animal Models of Thrombosis and Hemorrhagic Diseases.* HEW Publ #76-982, Nat Instit Health, Washington, DC, 1975.
2. Perman and Schall, in Ettinger: *Textbook of Veterinary Internal Medicine.* 2nd ed. WB Saunders, Philadelphia, 1983.
3. Feline Pract **7(5)** (1977) 29.
4. Pract Vet **50(1)** (1979) 14.
5. Kirk and Bistner: *Handbook of Veterinary Procedures and Emergency Treatment.* 2nd ed. WB Saunders, Philadelphia, 1975.
6. Comp Cont Ed Pract Vet **6** (1982) 521.
7. Thornton, in Kirk: *Current Veterinary Therapy IV.* WB Saunders, Philadelphia, 1972.
8. Proc Ann Mtg AAHA **47** (1980) 187.
9. JAVMA **163** (1973) 988.
10. JAVMA **167** (1975) 56.

BANDAGES AND DRESSINGS

by K. Kazmierczak

Uses

A bandage is a piece of gauze or other material applied to a limb or other portion of the body. If the animal is confined to a cage, a bandage can prevent contamination from urine, feces, dander and other contaminants. It can also prevent the animal from chewing and licking the affected area.

A bandage can maintain the proper environment for healing of an open wound by keeping the area clean and free of contaminants that could cause an infection and delay healing. A bandage can also provide support to weakened tissues or control edema associated with fractures or blunt trauma. Bandages can be used to limit or prevent use of a limb with a fracture or after joint surgery to aid healing.

A bandage can be applied to secure a catheter for IV fluid administration. Neck bandages are commonly used to secure a jugular catheter and limb bandages for a cephalic vein catheter. When large areas of skin have been undermined or large areas of tissue removed, a bandage can be applied to prevent seromas by compressing dead space.

Table 4. Materials Used in Bandages

Materials	Trade Name	Manufacturer
Adhesive tape	Zonas	Johnson & Johnson
	Orthalectic-Porous	Parke-Davis
	Curity Standard Porous	Kendall
Elastic gauze	Kling	Johnson & Johnson
	Stretch Gauze	Parke-Davis
	Kerlix Rolls	Kendall
Elastic tape	Elastikon	Johnson & Johnson
	Conform	Kendall
Gauze	Absorbent Gauze Roll	Parke-Davis
	Gauze Roll	Kendall
	Nu-Gauze	Johnson & Johnson
Adhesive elastic wrap	Vet-Wrap	3-M
	Coban	3-M
Nonadherent sponges	Curity Telfa Pads	Colgate-Palmolive
	Release	Johnson & Johnson
	Micro Pad	3-M
	Telfa "Ouchless"	Kendall
	Non-Stick Sterile Pads	Johnson & Johnson
Roll cotton	Absorbent Cotton	Parke-Davis
	Red Cross Cotton	Johnson & Johnson
	Curity Cotton Roll	Kendall
Roll padding	Sof-Rol	Johnson & Johnson
	Specialist Cast Padding	Johnson & Johnson
	New Webril Orthopedic	Kendall
Sponges	Topper	Johnson & Johnson
	Gauze Sponge	Parke-Davis
	Unisorb	Parke-Davis
	Kerlix	Kendall
	Sof-Wick	Johnson & Johnson
Stretch bandage	Ace	Becton Dickinson
	Dyna-Flex	Johnson & Johnson
	Rediflex	Parke-Davis
	Tensor Elastic Bandage	Kendall

Bandage Materials

The most commonly used bandage materials are gauze sponges, gauze, elastic gauze, roll cotton, adhesive tape, elastic tape, roll padding, nonadherent sponges, and nonadherent elastic wrap (Table 4). The type and purpose of a bandage determine the combination of materials used. For example, to prevent a seroma postoperatively, the bandage may consist of gauze sponges placed along the incision line for absorption, elastic gauze to hold them in place, and elastic tape or elastic wrap to apply slight compression. The same materials can be used for a granulating wound. However, nonadherent gauze sponges (*eg,* Telfa Pads: Colgate-Palmolive) can be used in place of gauze sponges. Nonadherent sponges cause less disturbance of a granulating tissue bed each time the bandage is changed than do other types of sponges.

Bandage Application

Application and care of the bandage are important if it is to achieve the desired results.

When bandaging a limb, the most important rule is to apply the bandage material in a spiral fashion to prevent development of pressure rings on the skin. A pressure ring occurs when bandage materials have been applied in a circular fashion or a bandage has slipped from its original position. A constrictive, encircling bandage can cause severe edema within 24 hours.

To ensure a bandage is not applied too tightly, it should be possible to easily slip 2 fingers under the edge of the bandage (Fig 40). This also applies when securing an IV catheter; if too tight, the bandage impairs flow of fluids. When the limbs have been bandaged, the toes should be checked at least twice a day for signs of edema or coldness.

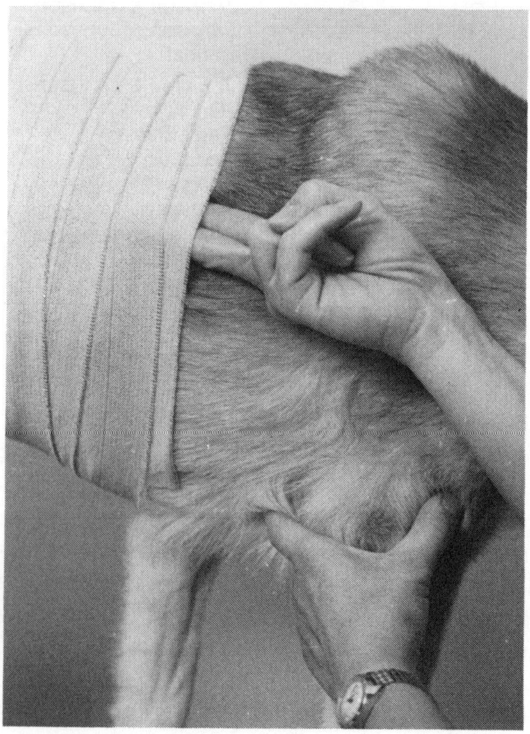

Fig 40. Testing bandage tension by inserting 2 fingers beneath the bandage.

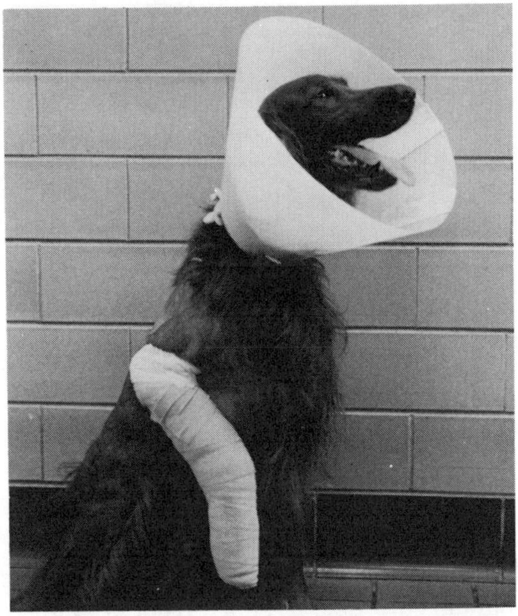

Fig 41. Use of an Elizabethan collar to prevent bandage removal.

If this occurs, the bandage should be removed immediately to restore proper blood circulation.

Elastic tape should be pulled off the roll and then laid onto the animal without any tension, unless mild compression is desired. If stretched and applied with too much tension, it can lead to edema of

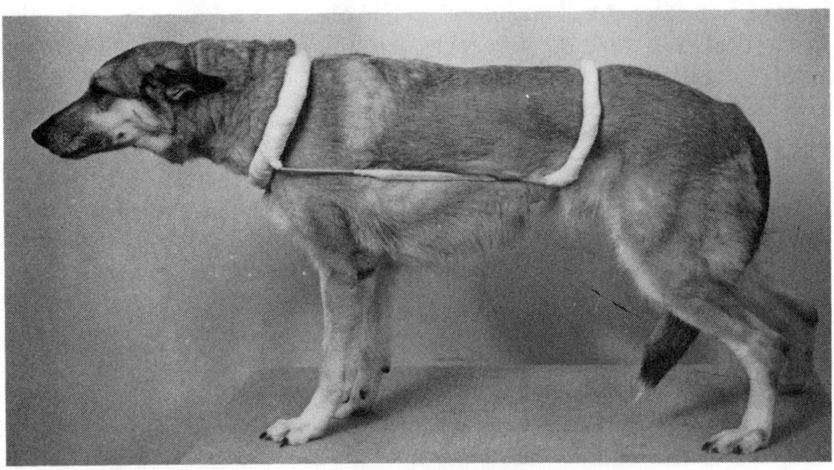

Fig 42. A side brace can be used to prevent self-mutilation.

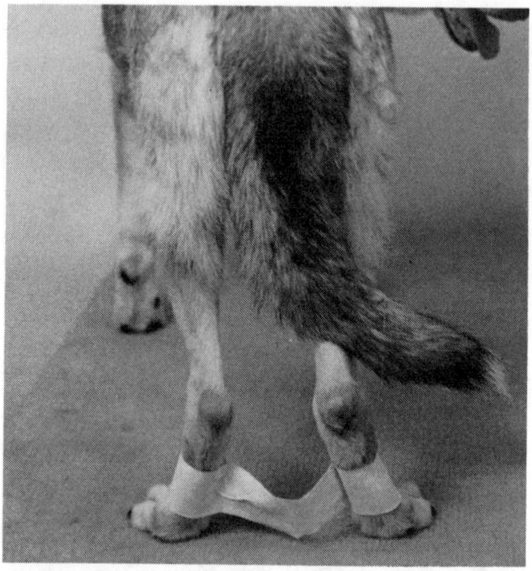

Fig 43. Hobbles made from bandaging material can be used to prevent injuries caused by excessive scratching.

bandaged limbs, dyspnea from a bandaged thorax, head or neck, or choking when applied to the head and neck region.

Chafing caused by bandages occurs most often in the axillary and groin areas. Talcum powder, medicated powder, or baking soda can be applied to relieve the irritation. Chafing may be prevented if the powder or baking soda is applied to the dry skin in these areas when the bandage is first applied.

The animal should be prevented from chewing, licking or scratching the bandage. Application of an Elizabethan collar (Fig 41) or side brace (Fig 42) may be necessary. Hobbles can be used to prevent scratching at a thoracic, abdominal, head or neck bandage (Fig 43). It should be noted that scratching may be a signal that the bandage is causing some discomfort.

Head and Neck

The head and neck region may be bandaged after ocular surgery, repair of an aural hematoma or cervical spinal surgery, or to secure a pharyngostomy tube or jugular catheter. Care must be taken not to restrict respiration, swallowing, eating or vision (this may be unavoidable under certain circumstances).

It should be easy to slip 2 fingers under each end of the bandage (Fig 40). If the bandage is too tight, the animal will show signs of dyspnea or difficulty swallowing, or may scratch at the bandage. To remedy this, the bandage can be cut to relieve the tension. Tape can then be laid over the cut bandage without any tension. This prevents having to replace the entire bandage.

If the bandage loosens, it most frequently slips caudad. If this occurs, the bandage should be removed immediately, as it can restrict respiration.

Occasionally an animal scratches at the bandage in an attempt to remove it. In such cases, it may be necessary to put hobbles or an Elizabethan collar on the animal.

Thorax

The thorax is most routinely bandaged when securing a chest drain, stabilizing fractured ribs, or protecting large thoracic wounds. The major concern when bandaging the thorax is not to impair respiratory movement. The tightness of the bandage can be checked by easily slipping 2 fingers under either end of the bandage (Fig 40). Tape, especially elastic tape, should be pulled off the roll and laid onto the animal without any tension. If the animal shows signs of dyspnea, remove the bandage immediately, as it may be too tight.

A common failure is slippage of a thoracic bandage. To help prevent this, be sure the tape is adhered to 1-1½ inches of hair at the cranial and caudal edges of the bandage.

If the animal scratches at the bandage in an attempt to remove it, hobbles will be necessary.

Abdomen

Indications for bandaging the abdomen are radical mastectomy or other extensive dissection of the abdominal region, hernia repair,

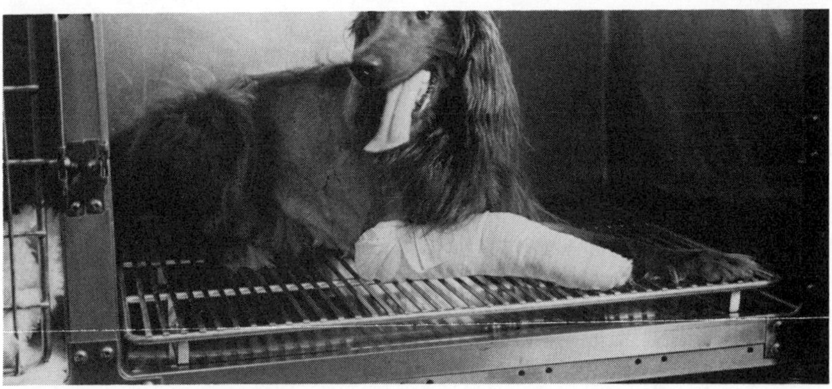

Fig 44. Use of a cage rack to elevate a patient from the cage floor and prevent bandage contamination.

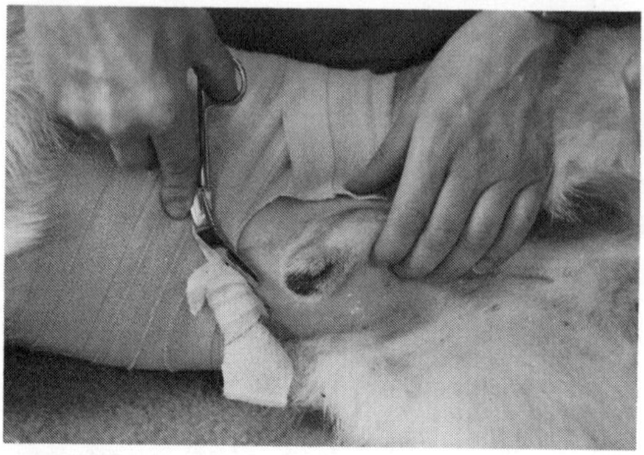

Fig 45. Modification of an abdominal bandage may be necessary in male dogs to prevent urine contamination.

placement of a drain, or securing a gastrostomy tube (a tube placed into the stomach through the abdominal wall).

To prevent the bandage from slipping caudad, it must be taped securely to the hair at the cranial end or even up on the chest.

It should be easy to insert 2 fingers at either end of the bandage to check that the bandage has not been applied too tightly. If the bandage is too tight, it can impair respiration or cause discomfort.

When an animal is confined to a cage and recumbent, the bandage becomes contaminated with urine and feces. This can be avoided by using a special rack to elevate the animal off the cage floor and allow for drainage of urine and feces (Fig 44).

The prepuce must not be included in a bandage on the abdomen of a male dog, as it can interfere with urination (Fig 45).

Limbs

Indications for bandaging a limb include postoperative immobilization of fracture repairs, protection of granulating wounds, and stabilization of a limb for fluid therapy.

A Robert Jones bandage is commonly applied to temporarily stabilize fractures before definitive treatment. This bandage consists of several layers of roll cotton compressed tightly with elastic gauze and elastic tape. Note that this is the only type of bandage in which elastic gauze and tape are applied tightly. The underlying layers of cotton prevent constriction of the limb.

When bandaging the thigh, knee, proximal (upper) forelimb or elbow, the entire limb should be included. Application of the bandage should begin at the paw and continue proximad in a spiral fashion (Fig 46). This allows even distribution of pressure along the limb and maintains venous return from the paw.

To ensure the bandage has not been applied too tightly, it should be possible to slip 2 fingers under the proximal end of the bandage. The toes should be checked twice a day for edema, coldness or an abnormal odor, which are signs of decreased venous return.

If the bandage has slipped from its original position due to the animal's movement or chewing, the bandage may cause a pressure ring. Remove the bandage immediately if it has slipped or the toes become edematous.

Keeping a limb bandage dry and clean presents special problems in regard to exercising an animal. A wet, soiled bandage presents a perfect environment for proliferation of microorganisms, which could lead to infection or moist dermatitis. This can be avoided by taping a plastic bag around the limb when the animal is exercised outside and then removing it when the animal is returned inside. It is not advisable to use a rubber band to secure the bag, as it can slip off and constrict blood flow. If the bandage becomes wet, it should be removed immediately and a dry dressing applied.

Paw

The paw is normally bandaged after declawing cats, dewclaw removal in dogs, and repair of lacerations to the toes or foot pads.

To ensure adequate venous return from the paw, 2 fingers should easily slip under the proximal end of the bandage. The tape should be applied in a spiral fashion to prevent pressure rings.

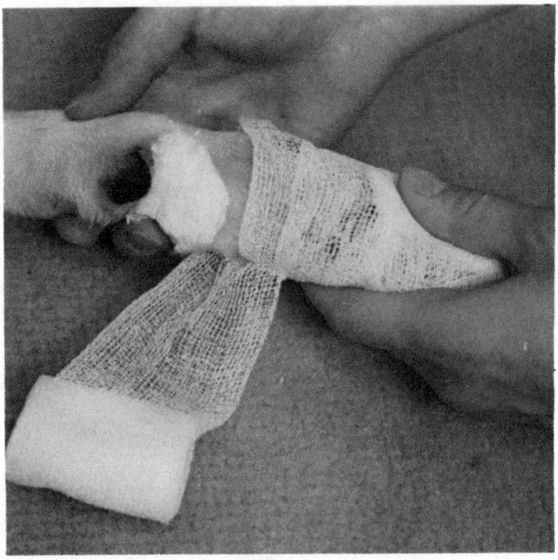

Fig 46. Starting a limb bandage at the distal end of the leg.

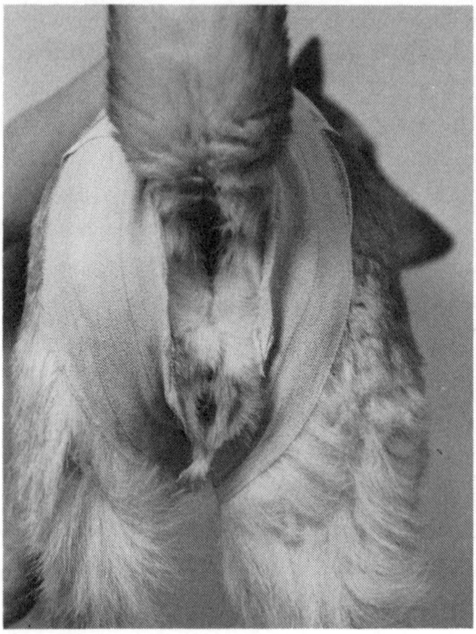

Fig 47. Proper placement of a pelvic bandage in a female dog.

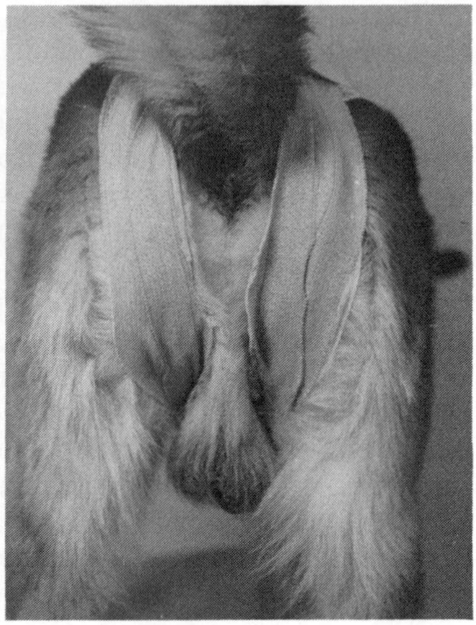

Fig 48. Proper placement of a pelvic bandage in a male dog.

When bandaging the paw, the accessory pad should also be included in the bandage. A small piece of cotton under the pad helps prevent irritation (Fig 46). Chafing could occur if the bandage were applied just under the accessory pad.

To keep the bandage dry when the animal is exercised outside, a plastic bag may be applied around the bandage and secured with tape. The bag should be removed immediately when the animal is returned inside. If the bandage becomes wet, it should be removed immediately to prevent possible infection and a dry bandage applied.

Pelvis and Groin

Mastectomy, repair of perineal hernias, abscesses, wounds with drains and pelvic surgery are a few situations requiring bandaging in this area. This is perhaps the most difficult area to bandage.

The bandage should not be applied tightly. Check by slipping 2 fingers under the cranial edge of the bandage and where it encircles the legs. The legs, vulva or scrotum may become edematous if the bandage is too tight.

The bandage must not include the vulva, prepuce, scrotum or anus so as not to impair the animal's ability to urinate or defecate (Figs 47, 48). The bandage should be checked at least twice a day for dryness. If the bandage becomes soiled with urine or feces, it must be changed. Placing the animal on a rack may aid in keeping the bandage dry (Fig 44).

To prevent the bandage from slipping caudad, apply tape to 1-1½ inches of hair around the cranial edge of the bandage.

Tail

Occasionally there may be a need to bandage the tail, as in partial tail amputation, granulating wounds or tumor removal. The major problem is securing the bandage.

In animals with a long tail, it may be necessary to apply the bandage 1 inch on either side of the lesion, or over the entire tail. In animals with a docked tail, tape should be applied loosely around the tail head.

An Elizabethan collar or side brace may be necessary to prevent the animal from chewing the bandage off (Figs 41, 42).

Home Care of Bandages

When an animal is discharged, the owner must be instructed on how to maintain the bandage. The bandage should be kept clean and dry. A plastic bag can be taped over the bandage when the animal is outside and removed when indoors, so the bandage may "breathe." The animal should be relatively confined, with exercise only on a leash.

Self-mutilation must be prevented and the animal observed twice daily for edema or coldness of the toes, or an odor from the bandage. If the bandage becomes wet or loose, the toes become edematous, or the animal removes the bandage, the client should notify the veterinarian immediately. It may be necessary to have the animal examined to evaluate the wound and possibly replace the bandage.

These home care instructions can be printed with the name of the clinic and veterinarian, and the telephone number and given to the client upon the animal's discharge. The technician should review this information with the client at the time the animal is discharged.

Recommended Reading

Routes of Drug Administration

Dodman, in Lane: *Jones' Animal Nursing.* 3rd ed. Pergamon Press, Oxford, England, 1980.

Firth, in Catcott: *Animal Health Technology.* 2nd ed. American Veterinary Publications, Santa Barbara, 1977.

Haskins, in Sattler *et al: Veterinary Critical Care.* Lea & Febiger, Philadelphia, 1981.

O'Hagen, in Lane: *Jones' Animal Nursing.* 3rd ed. Pergamon Press, Oxford, England, 1980.

Vet Tech **5** (1984) 340.

Tube Feeding

Firth, in Catcott: *Animal Health Technology.* 2nd ed. American Veterinary Publications, Santa Barbara, 1977.

Comp Cont Ed Anim Health Tech **1** (1980) 29.

JAAHA **19** (1983) 207.

Dental Prophylaxis

Frost: *Canine Dentistry: A Compendium.* Day Communications, 1982.

Tholen: *Concepts in Veterinary Dentistry.* Veterinary Medicine Publ, Edwardsville, KS, 1983.

Vet Tech **5** (1984) 286.

Vet Tech **5** (1984) 356.

Urine Collection

Bush, in Lane: *Jones' Animal Nursing.* 3rd ed. Pergamon Press, Oxford, England, 1980.

Osborne and Stevens: *Handbook of Canine and Feline Urinalysis.* Ralston Purina, St. Louis, 1981.

Eye Care

Anim Health Tech **4** (1983) 198.

Severin: *Veterinary Ophthalmology Notes.* 2nd ed. Colorado State Univ Press, Fort Collins, 1976.

Slatter: *Fundamentals of Veterinary Ophthalmology.* WB Saunders, Philadelphia, 1981.

Ear Care

Venker-van Hagen, in Kirk: *Current Veterinary Therapy VIII.* WB Saunders, Philadelphia, 1983.

Physical Therapy

Vet Clin No Am **5** (1975) 157.

Mod Vet Pract **58** (1977) 39.

Downer: *Physical Therapy for Animals.* Charles C Thomas, Springfield, IL, 1978.

Mod Vet Pract **60** (1979) 115.

Comp Cont Ed Anim Health Tech **2** (1981) 199.

Comp Cont Ed Anim Health Tech **2** (1981) 262.

Whittick: *Canine Orthopedics.* Lea & Febiger, Philadelphia, 1974.

Bandages and Dressings

Knecht *et al: Fundamental Techniques in Veterinary Surgery.* 2nd ed. WB Saunders, Philadelphia, 1981.

5

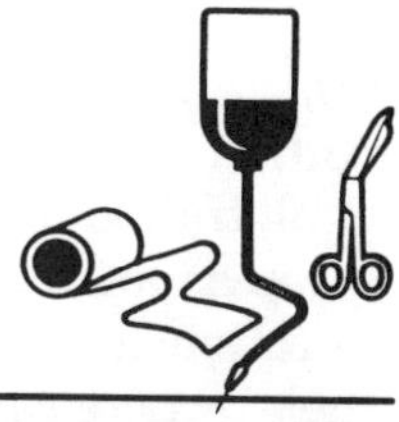

treatment technics for horses

A.M. LAMAR

The continual development of new drugs and drug vehicles has changed and will continue to change the methods by which horses are treated. But even with these changes, basic treatment technics remain essentially the same. This chapter describes several methods to give oral, parenteral and topical medication, to collect blood and urine specimens, and to apply many types of bandages.

Giving Medication

Oral Administration

Per os (PO) and oral are terms used to indicate medication given via the mouth. This is the most convenient and least painful method of giving medication. However, it has some disadvantages.

The effectiveness of oral medication depends on how well the drug is absorbed from the stomach or intestines. Absorption is much slower than with parenteral use (injection). It is also difficult to ensure that the total volume of medication is swallowed, even when the most adept person administers the treatment. Despite these drawbacks, the oral route is used frequently by veterinary personnel and horse owners.

Several types of medication can be given PO. Anthelmintics (worm medication) now come in various forms, such as powder, granules, liquid and paste, and are approved for use in feed or as a drench. Anti-inflammatory drugs, such as phenylbutazone and flunixin meglumine (Banamine: Schering) can be given as powder or granules in the feed,

Acknowledgment: The author thanks Dawn Christenson, LVT, for her assistance with the illustrations.

tablets by bolus, crushed tablets in a palatable medium, or pastes. Antibiotics are marketed in tablet, capsule, liquid and paste forms. Oral tranquilizers may be given with grain. Electrolytes may be given as an additive to drinking water. Animals that do not tolerate injections or gastric intubation (stomach tubing) or those treated by their owners can be medicated PO.

Oral medications may be given in several ways. The least reliable method is addition of the medication to the grain or drinking water. Many horses taste the additives and refuse to eat or drink entirely or, if the medication is in the grain, may pick out the grain and leave the drug, particularly if the grain and drug do not mix well.

Years ago, the balling gun was commonly used (Fig 1). It is still used for administering tablets or boluses but can cause problems. If the tablet or bolus is dry, it may become lodged in the esophagus. If the drug is irritating, it may erode through the pharyngeal or esophageal mucosa. Tablets or boluses given by balling gun should be lubricated well and placed as far back in the mouth as possible. The patient must be watched carefully after administration, as the medication may be dropped from the mouth if it is not deposited near the back of the tongue. The swallowing reflex can be stimulated by gently rubbing the roof of the mouth with the balling gun or allowing the horse to eat a small amount of grain after the tablet has been given.

Dose syringes are another common means of giving oral medication (Fig 1). They may be obtained as stainless steel syringes in vari-

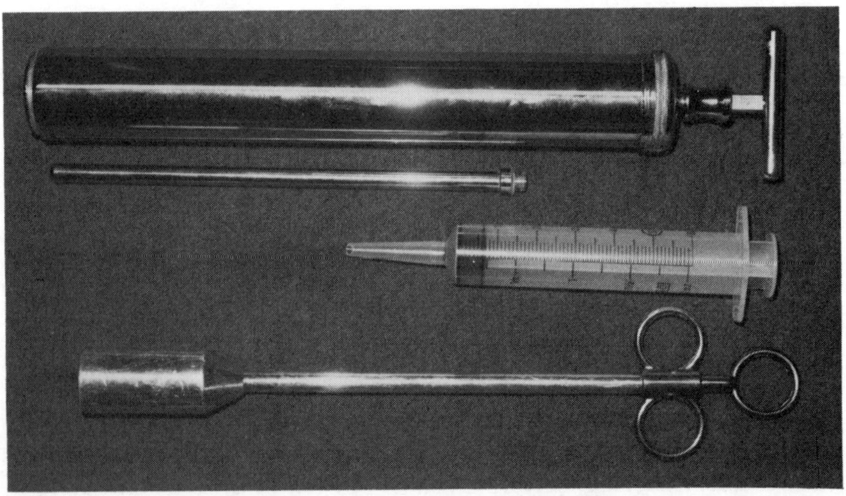

Fig 1. Oral medication devices. Top: 12-oz dose syringe with an 8-inch tip. Middle: 2-oz plastic catheter-tipped syringe. Bottom: balling gun.

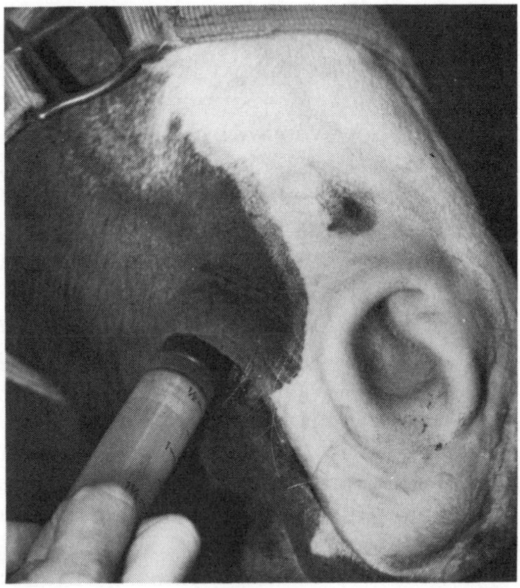

Fig 2. Use of a dose syringe. Introduce the syringe at the buccal commissure, avoiding the check teeth. Inject slowly, allowing the horse to swallow frequently during administration.

ous sizes (2-, 6- and 12-oz), with tips of different lengths (4- and 8-inch), or as catheter-tipped, plastic syringes (2-oz). Care must be taken when using the plastic variety, as they can be easily crushed by the horse's teeth. Premixed liquid medication and powders or crushed tablets mixed with molasses or syrup may be given by dose syringe. Water should not be used to dissolve oral medication because the resultant solution is too thin; a gruel or paste-like consistency is best.

To properly use a dose syringe, stand at the horse's head, holding the halter with one hand, and introduce the syringe at the buccal commissure (corner of the mouth) with the opposite hand (Fig 2). Advance the syringe as far back on the tongue as possible, avoiding the cheek teeth. Discharge the medication slowly, allowing the horse to swallow while it is being given. If the horse does not swallow on its own, rubbing the tongue or the roof of the mouth with the tip of the syringe often stimulates swallowing. Elevating the horse's head slightly also helps prevent the medication from trickling out of the mouth. If the head is held too high, however, some of the medication may be aspirated into the trachea, which could result in pneumonitis. Using drugs in paste form has helped resolve this problem. By thickening the consistency of the medication, the chance of aspiration is reduced and more of the drug is retained and swallowed.

Most horses do not object to this method, but some form of restraint may be necessary on those that do.

Nasogastric Intubation

Nasogastric intubation ("tubing") is used to deposit medication, fluids or nutrients directly into the stomach. It is more effective than the balling gun or dose syringe. Many horses object to this method of treatment; however, with proper restraint, medication can be given without difficulty. Even though the skill of "tubing" horses requires extensive practice and entails the danger of nasal, pharyngeal and esophageal trauma and inadvertent tracheal intubation, nasogastric intubation is commonly used to give anthelmintics, lubricants, astringents, fluids and nutrients to horses.

Selection of a tube of proper diameter is the first step in nasogastric intubation. Many types of tubes are available, from very small tubes for foals to very large tubes for draft horses. The length is generally the same despite the tube's diameter. If the tube is too small, it passes too easily, making it difficult to determine its location. If it is too large, it traumatizes the nasal turbinates and may cause epistaxis (nosebleed). An average 1000-lb horse requires a medium-sized tube (5/8-inch outside diameter).

Restraint is extremely important during nasogastric intubation. It is very difficult to pass a nasogastric tube if the horse is continually moving about. The nasal turbinates may also be damaged if the horse tosses its head while the tube is in the nasal cavity. If the horse is to be "tubed" in a stall, both restraint and intubation should be applied from the same side to decrease the possibility of injury to everyone involved. When using treatment stocks, restraint may be applied from either side during intubation. Generally, a lip twitch is sufficient restraint. If this is inadequate, tranquilization may be indicated.

Before intubation, the tube should be warmed in a bucket of clean, warm water so it is pliable. A lubricant, such as water or K-Y Jelly (Johnson & Johnson) should be applied to facilitate tube passage. The tube may be inserted into either nostril; technicians should be able to pass the tube from both sides. If standing on the left side of the horse, loop the tube over the left arm and place the palm of the right hand over the bridge of the horse's nose, with the thumb inserted into the nostril (left hand if standing on the right side), making certain the fingers do not occlude the opposite nostril (Fig 3). When holding the horse in this manner, lateral movement of the head can be controlled, the neck can be flexed, and the tube can be easily directed into the ventral meatus of the nasal cavity.

Insert the tube into the nostril with the left hand and advance it slowly and gently, at the same time pushing down on the tube with the thumb of the right hand. In an average horse, the tube should proceed about 12 inches caudad before it stops at the dorsal pharyngeal

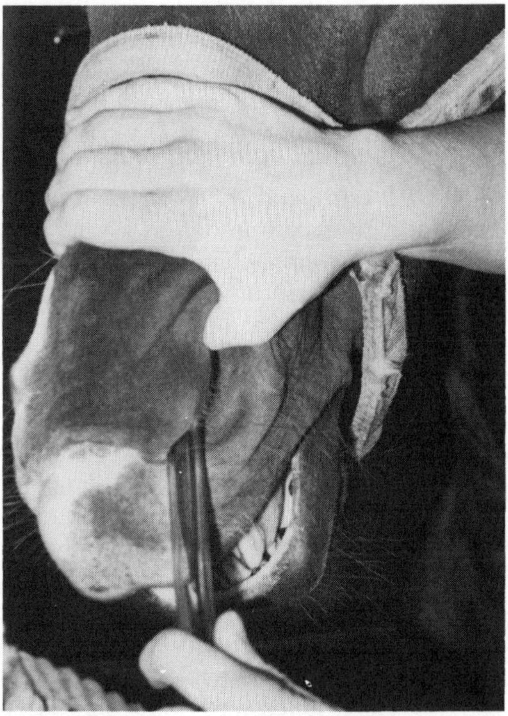

Fig 3. Passing a nasogastric tube. Place the palm of the hand over the bridge of the horse's nose, insert the thumb into the animal's nostril, and advance the tube under the thumb with the opposite hand.

wall. If the tube stops before this, it may be in the middle meatus. If this is the case, the procedure should be repeated and the tube directed ventrad into the ventral meatus. When the tube stops at the pharynx, gentle movement back and forth should stimulate the swallowing reflex. If this does not occur, slowly rotating or blowing into the tube may cause the animal to swallow. Throughout this portion of the procedure, the throat region should be observed. When the horse swallows, the tube should be advanced 4-6 inches. Once the tube is in the esophagus, passage of the tube may be enhanced by gently blowing into the tube to dilate the muscular wall of the esophagus.

Throughout this procedure, there are numerous ways to ensure that the tube is in the correct location. As mentioned previously, if caudal progression of the tube ceases before it is inserted to about 12 inches, it is more than likely in the middle meatus. Force applied at this point often produces epistaxis.

When the tube reaches the pharynx, it can enter either the esophagus or the trachea. If it enters the trachea, most horses cough; however, this is not a reliable indicator as to the location of the tube because horses with pharyngitis may cough even if the tube is in the esophagus. Also, if the tube is in the trachea instead of the esophagus, it advances very easily due to the open structure of the trachea as compared to the collapsed state of the esophagus. (Overly small tubes also pass easily in the esophagus.) Occasionally, the tube may rattle against the sides of the trachea, which indicates its location. This is determined by shaking the trachea at the ventral aspect of the neck with one hand. If respiration can be heard or felt through the nasogastric tube, it is definitely in the trachea and should be withdrawn and the procedure repeated.

If the tube passes into the esophagus as desired, the first thing observed is the amount of pressure required to advance the tube. The esophagus is a muscular structure that remains closed, except when an object is moving through it. For this reason, the tube is much easier to advance when air is gently blown ahead of the advancing tube. Another sign of correct tube placement is visualization of the tube passing through the esophagus. This may be observed in most horses over the left side of the neck, near the jugular furrow. In some horses, however, the esophagus may be located on the right side of the neck.

It is important not to confuse passage of the tube with the jugular pulse, which is present in many horses. By slowly advancing and withdrawing the tube while applying manual pressure over the area, the tube may be felt and its presence in the esophagus confirmed. In horses with very thick necks, the tube may not be seen at all. Two distinct tubular structures, *ie,* the esophagus with the tube in place and the trachea, may be felt in horses with very thin necks. These cannot be discerned in most horses, however.

The final sign observed when passing a nasogastric tube occurs when it enters the stomach. Gurgling sounds are heard in most horses and are often accompanied by a distinct gastric odor. Administration of medication must not proceed until the tube is, without a doubt, in the stomach.

When the tube is in the stomach, the medication may be administered with a stomach pump, dose syringe or funnel. After the medication has been given, give 12 oz of water then gently blow through the tube to force most of this fluid into the stomach. Before withdrawing the tube, cap the end or kink it to prevent material remaining in the tube from leaking out as it passes the trachea. Such leakage may cause aspiration, with subsequent pneumonitis. The head should be held very still as the tube is removed so as to prevent the end of the tube from striking the turbinates and causing hemorrhage.

One complication that may result from nasogastric intubation, no matter how carefully performed, is epistaxis. If this occurs, the patient should be kept quiet until the hemorrhage ceases (usually in 10-20 minutes). Towels held over the nostril absorb the blood, but some horses may resist this and hemorrhage even more. Because only a very small amount of blood is lost through intubation-related epistaxis, there is no great cause for alarm.

Intradermal Administration

The intradermal (ID) route of administration involves injection of a small quantity of medication between the dermis and epidermis. Medication given in this way is absorbed much more slowly than with SC, IM or IV injection. This route is used most often for allergy testing, though some vaccines may be given ID as well.

An ID injection may be given anywhere on the body, most commonly on the lateral aspect of the neck. Before injection, the skin should be cleansed with 70% alcohol and allowed to dry. A small area of skin may then be picked up by thumb and forefinger to isolate the area for injection

Select a small needle (25-ga, 5/8-inch) and introduce it into the dermis by pressing it against the skin at a slight angle, pushing it forward at the same time. Once inside the tissues, aspirate (withdraw the plunger of the syringe slightly) to make certain a vessel has not been entered and then inject slowly. Resistance should be felt as the solution is injected. A prominent bleb (raised area) rises shortly after the injection has begun. If this bleb is not seen immediately, withdraw the needle and repeat the procedure.

Subcutaneous Administration

Medication given by the subcutaneous (SC) route (beneath the skin) is absorbed faster than with the oral and ID routes but slower than with the IM and IV routes. Drugs commonly given SC include some vaccines, local anesthetics and any other drug for which slow absorption is required.

Subcutaneous injections are most frequently given on the side of the neck. The injection site is cleansed with 70% alcohol and allowed to dry. This area of skin is then firmly grasped between the thumb and index finger, forming a tent of skin into which the needle is introduced (Fig 4). A 20- to 25-ga, 5/8- to 1-inch needle is selected, inserted under the skin and advanced to the hub. Once the needle is in place, aspirate to make certain a vessel has not been penetrated; then inject slowly. The solution should flow easily and a bleb should be evident directly under the skin. Gentle massaging of the area after injection may increase circulation to that area and consequently increase the absorption rate.

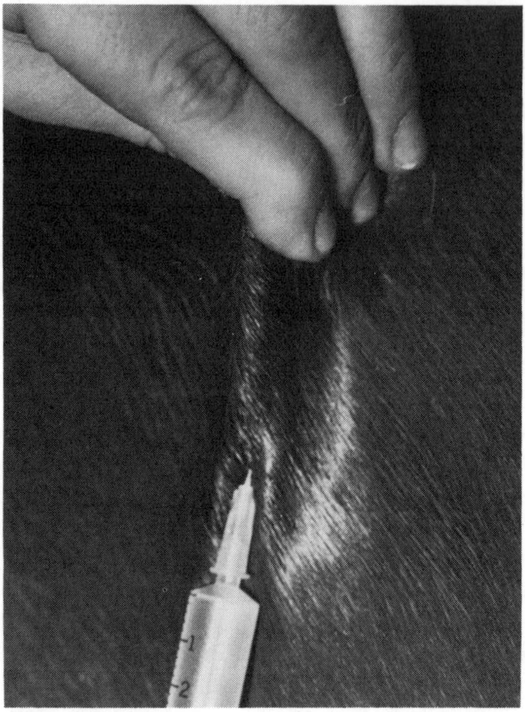

Fig 4. Subcutaneous injection. A "tent" is formed, into which the injection is given, when the skin on the lateral aspect of the neck is pinched.

Local anesthetics are given SC as diagnostic nerve blocks on the limbs, around lesions before potentially painful treatment or in areas on which surgery is to be performed under local anesthesia. These areas are usually cleansed thoroughly with a surgical scrub before injection of the anesthetic. If the anesthetic is to be deposited over the legs, abdomen or face, it is almost impossible to pick up a fold of skin. However, introducing the needle at an angle nearly parallel to the skin should result in proper needle placement. Sluggish flow of solution may indicate ID needle placement, necessitating repositioning the needle slightly deeper. If a bleb does not appear while injecting, the needle may be placed too deeply. If the injection is made into edematous tissues, however, a bleb is rarely seen.

Intramuscular Administration

Intramuscular (IM) injection, or injection of medication directly into a muscle, is commonly used in horses. Drugs given IM are absorbed relatively quickly. Intramuscular injection is usually easier for owners than ID, SC or IV injections. Care must be taken to make certain the drug is not inadvertently injected into a blood vessel, as severe reactions can occur if such drugs as procaine penicillin G enter the systemic circulation. This is more likely to happen using the IM route than with ID or SC injection.

Several sites can be used for IM injections in horses. A series of injection sites should be used, to minimize muscle damage and pain, if large amounts of medication are to be given over a long period. The largest muscle masses are located in the hindquarters. The gluteal muscle is located high on the rear limb, lateral to the vertebral column and caudal to the point of the hip (Fig 5). The disadvantage to using this muscle is that it is difficult to detect inflammation caused by the injection; any injection abscesses are difficult to drain from this location. It is a large muscle mass, however, and can be used when necessary.

The semimembranosus and semitendinosus muscle groups, located on the caudal aspect of the rear limb between the point of the

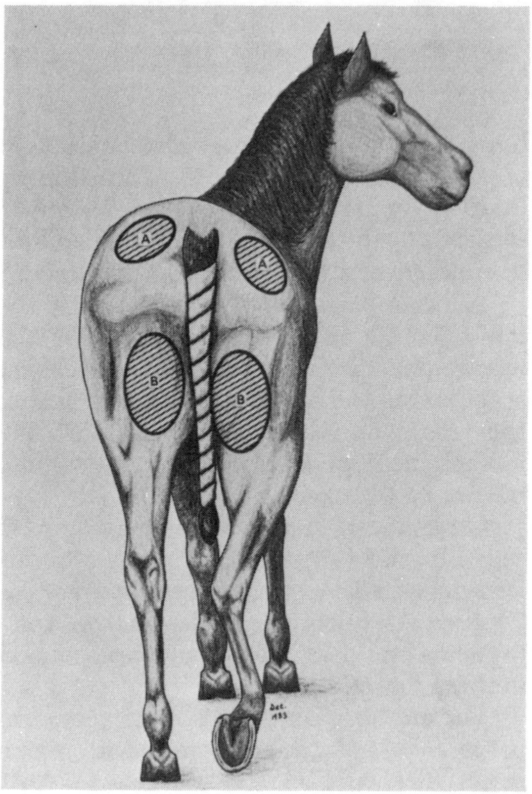

Fig 5. Intramuscular injection sites. A. gluteal muscles. B. semimembranosus and semitendinosus muscle groups.

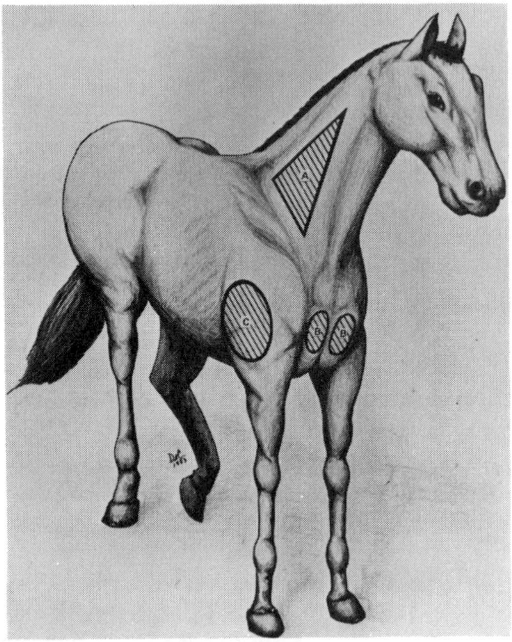

Fig 6. Intramuscular injection sites. A. lateral muscles of the neck. B. pectoral muscles. C. triceps muscle.

buttock and the hock, may also be used (Fig 5). This large muscular area can be used often, with minimal complications. It is the choice location for IM injections in foals because of its large size. Though repeated IM injections in the rear legs may cause some degree of lameness, this usually subsides over several days after the last injection.

Another location for IM injection is the group of muscles on the lateral aspect of the neck. This area is bordered dorsad by the ligamentum nuchae, ventrad by the cervical vertebrae and caudad by the scapula (Fig 6). Large volumes of medication should not be injected in this area due to the small muscle mass. Foals should not be injected in their neck muscles because the resultant soreness may inhibit nursing.

Other muscle masses that may be used are the pectoral and triceps muscles (Fig 6). However, these muscles are relatively small, even in well-developed horses, and are therefore used infrequently. Frequent IM injections in the pectoral and triceps groups may result in edema and pain. Nor should large amounts of medication be given in these muscles.

For an IM injection in a rear muscle mass, the animal should be properly restrained, according to its temperament, and the required materials should be readily available. An 18- to 20-ga, 1- to 1½-inch

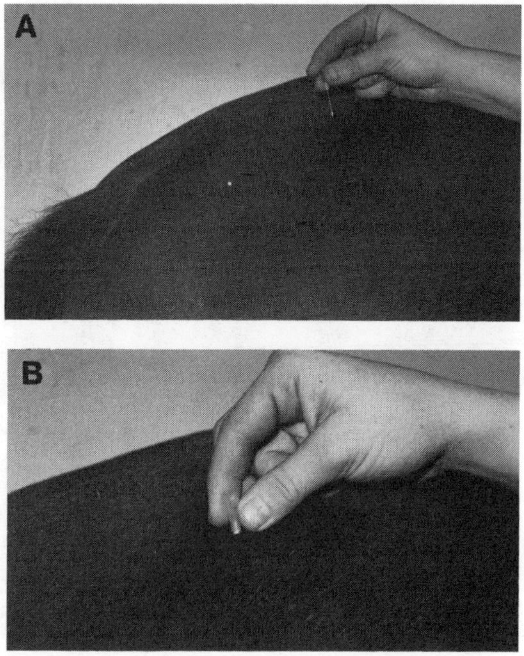

Fig 7. Injection into the gluteal muscle. A. When injecting into the muscles of the rear quarter, detach the syringe and hold the needle by the hub, with the point directed downward. B. Rhythmically tap the injection site with the side of the hand. On the third tap, insert the needle into the muscle to the hub.

needle is usually adequate. When injecting the gluteal muscle, the safest place to stand is very close beside the horse's hindquarters, facing caudad. If the horse attempts to kick while the operator is standing in this position, its movements can be felt and one can move aside before the kick.

The central area of the muscle is identified and the skin cleansed with 70% alcohol solution. The needle should be removed from the syringe for insertion because it is less awkward to place the needle into the muscle without the syringe attached. Also, if the horse reacts adversely to needle insertion, the needle usually remains in the muscle, should the horse move, if the added weight of the syringe is not present.

When inserting the needle in a rear muscle mass, hold it firmly between the thumb and index finger at the hub, with the point directed ventrad (downward) (Fig 7A). Immediately before introducing the needle into the muscle, the area should be tapped firmly with the edge of the fist (Fig 7A). This stimulates the nerve endings in the area, thereby decreasing the initial pain of needle penetration. After 2 quick, rhythmic taps, the needle is thrust through the skin and into the muscle on the third tap (Fig 7B). Very few horses react adversely to this method.

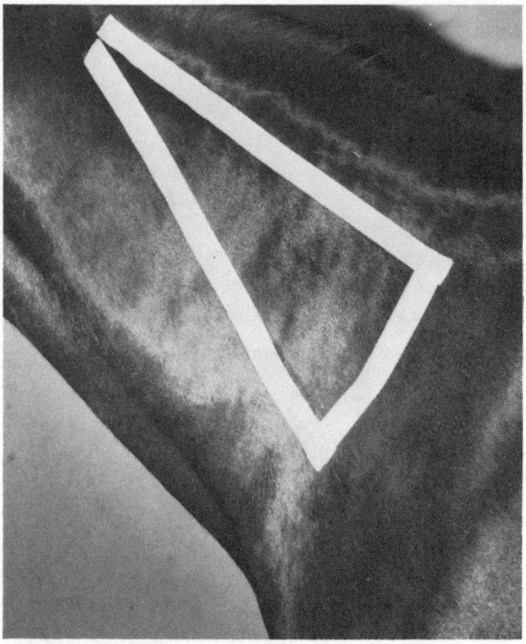

Fig 8. The muscular area of the neck is bordered dorsad by the ligamentum nuchae, caudad by the scapula, and ventrad by the cervical vertebral column.

After insertion, the needle should be sunk to the hub and the syringe attached. Before injecting the medication, aspirate (slightly withdraw syringe barrel) to make certain a vessel has not been penetrated. If blood is withdrawn into the syringe, remove the needle and repeat the procedure 2-3 inches from the original site or select a different muscle group altogether. Inject the drug slowly after the needle is properly placed. Do not inject more than 10-15 ml into one site, as excessive tissue distention by large volumes of injected liquid can result in tissue necrosis. If more than 15 ml is to be given, divide the dose and use 2 or more sites 2-3 inches apart. These divided doses should be given as separate injections rather than withdrawing the needle slightly and redirecting it. Moving the needle around once it is in the muscle causes excessive tissue trauma. Once the injection has been completed, the needle is withdrawn and properly disposed of.

The technic used for injecting into the semimembranosus and semitendinosus muscles is similar to that described for the gluteals. The recommended injection site is about halfway between the gastrocnemius tendon and the point of the buttock, in the thickest portion of the muscle. The needle is introduced in the manner previously described. To safely inject an unruly horse, reach across the horse and inject into the opposite leg; most horses that kick will do so with the

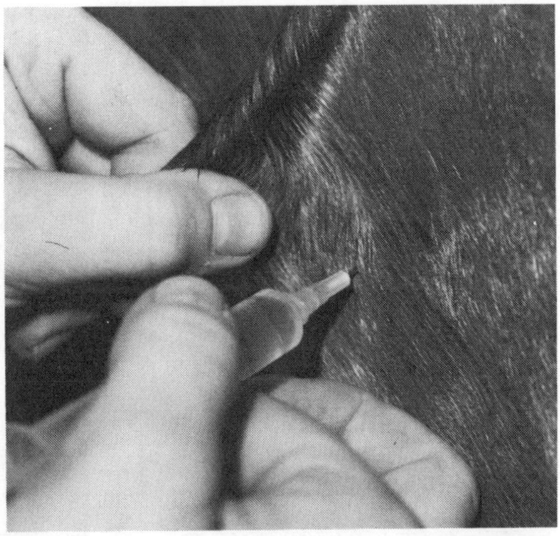

Fig 9. Injection into the lateral muscles of the neck. Grasp a fold of skin, introduce the needle perpendicular to the muscle, aspirate, inject, remove the needle and release the skin.

leg being injected. The same technic can be used when injecting into the gluteal muscle of a kicking horse, provided the animal is short enough that the opposite side can be seen.

Though the restraint technics are similar, the method for injections into the lateral muscles of the neck differs significantly from that used in the hindquarters. The best injection site is located by drawing an imaginary triangle on the neck, with the ligamentum nuchae, cervical spine and scapula as the borders (Fig 8).

A small area within this triangle is cleansed with 70% alcohol and allowed to dry. A portion of skin immediately adjacent to the selected injection site is then picked up between thumb and index finger (Fig 9). This acts as a form of restraint, transferring painful sensations elsewhere while the needle is inserted. Also, after the injection has been given and the skin is released, the needle holes in the skin and muscles are several inches apart, preventing leakage of the drug to the exterior, as so often occurs in the hindquarters. The slapping technic used for IM injections in other muscle groups may cause some skittish horses to become head shy after repeated injections into cervical muscles. For this reason, many technicians and veterinarians avoid "slapping" a needle into this area.

After the skin has been elevated, the needle is inserted gently to the hub, with or without the syringe attached (Fig 9). After aspiration to avoid inadvertently injecting into a vessel, the medication is given slowly. After the injection, the needle is withdrawn and the skin released. Premature release of the skin may bend the needle, traumatizing surrounding tissues.

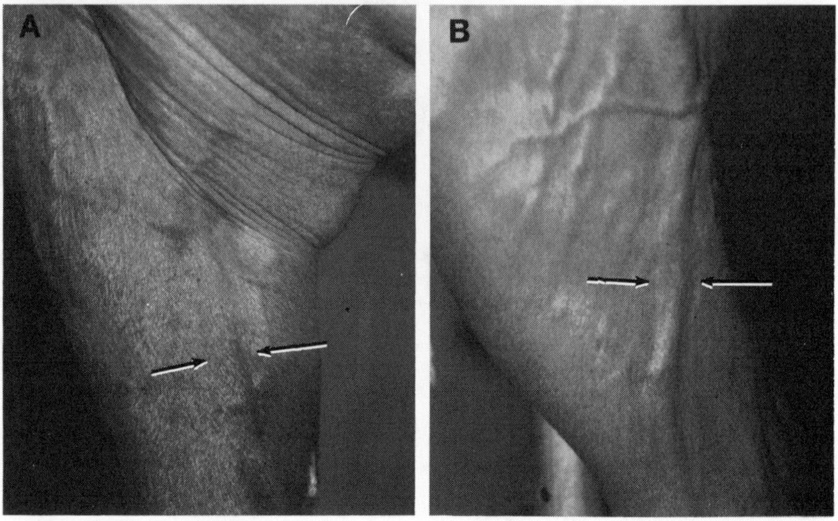

Fig 10A. The cephalic vein (arrows) on the equine forelimb. B. The saphenous vein (arrows) on the equine hindlimb. In both of these photos, the horse's head is to the left.

Other muscle groups that may be used for IM injections are the triceps and the pectoral muscles (Fig 6). The technic used in these areas is identical to that used in the hindquarters.

Intravenous Administration

Intravenous (IV) injection allows the drug to bypass the absorption process and enter the bloodstream directly, rapidly providing high blood levels of the drug given.

Several veins are used for IV injections in horses. The most common vein used is the jugular vein, a large vein located on the ventrolateral aspect of the neck in what is termed the "jugular furrow" (Figs 11, 13). In most horses this can be recognized as a depression, 1-2 inches wide, extending bilaterally along the entire length of the neck from the angle of the jaw to the shoulder.

Other vessels that may be used include the cephalic and saphenous veins. The cephalic vein is located on the medial aspect of the forearm, proximal to the carpus (Fig 10A). The saphenous vein is on the medial aspect of each rear limb, extending from the inguinal region to the distal tarsus (Fig 10B). Though they are both rather prominent vessels, it takes skill to penetrate them because they move freely under the skin and most horses resent being injected in these areas.

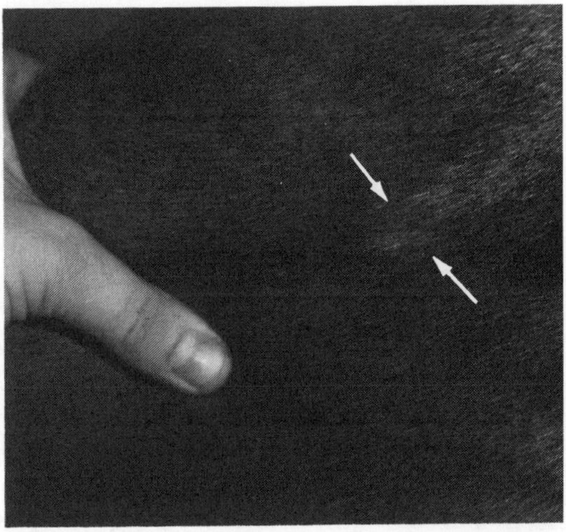

Fig 11. Occlusion of the jugular vein midway down the jugular furrow allows the vein to fill. A distinct distension of the vein (arrows) is evident cranial to the thumb.

The size of the needle used for IV injections should be proportional to the size of the vein. In the cephalic and saphenous veins, a 20- to 22-ga, 1-inch needle is used, while an 18- to 20-ga, 1- to 1½-inch needle is used in the jugular veins. Smaller needles may be required when working on ponies and foals. If repeated injections are to be given, a smaller needle should be used to minimize the tissue trauma associated with venipuncture.

The technic used for venipuncture is essentially the same for all veins. To locate (raise) the jugular vein, digital pressure is applied with a thumb over the jugular furrow about two-thirds of the way down (caudal on) the neck. With blood flow obstructed, the distended vein is seen immediately above (cranial to) the thumb (Fig 11). If the vein is not readily identified, alternate application and release of pressure over the jugular furrow to detect filling of the vein with blood. "Strumming" or lightly tapping the vein cranial to the thumb with the opposite index finger may cause waves in the jugular vein, which assist in identifying the vessel. Because the cephalic and saphenous veins are very superficial in most horses, raising of these veins is usually unnecessary.

In horses with very thick necks, it may be very difficult or nearly impossible to see the jugular vein. Palpating the muscles on either side of the jugular furrow may be the only means of locating the vein in such horses. Once the vein is identified, the overlying skin is cleansed thoroughly with 70% alcohol. This not only cleans the skin but also smoothes down the hair, making the vein more visible. The needle is inserted, bevel up, at a 30° angle to the vein. It may be inserted toward the heart or toward the head, depending on personal preference.

Whether or not the syringe should remain attached during venipuncture is open to discussion. When the syringe is in place during the procedure, very little manipulation of the needle is required to complete the injection; however, it is more difficult to determine if the blood aspirated into the syringe is venous or arterial. This problem may be remedied by inserting the needle alone and observing the character of the blood exiting the needle. If, however, a very small-bore needle is used, the characteristic "arterial spurt" may not occur, which may lead to an intraarterial injection that could have serious side effects. The technic used is based on personal preference.

The venipuncture method selected depends on the behavior of the patient. One successful method involves pressing firmly, with the needle, on the skin over the vessel while slowly sliding the needle forward and into the vein. This eliminates the possibility of surprising the animal, thereby dislodging the needle. The needle is more accurately placed and trauma to surrounding tissues is minimized. If the patient reacts adversely to this approach, a quick thrust with the needle through the skin may be required for venipuncture. With the quick-thrust method, the needle may not adequately enter the vein, and may require redirection once it is through the skin and the patient quiets down.

When the needle is believed to be in the vein, aspirate to ensure a good backflow of blood. If this is not observed, slightly advancing, withdrawing or rotating the needle may position it so it is directed into the vessel's lumen. Once the needle is properly placed, release the vessel and inject slowly and evenly. Aspirate frequently throughout the injection, especially after any movement of the animal, to ensure that all of the medication is given IV. After the injection, remove the needle and apply digital pressure (with fingers) to the injection site until all hemorrhage has ceased.

Complications: The most common mistake made during IV injections is injecting medication into the perivascular tissues (around, rather than in, the vein). Severe irritation by such drugs as phenylbutazone or sodium pentothal may lead to sloughing of the overlying skin. If a caustic drug is injected outside a vein, infiltrate the SC tissues at the site with saline and lidocaine. This dilutes the drug and relieves the pain an irritating drug may cause.

Another complication of improper IV injection is phlebitis, which may result from perivascular injection but is also associated with undue trauma to the vessel during venipuncture. Dull or barbed needles can extensively damage the vessel wall, as can repeated attempts to enter the vessel. Progression of this condition into thrombophlebitis may result in complete occlusion of the vessel. If this occurs bilaterally, the head may swell due to poor venous return.

A very serious complication of improper IV injection is intraarterial injection. Medication given in this way may produce mild disorientation, convulsions and possibly death within a few seconds after beginning the injection. If the animal does recover, it may take only a few minutes or several days. Intraarterial injections are best avoided by working in a well-lit area, applying adequate restraint, using an appropriately sized needle, observing the character of the blood aspirated and recognizing the early signs of intraarterial injection so that immediate steps can be taken to treat the patient.

Intravenous Catheterization

Intravenous catheterization is commonly used in horses requiring extensive fluid therapy. If properly cared for, indwelling catheters may remain functional for several days. However, when IV catheters are improperly placed or poorly maintained, several complications may result. These may range from local infections at the catheter exit site, to thrombophlebitis and embolus formation, which could eventually lead to death. Therefore, proper aseptic technic is required for this avenue of therapy.

The jugular veins are most frequently used for IV catheterization. The cephalic and saphenous veins may also be catheterized, but limb movement often results in excessive movement of the catheter, which

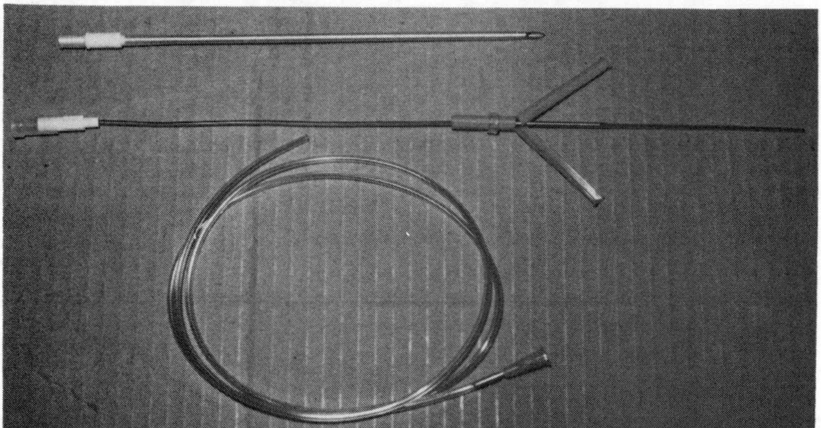

Fig 12. Intravenous catheters. Top: over-the-needle catheter. Middle: through-the-needle catheter. Bottom: polyethylene tubing with blunt needle adaptor.

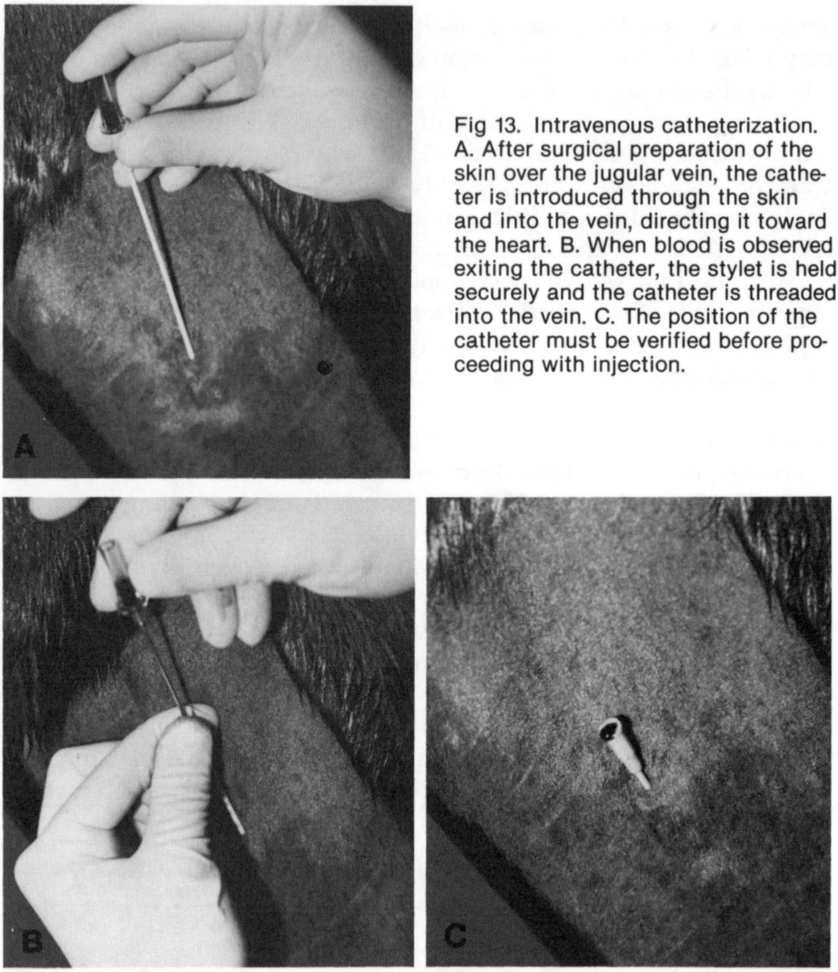

Fig 13. Intravenous catheterization. A. After surgical preparation of the skin over the jugular vein, the catheter is introduced through the skin and into the vein, directing it toward the heart. B. When blood is observed exiting the catheter, the stylet is held securely and the catheter is threaded into the vein. C. The position of the catheter must be verified before proceeding with injection.

may lead to thrombosis of these vessels. The lateral external thoracic vein is used occasionally but only when the previously mentioned veins are no longer patent (open or clear). This vein is located on the lateral thorax, immediately caudal to the elbow; it is not easily discerned, making a "cut down" (incision and retraction of overlying skin) necessary before catheterization.

Many types of catheters are available for use in horses (Fig 12). The selection of catheter size is based on vessel size and the rate at which the fluids must be given. Over-the-needle catheters are most often used in adult horses due to the large diameter and durable construction of these catheters. Through-the-needle catheters come in

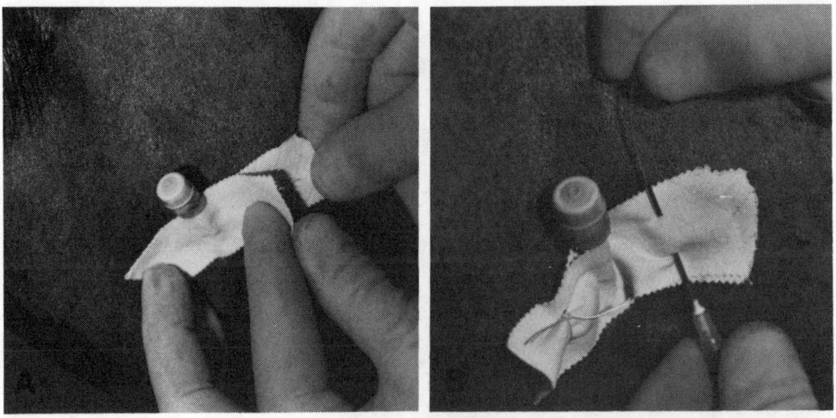

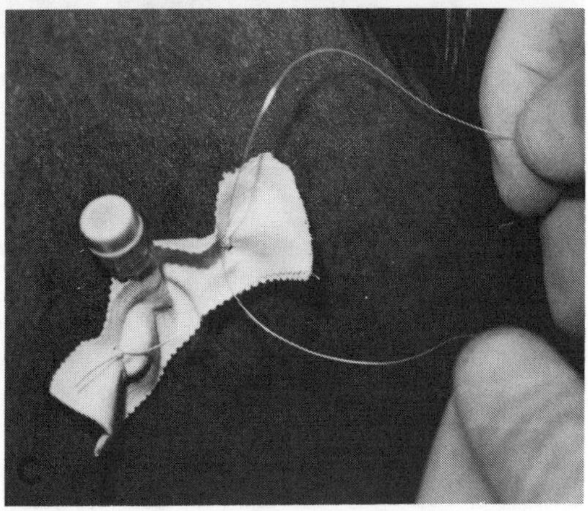

Fig 14. Securing the IV catheter with a tape butterfly. A. A 4-inch section of adhesive tape is folded in half and secured to itself around the catheter. B. A piece of suture material is placed through the tape and skin, using a hypodermic needle as a guide. C. The sutures are tied over the tape.

smaller sizes that are ideal for ponies and foals. These smaller catheters are less rigid, however, and caution is required to prevent bending upon insertion.

Commercially prepared sterile catheter units are most often used. Catheters may also be prepared from polyethylene or Silastic tubing, and fitted with a needle adaptor. These pieces of tubing are sterilized and inserted through a large-bore needle.

The area chosen for catheterization should be clipped and surgically scrubbed, with local anesthetic injected if desired. Wearing sterile gloves, locate the vein and insert the needle through the skin and into the vein, toward the heart. Before removing the needle from the catheter and threading the catheter down the vein, aspirate with a syringe or hold off the vein securely to ensure a backflow of blood, signifying proper placement. Advance the catheter off the needle and down the

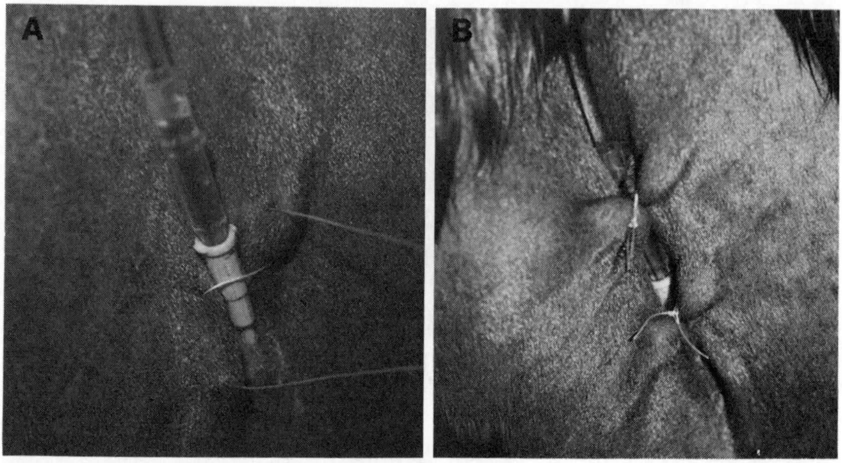

Fig 15. Catheters may be secured by suturing the skin over the catheter hub and extension lines. A. Place the suture through the skin on each side of the catheter so the free ends are in opposite corners. B. Tie the sutures to pull the skin over the catheter and extension lines.

vein gently until its entire length is in the vein. Catheter placement must again be verified before continuing (Fig 13). Once the catheter is in its proper position, cap it and then flush it with heparinized saline. To prevent the catheter from moving about within the vessel, the catheter's end should be sutured to the underlying skin. Securing the catheter by bandaging is inadequate if it is to be left in place for an extended period. Catheters may be secured by various methods. Using a tape "butterfly" is one method (Fig 14). There are some disadvantages with this technic. The tape is not sterile and may increase the possibility of infection at the catheter's exit from the skin. Also, if the catheter becomes wet, the tape may loosen, which reduces its holding power. It is a relatively easy procedure, however, and works well under most circumstances.

Another method used to secure an IV catheter involves lifting and suturing the skin across the catheter hub (Fig 15). A piece of suture material is placed through the skin dorsal to the catheter. Before tying it, take the suture across the catheter hub and place it through the skin on the ventral side of the catheter in the same direction used on the dorsal suture. The free ends should be in opposite corners. Tying these ends pulls the skin over the catheter hub and holds the catheter more securely than the butterfly method.

Once the catheter is secured, antibacterial ointment is placed at the catheter's exit from the skin, with a piece of sterile gauze and

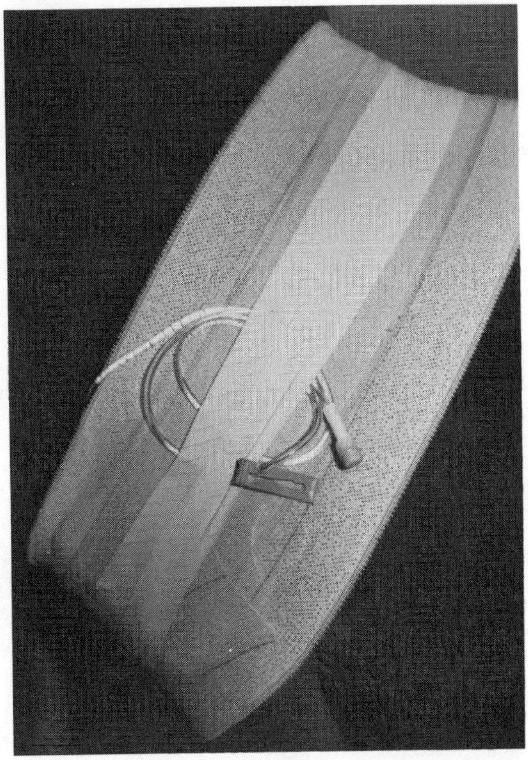

Fig 16. Apply a sterile dressing and gauze over the catheter's exit from the skin and bandage with an adhesive bandage. Loop the extension lines and secure with adhesive tape.

adhesive bandage material (*eg,* Elastikon: Johnson & Johnson) used to hold it in place. The IV drip extension line should be looped into or on top of the bandage and held in place with adhesive tape (Fig 16). Use of a loop in the extension line prevents direct traction on the catheter when the animal moves.

A method of inserting an IV catheter in foals may also be applied to adults. It involves running the catheter through a SC tunnel so that it exits on the side of the neck (Fig 17). This method reduces the possibility of infection and ensures secure catheter attachment.

Polyethylene or Silastic tubing, about 24 inches long and of appropriate diameter for the vein to be catheterized, is passed through a large (8- to 12-ga, 3- to 4-inch) needle. Material for incising and suturing skin should also be available.

Once the supplies have been selected, an area of about 3x3 inches over the jugular vein and another area of equal size, 3-4 inches dorsal to the first site, are clipped, scrubbed and infiltrated with a local anesthetic. A small incision is made over the jugular vein and the nee-

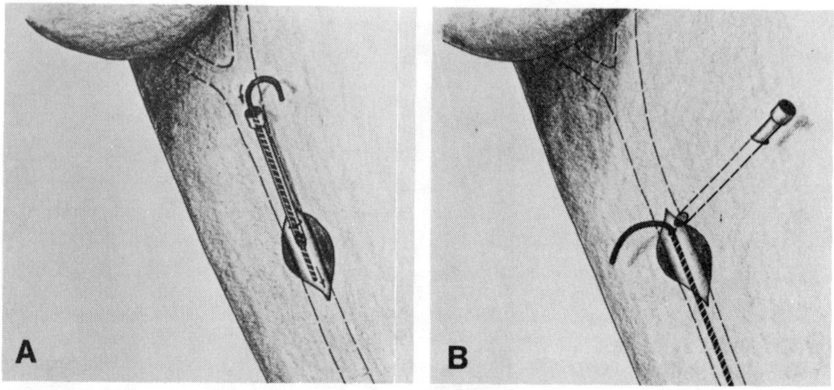

Fig 17. TUNNEL TECHNIC OF JUGULAR VEIN CATHETERIZATION.
A. After surgical preparation, make a small incision over the jugular vein, introduce a large-bore needle into the vein, and thread the catheter through the needle until 6-8 inches of the catheter lie in the vein. B. Remove the needle from the vein and thread the needle SC from the prepared dorsal site to the original incision.

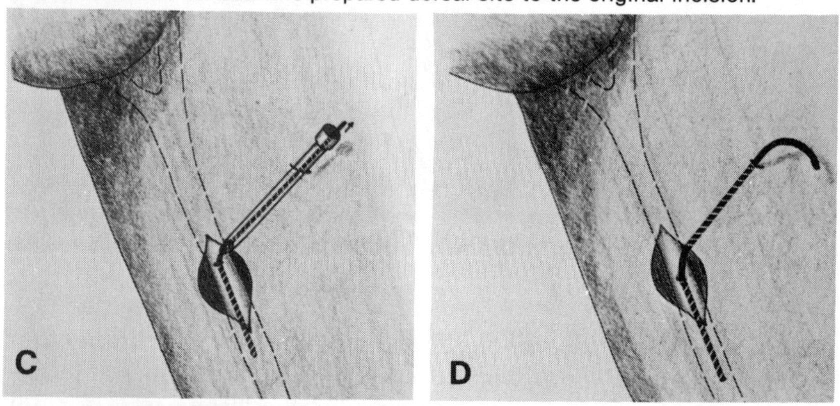

C. Thread the catheter back through the needle until the catheter lies smoothly in the SC space. D. Remove the needle.

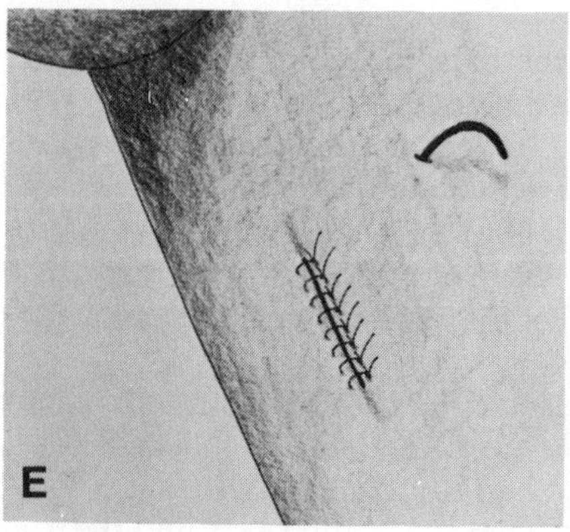

E. Suture the incision over the jugular vein and secure the catheter to the skin with a tape butterfly.

dle is inserted into the vein. The catheter is threaded down (toward the heart) this needle until 6-8 inches of it are within the vein. After the needle is withdrawn over the catheter, another small incision is made in the mid-cervical site and the needle is passed SC from this incision to the initial incision at the jugular vein. The catheter is then passed through the needle until it lies smoothly in the SC tissues. The needle is then removed. After both incisions are sutured, the catheter is secured at the exit and a bandage applied as previously described.

Complications: Complications can be minimized by using aseptic technic during catheterization, and by frequent examination and appropriate maintenance of the catheter and associated equipment. All supplies required must be sterile before use, and needles and catheters must be free of barbs and frays that could damage the vessel wall. Because the likelihood of thrombophlebitis increases the longer a catheter is left in place, the catheter should be changed at least every 72 hours. All associated IV tubing should be changed every 24-48 hours and the dressing replaced every 24 hours to decrease the possibility of contamination and resultant infection.

Intrauterine Infusion

Intrauterine infusions involve injection of liquid medication through an infusion pipette or catheter passed through the vulva, vagina and cervix, into the uterus (Fig 18). Indications for this procedure include treatment of intrauterine infections, and prophylactic medication after diagnostic procedures or artificial insemination.

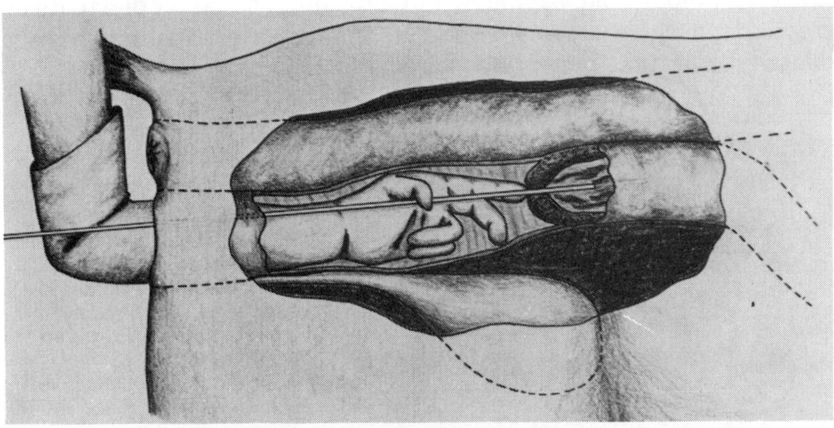

Fig 18. Intrauterine infusion. After thoroughly cleansing the perineal area, insert a sterile-gloved, lubricated hand through the vulva and into the vagina, guarding the tip of the catheter with the index finger. Insert the finger into the cervix and advance the catheter under the finger and into the uterus.

Because technicians are not permitted to give intrauterine infusions in some states, the clinician should be consulted before such treatment is given.

Proper preparation of the mare is important to avoid introducing microorganisms into the reproductive tract during the procedure. The tail should be wrapped with gauze or a clean bandage, after which it is held or tied up out of the way. The vulva must be scrubbed and rinsed thoroughly to remove contaminants, after which a small piece of wet cotton is used to swab the inner surface of the dorsal labial commissure (dorsal, inner aspect of the vulva) to remove fecal material that often collects there, particularly after rectal palpation.

Use of sterile equipment is essential. Disposable obstetrical (OB) sleeves may be gas sterilized or a sterile surgeon's glove may be placed over a nonsterile OB sleeve. An infusion pipette or Chambers intrauterine catheter (Wellcome) is placed in the palm of the hand, with the index finger covering the opening. A sterile, water-soluble lubricant, such as K-Y Jelly (Johnson & Johnson) or Ster-L-Jel (McCullough Cartwright), is applied to the dorsal surface of the hand and arm, which are then inserted through the vulva. Rotation of the hand and arm during insertion distributes the lubricant evenly and minimizes reproductive tract irritation. If the mare strains when the arm is inserted, wait until the animal relaxes and then proceed. At the cranial wall of the vagina lies the cervix.

In an estrual mare (in estrus), the cervix is relaxed and lies near the vaginal floor. Diestrual mares have a firm cervix located near the center of the cranial aspect of the vagina. During diestrus, digital (finger) manipulation may be required to enter the cervix due to its increased muscular tone. Postpartum mares (after foaling) have a dilated cervix that may allow passage of the entire hand.

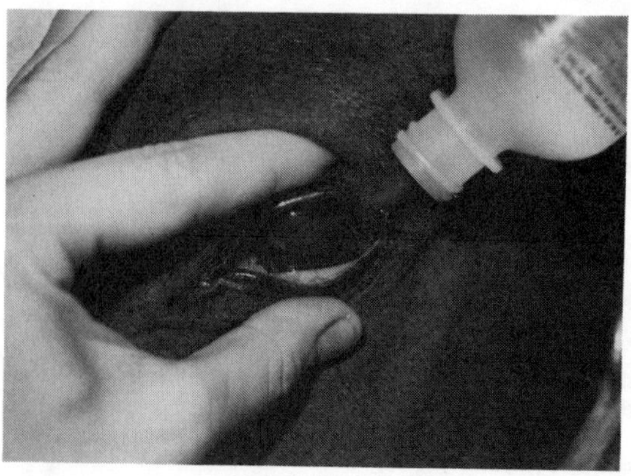

Fig 19. Topical application of ocular medication. Place the index finger dorsal to the margin of the upper eyelid and direct it dorsomediad, ventral to the supraorbital process. Evert the lower lid with the thumb of the same hand.

Once the cervix is located, advance the index finger through the os (opening) and slide the pipette under (ventral to) the finger until the pipette is 3-4 inches inside (cranial to) the cervix, near the uterine body. The medication is then infused through the pipette. If resistance is met during fluid infusion, withdraw or advance the pipette slightly, as its opening may be against the uterine wall. After the infusion, withdraw the pipette and cleanse the mare's vulva to remove excess lubricant.

Ocular Therapy

Diseases of the cornea, such as keratitis, ulcers, abrasions and lacerations, are often treated by topical application of ointments or solutions. A horse's cornea may be exposed by placing the index finger immediately dorsal to the margin of the upper eyelid and pushing it dorsomediad until it contacts the supraorbital process. The lower lid is everted by rolling it into position with the thumb of the same hand (Fig 19). A thin "ribbon" of ointment or a few drops of solution is then applied to the ventral conjunctival fornix. If ointment and solution must be used together, the solution should be applied first to prevent it from running over the ointment and out of the eye, wasting the solution and reducing its efficacy. Ophthalmic solutions must be

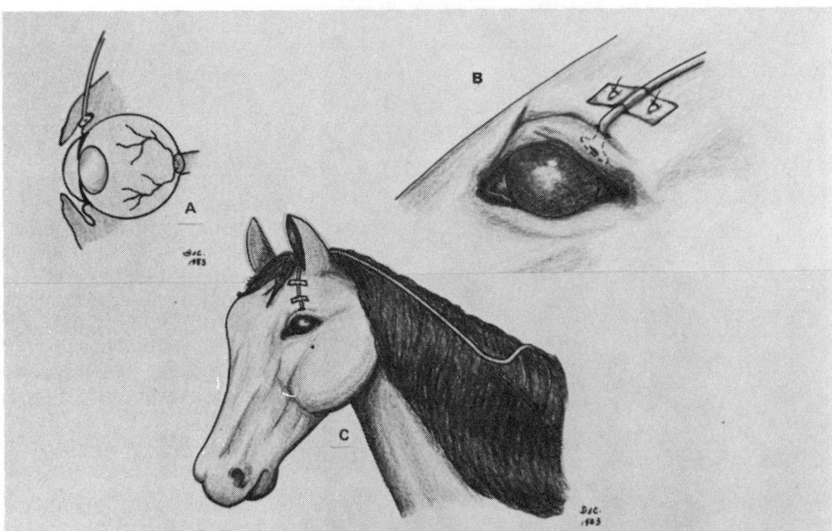

Fig 20. Subpalpebral catheter. A. Lateral section of the eye shows the flared end of the catheter fitted into the conjunctival fornix. B. The catheter sutured in place. C. Overall view of the subpalpebral catheter system. The catheter should be long enough to reach the withers, where it is secured with adhesive tape.

instilled often to maintain an effective concentration of the drug; ointments can be applied less often because of their prolonged contact time. The veterinarian should be consulted on which form to use.

Subpalpebral catheters are often used in uncooperative patients that require ocular therapy for extended periods. Most horses tolerate placement of these catheters under local or regional anesthesia; however, extremely fractious animals may require general anesthesia. Polyethylene tubing (PE 160 or 200) is prepared by applying heat to one end to create a flange (flared end) at the opening. The tubing should be long enough to reach from the eye to the withers.

A large (12-ga), hubless needle is introduced into the dorsal conjunctival fornix at the dorsolateral aspect of the upper eyelid. The plain (unflared) end of the catheter is threaded through the needle until the flange is fitted snugly into the conjunctival space (Fig 20), after which the needle is removed. The catheter is sutured to the skin dorsal to the eyelid with the aid of a tape butterfly (Fig 20). The free end of the catheter is fitted with a needle adaptor and injection cap (Becton-Dickinson), through which the medication is injected, and is

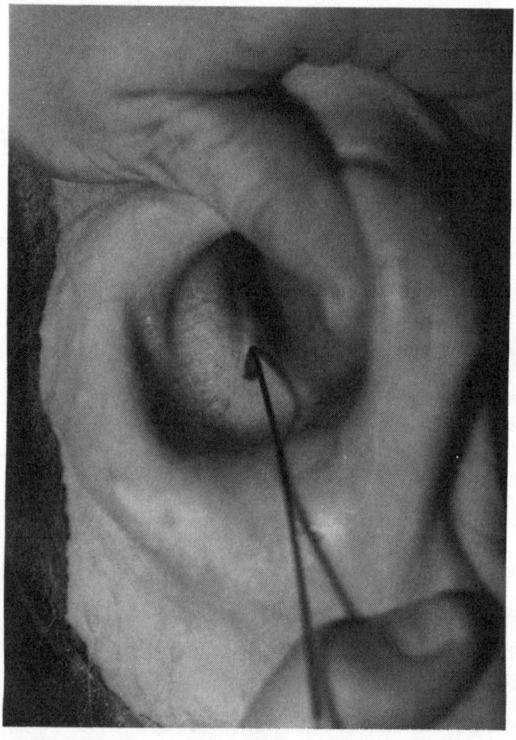

Fig 21. Retrograde catheterization of the nasolacrimal duct. The duct opening is located on the floor of the nasal cavity, near the junction of the skin and mucous membrane. Insert a smooth-tipped catheter into the duct, occlude the surrounding duct opening and gently inject the irrigating solution.

then secured to the mane at the withers with adhesive tape. After injecting solutions through the system, it is important to then inject air so that the medication is flushed out of the catheter and over the eye.

Nasolacrimal Duct Irrigation

Obstruction of the lacrimal apparatus (tear ducts) of the horse is usually unilateral (only on one side) and may be identified by epiphora (constant tearing) on the affected side. Retrograde (nose to eye) irrigation of the nasolacrimal duct is the most common means used to open obstructed ducts. A smooth tipped catheter such as a 5 French polyethylene catheter is most commonly used for this procedure.

With the horse properly restrained, the nasolacrimal duct opening in the nostril is identified on the floor of the nasal cavity near the junction of the skin and mucous membrane. A smooth-tipped, 5-Fr polyethylene catheter is gently threaded 2-3 inches inside the duct (Fig 21). The opening of the nasolacrimal duct is sealed around the catheter by applying digital pressure over the area to prevent backflow of the irrigating solution. The duct is considered patent (open) when irrigation fluid flows easily and exits readily at the medial canthus (inner corner) of the eye.

The ventral palpebral punctum at the medial canthus of the eye may be catheterized in cooperative horses. Because this opening is significantly smaller than the opening in the nostril, a smaller-gauge catheter is required than for retrograde flushing. The catheter is introduced through the punctum and into the nasolacrimal duct, after which irrigating solution is injected slowly and gently. The duct is considered patent when the solution flows easily from the opening in the nostril.

BLOOD COLLECTION AND ADMINISTRATION

Collecting Blood Samples for Diagnostic Tests

Blood samples are required for diagnostic tests, such as complete blood count (CBC), packed cell volume (PCV), blood chemistry analyses, blood gas studies, coagulation profiles, equine infectious anemia tests and many others. The amount of blood needed for these tests varies from less than 1 ml to 10 ml. The type of sample collected (*ie,* coagulated or anticoagulated) depends on the requirements of the test. These samples may be with a needle and syringe or with vacuum tubes and their needles (*eg,* Vacutainer: Becton-Dickinson).

The jugular vein is most commonly used to obtain venous blood samples, though the cephalic and saphenous veins may be used if necessary. An arterial sample may be obtained from the carotid artery,

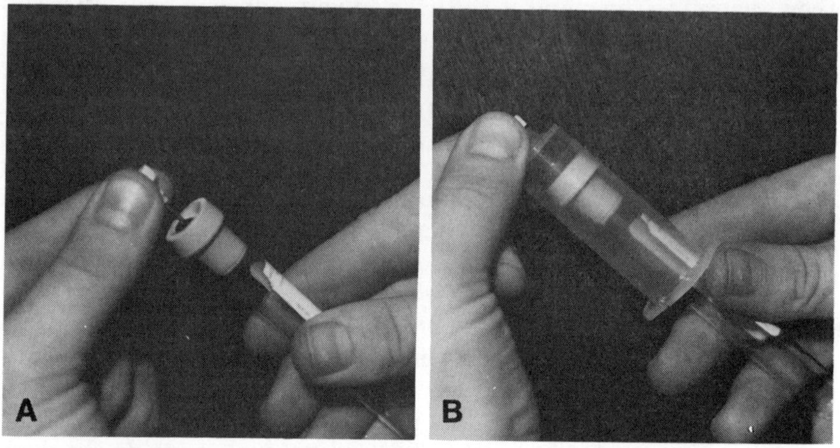

Fig 22. Blood collection. A. Using the Vacutainer system to collect blood, hold the hub of the needle securely, while advancing the tube onto the needle so that the other end of the needle remains in the vein's lumen. B. Use of a vacutainer needle holder allows the tube to be attached to the needle with very little manipulation.

located dorsomedial to the jugular vein in the jugular furrow, or the great metatarsal artery, found along the cranial aspect of the fourth metatarsal bone. The skin overlying the vessel should be prepared as for IV injections.

A 20- to 22-ga, 1- to 1½-inch needle is used for venous samples. The needle is introduced into the vein as for IV injections. If the Vacutainer system is used, the needle must be threaded into the vein and advanced to its hub. Failure to do so may result in penetration of the opposite wall by the needle or withdrawal of the needle from the vein when the tube is attached. When a backflow of blood is observed, digital pressure on the vein is released. The needle hub is held firmly between the thumb and index finger and the external end of the needle is forced through the center of the rubber stopper and into the tube (Fig 22). Use of a Vacutainer needle holder provides more accurate placement of the needle into the tube, with minimal manual manipulation (Fig 22).

If blood is not flowing adequately once the tube and needle are connected, withdraw, advance or rotate the entire unit slightly. The tube quickly fills with blood until the vacuum is depleted. Because the amount of anticoagulant present in each vacuum tube corresponds to the volume of blood the tube accommodates, it is important to allow these tubes to fill until the vacuum is depleted or the sample will be incorrectly diluted.

When the tube has filled, remove the needle from the vein, rotate the tube to mix the blood with the anticoagulant (if present in the tube), and apply digital pressure over the venipuncture site to prevent hemorrhage.

If Vacutainer needles are not used, blood may be collected with a needle and syringe and immediately transferred to an appropriate tube. Hemolysis may occur if the blood is rapidly injected into the tube through the needle. Hemolysis may be prevented by detaching the needle and depositing the blood directly from the syringe into the open tube.

When collecting small amounts (0.5-2 ml) of blood for such tests as a PCV or blood gas analysis, use of a needle and small syringe is adequate. Before collecting the blood, the syringe should be flushed with a small amount of heparin to prevent coagulation of the sample. When collecting a sample for blood gas evaluation, expel all air from the syringe after the blood is obtained so the values obtained are accurate. Insertion of the needle end into a rubber stopper prevents air from entering the blood-filled syringe during transport.

Palpation of an arterial pulse is the only indication as to the location of an artery. When attempting to obtain blood from the carotid artery, an 18- to 20-ga, 1½-inch needle attached to a heparinized syringe is used, as previously described. The arterial pulse may be detected by palpating the distal third of the jugular furrow. The carotid artery is more superficial in this area than at any other point along its course. It is located dorsal to the jugular vein and trachea.

Once the pulse is identified, the needle is inserted at a 90° angle (perpendicular) to the skin and advanced slowly toward the artery. Because the carotid artery moves rather freely in this location, several attempts may be required before the sample is collected. A bright-red spurt of blood exits the needle once the arterial lumen has been entered. After withdrawal of the needle, digital pressure must be applied over the site for as long as 5 minutes to prevent hematoma formation, a common event after arterial puncture.

The great metatarsal artery is much smaller than the carotid artery; therefore, a smaller (22- to 25-ga, 1-inch) needle is required for collection of blood from this artery. Due to its location, this artery is not often used because very few horses stand quietly while it is punctured. The arterial pulse may be detected along the cranial aspect of the fourth metatarsal bone. The needle is introduced at a 15-30° angle and blood collected in a heparinized syringe. Digital pressure must be applied to the area after collection, as in carotid artery puncture, to avoid hematoma formation.

Blood Transfusions

Severe blood loss, anemia, hypoproteinemia, hypogammaglobulinemia and neonatal isoerythrolysis are some conditions for which transfusions may be indicated in horses. Transfusions may consist of only blood cells, whole blood or plasma, depending on which deficiencies are present. Before blood is transfused, it should be crossmatched to assess the compatibility of the donor's and recipient's blood. Failure to do so may result in administration of incompatible blood, with a subsequent transfusion reaction. If whole blood is to be given, it must be compatible in both major and minor phases; that is, agglutination must not be observed when the donor's cells are added to the recipient's plasma (major) or when the recipient's cells are added to the donor's plasma (minor). When only plasma is to be given, compatibility is necessary only in the minor phase.

Blood Collection for Transfusion

After selecting a healthy, compatible blood donor, prepare the equipment used to collect large volumes of blood. Blood collection bottles containing acid-citrate-dextrose (ACD) may be purchased with accompanying blood collection and administration sets (Diamond Labs, Des Moines, IA). Empty evacuated containers (Fenwal Labs, Deerfield, IL), designed to accept plasma from the original collection bottle, are also prepared before plasma collection. Plastic bags are available as single or multiple Blood-Pack units (Fenwal), which have a detachable collection set containing citrate-phosphate-dextrose-adenine (CPDA-1), with or without an attached empty bag (transfer pack) (Abbott) that receives the cells or plasma from the original container.

The donor horse's jugular vein should be thoroughly scrubbed, after which a large (10- to 12-ga, 2- to 3-inch) needle is inserted into the vein, toward the heart. The collection tube is then attached to the needle and the opposite end inserted into the collection container. The jugular vein must be occluded (held off) continually throughout the procedure to enhance flow of blood into the container and prevent collapse of the vessel during collection, particularly when vacuum containers are used. During collection, the collection container should be rocked gently back and forth to mix the blood with the anticoagulant. Hemolysis may result if this is not done carefully. After the blood is collected, the needle is removed and digital pressure is applied to the site until all hemorrhage has ceased. The container of blood should immediately be labeled with donor identification and the date and time of collection

Whole blood may be given immediately after collection, but plasma may be given only after centrifugation or sedimentation to remove blood cells. The cells usually settle to the bottom of the container within 2 hours at room temperature. If plasma is not to be immediately transfused, the whole blood may be refrigerated for 12 hours, after which the blood cells may be separated. After cells are separated, plasma may be siphoned off or aspirated into a vacuum container.

The transfusion recipient must have an IV catheter inserted before the transfusion. The transfusion should be given through an administration set containing an in-line filter to prevent infusion of fibrin and blood clots. The first 100-200 ml should be given very slowly and the patient watched closely for signs of a transfusion reaction. The first sign of such a reaction is uneasiness, followed by dyspnea, tremors, and a fast, weak pulse. Collapse and apnea may result if the condition is not treated immediately. The transfusion should be immediately discontinued after the first signs of a reaction. Epinephrine and antihistamines may be required to treat horses with a transfusion reaction; therefore, these emergency drugs should always be immediately available when transfusions are given. The patient should be monitored throughout the transfusion; if no abnormalities are initially evident, the flow rate may be slowly increased and the transfusion completed.

URINE COLLECTION

Urine may have to be collected from a horse for several reasons. A urinalysis may be part of a routine physical examination. Such conditions as myositis, azoturia and urolithiasis may be diagnosed and monitored by urinalysis. The response to treatment of such conditions as cystitis may also be monitored by urinalysis. Finally, testing of the urine for the presence of certain drugs is now required at many race tracks and competitive horse shows.

Urine specimens may be obtained by catching a mid-stream sample during urination or by catheterizing the bladder. Catheterization provides a sterile sample, more suitable for microbial analysis than "free catch" samples.

Collecting Urine from Male Horses

A urine sample may be obtained easily from some male horses by placing the animal in a stall with fresh straw bedding. If the horse does not urinate within a short time, urination can occasionally be hastened by kicking the straw about. If a urine sample is required in a

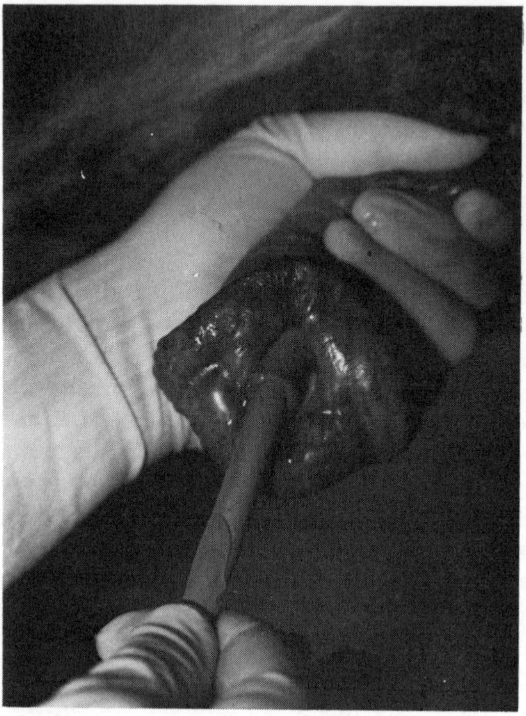

Fig 23. Urethral catheterization of the male horse. After thorough cleansing of the glans penis, a sterile, lubricated plastic or rubber catheter is introduced into the urethra and advanced into the urinary bladder.

short period, an injection of furosemide (a diuretic) promotes urination. When collecting a voided sample, allow the horse to urinate a small amount before collection, as the initial flow of urine may contain urethral debris, which may alter the results of the urinalysis or drug test. The mid-stream sample should be collected in a clean, labeled container and refrigerated until the analysis can be performed.

Male horses usually must be tranquilized for bladder catheterization. Acepromazine maleate relaxes the retractor penis muscle, allowing the penis to protrude from the prepuce. Once this has occurred, the penis is grasped caudal to the glans penis and is washed with a mild soap and rinsed thoroughly. Primary attention while washing the penis should be directed to the glans penis, urethral process and urethral diverticulum. The diverticulum is a blind pouch, dorsal to the urethral process, that collects smegma. This collection of smegma has been referred to as a "bean" due to its shape.

Once these areas have been cleansed, a lubricated, sterile plastic or rubber stallion catheter is introduced into the urethra, and advanced slowly and gently to avoid traumatizing the urethra (Fig 23). As the catheter reaches the ischial arch, just ventral to the anus, slight force may be required to pass the catheter through the curvature of the urethra in this area. As the catheter passes over the ischial arch, the horse usually raises its tail, indicating the catheter is near the bladder. Gentle aspiration with a sterile syringe may be required to start the flow of urine unless the bladder is full. A mid-stream sample of urine passively exiting the catheter is then collected in a labeled, sterile container and refrigerated until it is analyzed.

Collecting Urine from Female Horses

Urine collection is comparatively difficult in mares. Mares generally do not react in the same manner as geldings or stallions when placed in a freshly bedded stall. A voided sample is often obtained, however, during catheterization, as manipulation of the urethral orifice often results in urination. If a sample is not collected during catheterization, most mares attempt to urinate when taken back to their stalls. A mid-stream sample is collected in a labeled, sterile container and refrigerated until it is analyzed.

Catheterization of a mare's bladder does not generally require tranquilization. Sterile equipment must be used to obtain a sterile sample and avoid contamination of the urinary tract. The perineum should be thoroughly cleansed before catheterization (see Intrauterine Infusion).

Several types of catheters are available for use in mares, the one selected is determined by personal preference (Fig 24). The metal mare urinary catheter (Wellcome, Kansas City, MO) is used most frequently. A rubber stallion catheter may be used, though greater manipulation of the catheter may be required to complete the procedure.

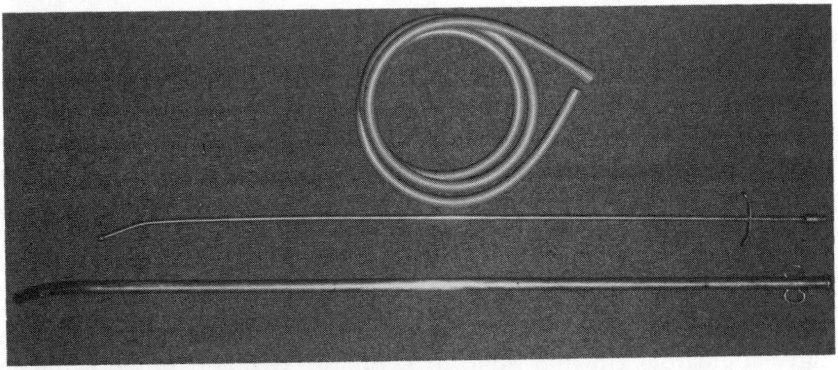

Fig 24. Urinary catheters. Top: rubber stallion catheter. Middle: Chambers' catheter. Bottom: metal mare urinary catheter.

Uterine pipettes or Chambers' catheters (Wellcome) may be used in fillies and small mares when a smaller-diameter catheter is required.

Sterile surgeon's gloves should be used to manually guide the catheter, if necessary. Sterile lubricant is applied and the hand is inserted through the vulva and into the vaginal vestibule. The urethral orifice may be palpated on the floor of the vestibule 4-6 inches from the ventral vulvar commissure (ventral aspect of the vulva). To enter the urethral orifice, the catheter is passed ventral to the hand and guided into the urethra by the index finger. Gentle aspiration with an attached sterile syringe may be required to obtain the urine. If this is unsuccessful, gently manipulate the catheter craniad and caudad, making certain the catheter does not leave the urethra. Such stimulation of the urethra often causes the mare to urinate. Once urine is obtained, the catheter is removed and the mare's vulva is rinsed with clean water to remove excess lubricant.

The mare urinary catheter may be passed into the bladder without manual guidance. The mare is prepared in the same manner as above. The catheter is inserted through the vulva and into the vaginal vestibule, with the tip remaining in contact with the floor of the vagina. A small amount of resistance is felt when it reaches the urethral orifice. At this point, turn the tip of the catheter slightly to one side and advance it slowly. The catheter should slide directly into the bladder. The procedure used to obtain the urine is the same as above.

ENEMAS

Enemas are used to facilitate passage of feces from the terminal colon and rectum. Constipation that is not corrected by oral administration of lubricants often requires use of an enema. The fluid volume and equipment used differ significantly between mature horses and foals.

Enemas in Foals

In foals, enemas are most often used to relieve meconium (fetal feces) impactions. Meconium is normally passed 3-12 hours after birth. Foals that experience difficulty in expelling this firm, tenacious material show abdominal straining, anal protrusion and frequent tail raising when attempting to defecate. Many breeding farms routinely give enemas to all newborn foals to prevent meconium retention.

Fleet enemas (Fleet Co., Lynchburg, VA), available in most drug stores, may be used safely in foals (Fig 25). These squeeze bottles have a flexible tip and contain a premixed liquid (mineral oil or phosphate solution). The tip is inserted into the foal's rectum and the contents of the bottle are slowly infused, after which the container is discarded.

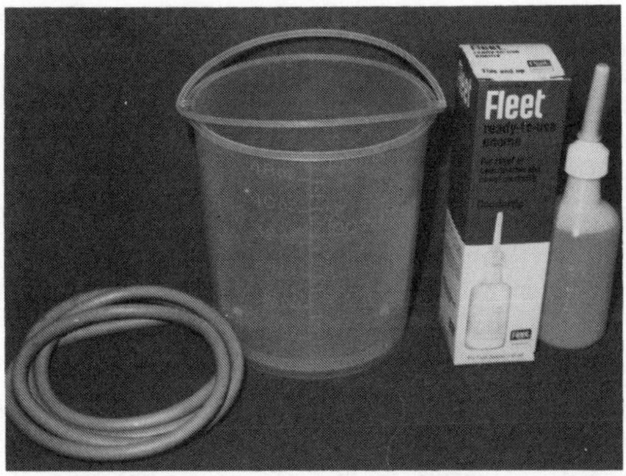

Fig 25. Enema units for use in foals. Left: enema bucket with attached rubber tube. Right: fleet enema.

Warm water may also be used in enemas. The fluid may be delivered through a plastic or rubber catheter or IV line attached to a bottle or dose syringe. Enema buckets (Haver-Lockhart, Shawnee, KS), manufactured with an outlet valve, to which rubber tubing may be connected, are ideal for warm-water enemas (Fig 25). The lubricated tubing is inserted into the rectum and advanced slowly and gently while the fluid is infused. The foal's fragile rectum may be torn or punctured if undue force is used during the procedure. Only a small amount (2-4 oz) of fluid should be infused, to prevent over-distention of the rectum. After infusion, wait until the foal expels most of the fluid and repeat the procedure, if necessary.

Enemas in Adult Horses

Adult horses rarely need enemas, but enemas can be used to soften and remove feces in mares with perineal laceration repairs. Fecal material often collects cranial to the repair due to the discomfort during attempts to defecate. Warm water is infused through a medium-sized nasogastric tube, using a funnel or stomach pump for delivery. Large quantities (1-3 gal) of fluid can be infused, but administration should be intermittently interrupted to allow evacuation of feces. It may be necessary to repeat these enemas for several days until the discomfort subsides and the mare defecates unassisted.

BANDAGE APPLICATION

Limb Bandages

Bandages are commonly applied to the legs of horses to protect wounds and surgical incisions and prevent self-inflicted injury during training, racing, work or trailering. They provide support to the tendinous structures of the opposite weight-bearing limb when an injured leg cannot bear full weight. In emergency situations, bandages are used to control hemorrhage and support fractures until definitive treatment. Certain types of bandages, in conjunction with sweats and poultices, help control limb edema. Due to their extensive use, it is important to be able to select appropriate materials and properly apply different types of bandages.

Bandage Materials

The foundation of every leg bandage consists of good padding material. Failure to apply adequate padding under a bandage could result in injury from excessive pressure. Roll cotton is ideal as a bandage foundation. It is very soft and absorbent, and conforms well to the limb. It is available in 1-lb rolls and is relatively inexpensive. Sheet cotton is also used extensively. These broad, thin sheets of cotton may be layered to produce the amount of padding desired. Quilted pads may be purchased or prepared from mattress pads and used as shipping bandages. This type of padding is washable and may be reused numerous times.

The form of wrapping material used is based on the type of injury, cost of bandage materials, frequency of bandage changes, and personal preference. Roll gauze, available in several widths, does not stretch, and is relatively inexpensive. Elastic bandages (*eg,* Ace Bandage), also available in various widths, stretch and are washable, and conform well to the limb. "Derby" bandages, commonly used as shipping bandages, are made of cotton-knit material that stretches and is washable, and are available with ties or Velcro closures. Disposable elastic bandages (*eg,* Vetrap: 3M, Elastikon: Johnson & Johnson) are commonly used on equine limbs. Vetrap is made of crepe material that adheres to itself, while Elastikon adheres to nearly any surface. Kling (Johnson & Johnson) is a disposable, double-layered stretch gauze that conforms well to the limb and clings to itself.

Flannel is an inelastic, reusable material available in large sheets and is ideal for spider or many-tail bandages. Stockinette (Johnson & Johnson), a knit material manufactured as a tube bandage, is available in many sizes. It is often used under casts and is excellent for bandaging the head and neck. Adhesive tape is used primarily to secure the ends of bandages. It should not be used as the primary bandage material because of its tendency to tighten around the limb if the bandage shifts in position.

Bandaging Principles

The principles of bandaging should be followed closely to prevent pressure injuries, strictures, or loosening of the bandage. As previously mentioned, failure to use adequate padding could produce tendinitis, particularly if the wrap is applied tightly. Pressure sores may occur, for the same reason, over bony prominences, such as the accessory carpal bone or tuber calcis. Even if the proper amount of padding is used, irritation may develop if wrinkles or folds are formed during bandage application. This may be prevented by applying both padding and wrapping material smoothly, snugly and in one (the same) direction. About an inch of padding must be left at the top and bottom of the bandage to avoid impairing blood circulation, which may occur if the wrapping material binds around the limb.

Derby bandages should be tied on the lateral aspect of the limb to prevent excessive tension over the extensor and flexor tendons. When knots are tied on the medial aspect of the limb, the horse may accidentally step on the ties and loosen the bandage. The ends of the bandage should be secured by taping them to the bandage. Adhesive tape should be applied, without tension, in a spiral around the bandage. If the tape is wrapped around the leg and reattached to itself, it could tighten and bind if the bandage slips, resulting in severe tendinitis. It is advisable to make a tab at the end of the tape by folding the end on itself so it may be easily located to facilitate bandage removal.

Bandage Types

Standing Bandage: A standing or support bandage is applied to the lower limb, from the distal carpus or tarsus to the hoof. Many trailering injuries occur at the level of the coronary band; therefore, it is imperative that this area be protected. Cotton should be wrapped securely around the limb and any wrinkles must be smoothed out to prevent irritation to the underlying tissues (Fig 26A). Gauze application is started at the level of the fetlock. It is wrapped snugly around the limb, working distad (toward the hoof) (Fig 26B). Including the bulbs of the heel in the bandage holds it more securely in place. The gauze is then worked proximad (upward), toward the carpus or tarsus, relaxing the tension somewhat over the tendons. The bandage is completed with adhesive tape applied in a spiral around the bandage (Fig 26C). The standing bandage is often used as a base, upon which other bandages are built; therefore, application of this bandage must be mastered before attempting to apply other types.

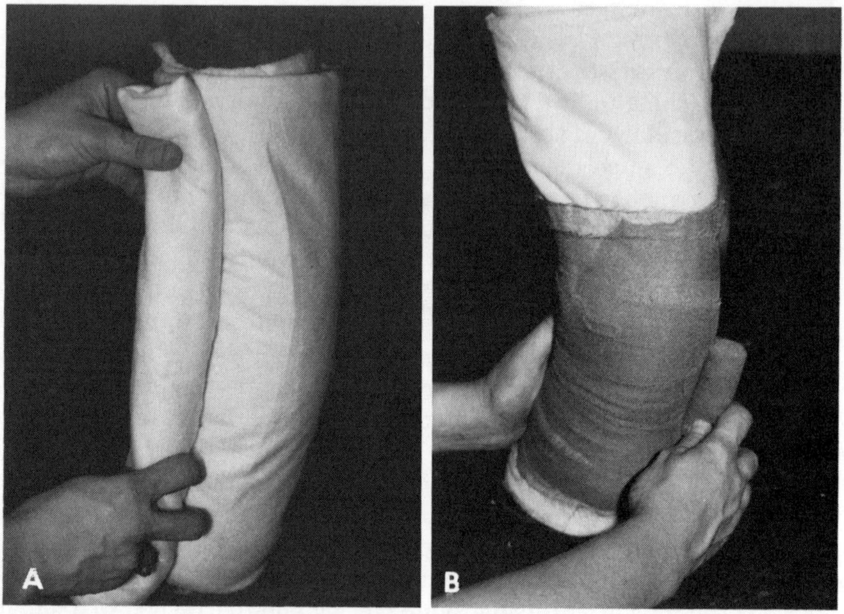

Fig 26. The standing bandage. A. Padding material is wrapped smoothly and snugly around the limb, from the proximal metacarpus/metatarsus, distad to the ground. B. Gauze application is started at the level of the fetlock and progresses toward the hoof, leaving at least 1 inch of cotton uncovered.

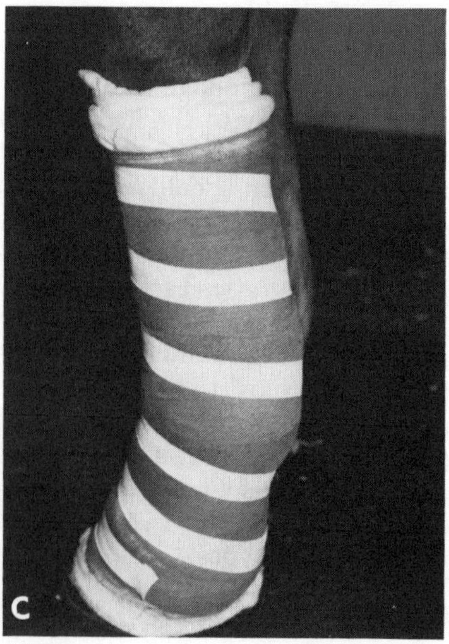

26C. Gauze is wrapped proximad toward the carpus/tarsus, somewhat relaxing the tension over the tendons. Adhesive tape is then applied over the gauze in a spiral fashion, ending with a tab on the lateral aspect of the bandage.

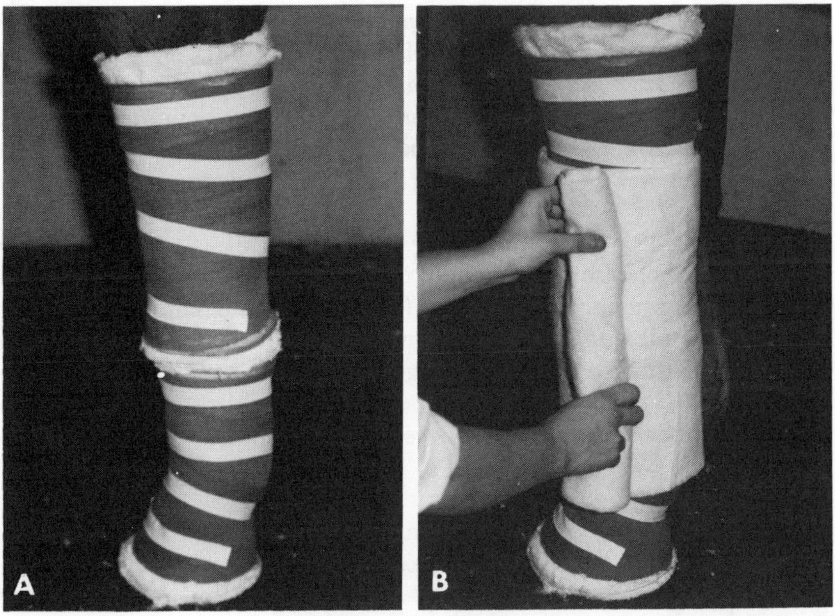

Fig 27. Carpal bandage. A. A standing bandage of cotton and gauze is applied to the lower limb and a similar bandage is applied proximal to it. B. These 2 bandages are "tied in" by applying sheet cotton over the junction of the underlying bandages.

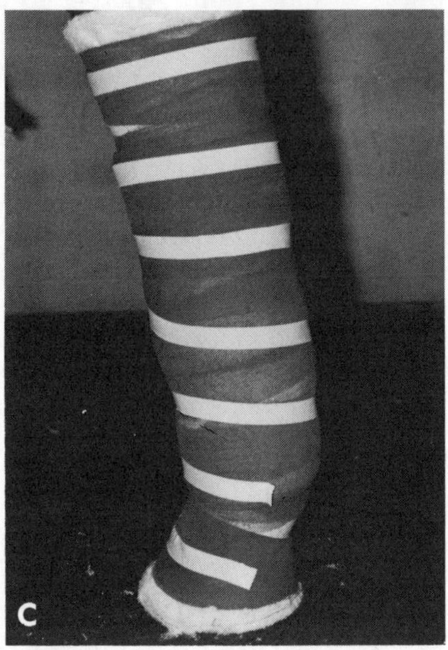

Fig 27C. The bandage is completed by wrapping another roll of gauze over the bandage. Adhesive tape is applied in a spiral, avoiding the accessory carpal bone area. Note the tape tabs left on the lateral aspect of the leg.

Carpal/Tarsal Bandages: Extensive practice is required to properly apply bandages over the carpal and tarsal joints so that they remain secure, without producing pressure sores over the bony prominences in these areas. To prevent slippage of these bandages, a standing bandage is applied as previously described. A "stovepipe" bandage, which overlaps the standing bandage by several inches, is then applied.

Another method of bandaging the carpus/tarsus uses roll cotton and gauze (or elastic bandages) in the standing bandage, with a similar bandage applied proximal to it (Fig 27A). The 2 bandages are then "tied in" by placing a sheet cotton bandage over the junction of the original 2 bandages and wrapping the entire leg with a third gauze roll (Figs 27B, 27C). Excessive pressure over the accessory carpal bone and tuber calcis must be avoided when applying adhesive tape.

Spider Bandage: Pressure may be applied evenly throughout the entire leg with a "spider" or "many-tail" bandage. This bandage usually also inhibits excessive flexion of joints over which it is applied. It is most commonly used over the carpus, but is also used on the tarsus.

A carpal/tarsal bandage is applied as previously described as the foundation of the "spider" bandage. A section of flannel is measured according to the length of the bandaged region and the circumference of the wrapped limb. Another 10-12 inches are added to the width to compensate for the ties. The flannel is then folded lengthwise and 5- to 6-inch-long strips are cut or torn, at 1-inch intervals, along both edges of the flannel to form the ties. The flannel is placed around the limb so the ties may be fastened on the lateral aspect. Beginning at the top, securely tie the strips of flannel together and intertwine each new tied set with the ones preceding it. Continue this down the bandage, smoothing it out frequently. Tie a knot in the final tie and cover all loose ends with adhesive material (Fig 28).

Support Bandages: The prognosis of a fractured leg may be affected by the type of support bandage applied before transportation of the patient; therefore, knowledge of emergency bandage application is important. With a compound fracture (bone exits the skin), the wound should be covered with a very clean or, preferably, a sterile wrap. Soaps or detergents should not be used to clean such wounds, nor should ointments be applied if surgical intervention is being considered.

When a fractured limb is bandaged, the joints proximal and distal to (above and below) the fracture site must be immobilized by application of large amounts of padding and tightly wrapped bandages. Up to 12 1-lb rolls of cotton may be used in these bandages. If the usual bandage materials are not available, several large pillows and 4- to 6-inch strips of a bed sheet may be used. The leg may be further stabilized by incorporating broom sticks or small boards into the ban-

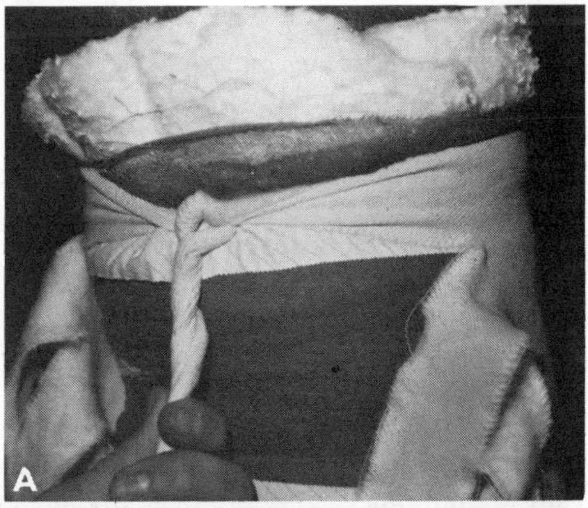

Fig 28. Spider bandage. A. The spider bandage is started by placing flannel around the limb so the ties can be secured on the lateral aspect of the leg. The first tie is fastened securely and twisted.

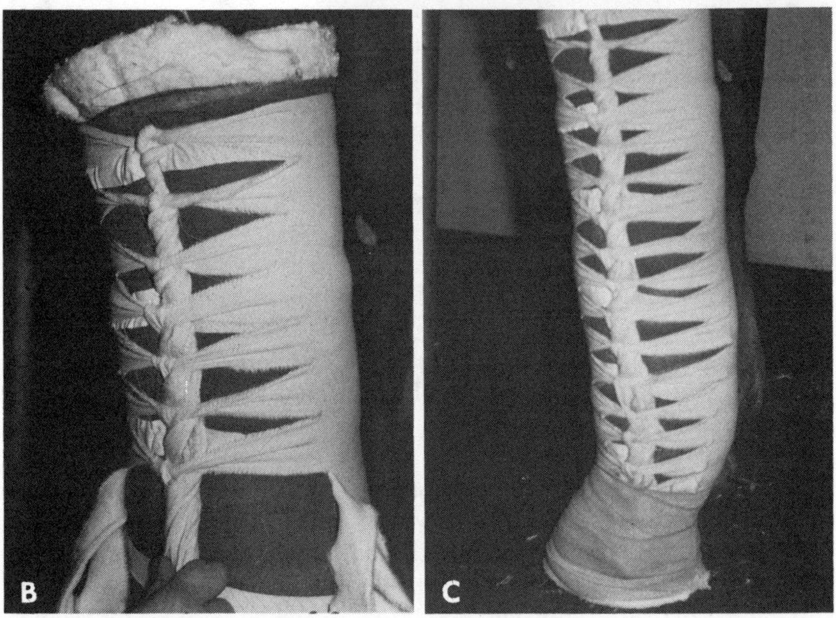

Figs 28B,C. After each tie is completed, it is entwined with the previous sets of ties. The spider bandage is completed by securing the ends with an adhesive bandage.

dage. This type of emergency bandage is referred to as a Robert Jones bandage.

Ointments, powders, dressings or sterile wound dressings may be applied beneath the previously mentioned bandages. A leg sweat may be applied to the skin beneath a bandage to "sweat out" fluid that may accumulate in interstitial tissues. Such sweats often contain equal parts of alcohol and glycerin. After this substance is massaged into the leg, an impermeable wrap, such as Saran Wrap or a plastic OB sleeve, is applied smoothly and evenly, followed by a standing bandage. This sweat bandage is left in place for 12-24 hours after which it may be removed or reapplied.

Poultices: Poultices are also used to remove excessive fluid from inflamed tissues. Poultice application involves applying a thick layer of the poultice material over the affected area, smoothing it on gently with damp hands and covering it with a plastic wrap and then an appropriate bandage. The poultice is left in place for 12-24 hours, after which it is rinsed off and reapplied if necessary.

Casts: Casts are sometimes used instead of bandages. They are most frequently used to stabilize fractures following fracture reduction (manipulative realignment) and/or surgical fixation. Foals with angular limb deformities may have casts applied. Because most foals adjust to casts very well, this form of stabilization may be superior to bandages, especially when pressure sores develop from bandaging these young patients. Casts may also be used on horses with chronic, slow-healing wounds, for which repeated bandage changes could be very expensive.

Before cast application, the leg is cleaned and covered with a double layer of stockinette, and orthopedic felt is fastened around the coronary band and the point at which the cast will terminate. Many types of cast material are available; selection is based on the desired weight of the completed cast, frequency of cast changes and personal preference. Though the veterinarian usually applies the cast, the technician should be able to prepare the limb and the materials required for completion of the procedure.

Splints: Splints may be applied over bandages to further reduce limb flexion or extension. It is very important to apply adequate padding beneath the splint to prevent severe pressure sores. Splints may be prepared from broom handles, boards or longitudinal halves of PVC (plastic) drain pipe. The PVC pipe is available in many sizes at most plumbing or hardware stores and may be cut to an appropriate length and width with a cast-cutting saw. The selected splint material

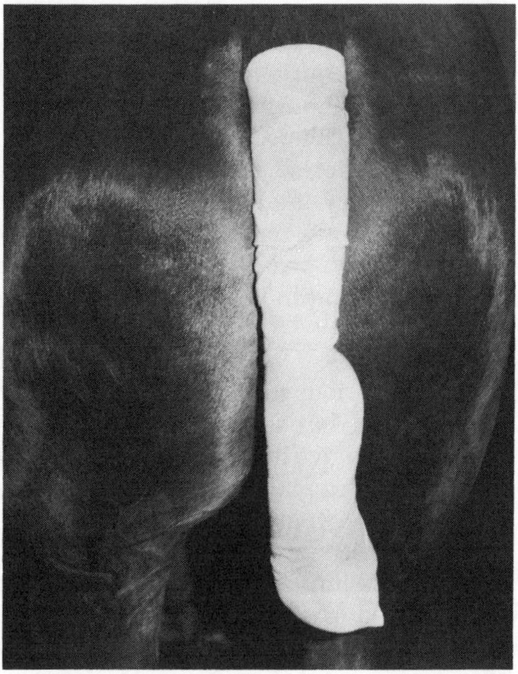

Fig 29. Tail wrap. This bandage incorporates the folded distal ends of the tail hairs.

is then applied over the well-padded bandage with adhesive bandage or tape.

Abdominal Bandages

Abdominal bandages are most frequently applied to support and protect incisions after abdominal surgery. These bandages usually consist of a sterile bandage applied over the incision, padding over the backbone to prevent pressure sores, and gauze wrapped around the abdomen, followed by an adhesive bandage material. The bandage should be applied tightly to support the abdomen during healing. Because bandages are very expensive, they are changed only when necessary. Many horses resent having their hair pulled upon removal of an adhesive bandage. For this reason, nonadhesive gauze is applied beneath an adhesive bandage, except at the cranial and caudal ends to facilitate removal. If the patient continues to object, application of ether to the sticky underside of the adhesive bandage during removal helps loosen it with little discomfort to the horse.

Tail Bandages

Tail wraps may be applied to prevent the hair from being soiled with loose feces and to retract the tail during breeding, genitourinary tract or rectal examinations or when working on the hind limbs. Using gauze or elastic bandage material, the wrap is started at the tailhead and continued caudad to the last coccygeal vertebra. The bandage may be completed at this point or the tail may be folded craniad and included in the bandage (Fig 29). If the bandage must stay in place for several hours or days, it may be further secured by including a few tail hairs in the first few wraps of the bandage.

Tail bandages must not be applied too tightly, especially if they are to be left in place for several hours, as the circulation may be impaired, resulting in ischemic necrosis and sloughing of the tail.

Preventing Self-Mutilation

Complications may result from improper bandaging, as previously mentioned, but self-mutilation may also occur when the patient attempts to remove its own bandage. This may be prevented by the use of bibs, cradles and cross-ties (see Chapter 2). Bibs allow free movement while preventing the animal from reaching the bandage with its teeth. Cradles restrict flexion of the neck, preventing the horse from reaching its limbs. Cross-ties, attached to the stall walls, hold the horse's head in a central location so that lateral movement is nearly eliminated and flexion is severely restricted. Some horses may work their way around these obstacles, however. In these instances, application of a red-pepper paste or tabasco sauce to the external surface of the bandage often prevents chewing on it.

Recommended Reading

Anon: *Giving Medication: A Nursing Photobook.* Intermediate Communications, Horsham, PA.

Compend Cont Ed Pract Vet **4** (1982) S237.

6

treatment technics for food animals

L.R. KRCATOVICH

There are many routes for administering the various forms of medication used to treat food animals. Technicians must become proficient in all forms of treatment technics so they may medicate animals in the most efficient, humane and safe method. It is important, especially when treating large herds, for the veterinary team to choose the least expensive and most effective route to medicate the animals.

INTRAVENOUS INJECTIONS

Intravenous (IV) administration of medication results in high blood levels of the drug in a short time. Though farm personnel may learn to give IV injections, most veterinarians prefer that laymen use the intramuscular (IM) or oral route to avoid possible phlebitis and thrombosis caused by poor venipuncture technic.

Cattle

The veins most often used for IV injections in cattle are the jugular veins, coccygeal (tail) vein and the subcutaneous abdominal (milk) veins. The jugular veins are most often used for large-volume IV injections; in addition to their accessibility, there is less chance of being kicked when using these veins. The jugular vein is always used for IV injections in calves because it is the largest accessible vessel.

The coccygeal (tail) vein is used for IV injection of small volumes (3-5 ml) of drugs. Though most cows are more tolerant of tail veni-

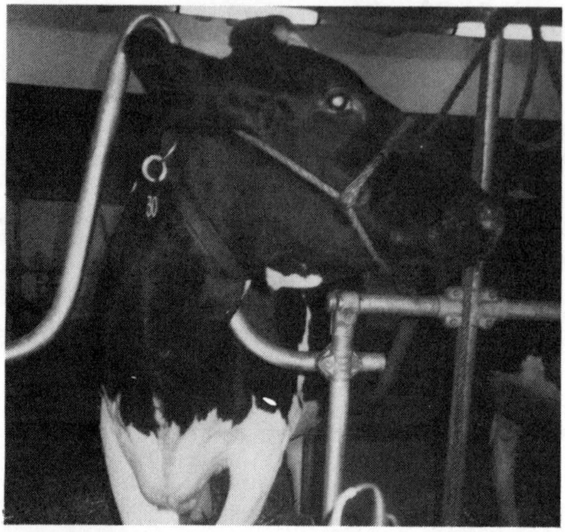

Fig 1. Correct restraint of the head for jugular venipuncture.

puncture than jugular injections, there is a greater chance of being kicked. This can be minimized with proper restraint.

The subcutaneous abdominal vein, also called the "mammary" or "milk" vein, is used mainly when the jugular veins are thrombosed (occluded) or cannot be located. There are several disadvantages to milk vein injections. The technician must position him- or herself so that there is increased danger of being kicked. A second person may be required to provide additional restraint. The milk vein rolls easily under the skin, making it hard to puncture and to thread the needle. Finally, hematomas are easily formed and may result in thrombosis of the vein.

Preparation for venipuncture is similar for all 3 veins. A disinfectant, such as 70% alcohol, should be applied to the injection site to remove gross contamination, provide antibacterial activity, and increase visibility of the vein. Venipunctures should not be made through dirt or fecal material, as phlebitis, septicemia and/or contamination of medication and samples may result.

Jugular Venipuncture

Good restraint is necessary when attempting any venipuncture. Ideally, the cow should be restrained in a head gate stanchion. Injecting medication into the jugular vein of an animal that is not properly restrained is difficult and dangerous. Therefore, never attempt venipuncture on a free, moving large animal. A halter should be applied and the head raised and pulled to one side (Fig 1). A quick-release knot should be used when tying an animal to a stationary object. If the cow should fall during infusion of medication, the head can be released immediately to prevent injury to the cow. If a recumbent cow must be treated, its head can be secured by tying the free end of the halter back above the hock with a quick-release knot (see Chapter 2). Tying the head to one side secures it, making the vein accessible, but it may also make it more difficult to distend the vein. Nose tongs (nose lead) may be applied to help quiet fractious cattle.

A standing calf may be restrained by pulling it close to your body, immobilizing its head. Older calves can be restrained like adult cattle, but application of nose tongs is usually not necessary. A recumbent calf should have its head firmly held with the neck extended. If the calf moves excessively, a second person should aid in restraint.

All required materials should be assembled before attempting venipuncture. The needle selected for IV injection of large volumes of fluids varies according to personal preference and the flow rate desired. A 12- to 14-ga, 2- to 3-inch needle is best for giving large volumes to adult cattle. Needles less than 2 inches long should not be used. A correctly threaded 3-inch needle is not likely to slip from the vein if the cow thrashes around, decreasing the chances of perivascular infiltration of irritants and hypertonic solutions. For injections of small volumes into the jugular vein, use of a 16-, 18- or 20-ga, 1½-inch needle is recommended for cows and calves. These small-gauge, disposable needles are easier to insert than the reusable, large-bore

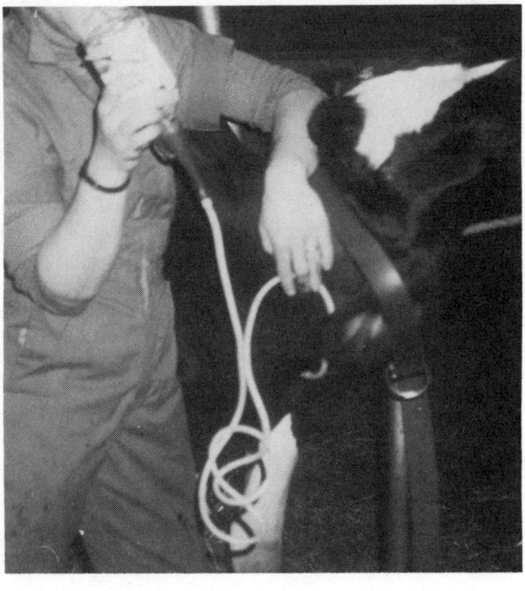

Fig 2. A simplex IV unit is attached to the bottle of medication for jugular vein administration.

needles, as disposable needles are used only once and are very sharp, whereas reusable needles tend to become dull.

A rubber IV line, referred to as a simplex, is used for IV infusions. This is commonly referred to as "jugging" (Fig 2). A syringe may also be used to inject medication. Its size depends on the volume of medication to be injected.

Figure 3 shows the proper positioning of the technician for jugular venipuncture. One should never kneel or stand directly in front of the animal during jugular venipuncture. To distend the jugular vein, apply pressure at the jugular furrow, about two-thirds of the way caudad on (down) the neck (Figs 3, 5). Allow time for the vein to fill. Briskly stroking the vein with a finger in a downward motion (toward the heart) helps raise it for easy visualization. Unless the animal is in shock or is severely dehydrated, a jugular venipuncture should not be attempted without sufficiently raising the vein. Though the jugular vein is quite large when raised, it is easily missed by inexperienced technicians.

Bovine skin is thick and difficult to penetrate with a large-gauge needle; therefore, the needle must be inserted with considerable force. Grasp the needle by the hub, using the thumb and first knuckle of the forefinger (Fig 4). Warn the cow of the impending needle insertion by hitting her on the neck, near but not over the injection site, with the

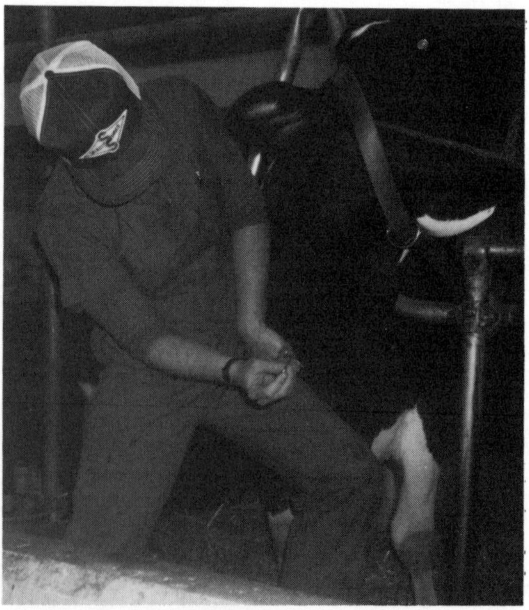

Fig 3. Proper position for jugular venipuncture.

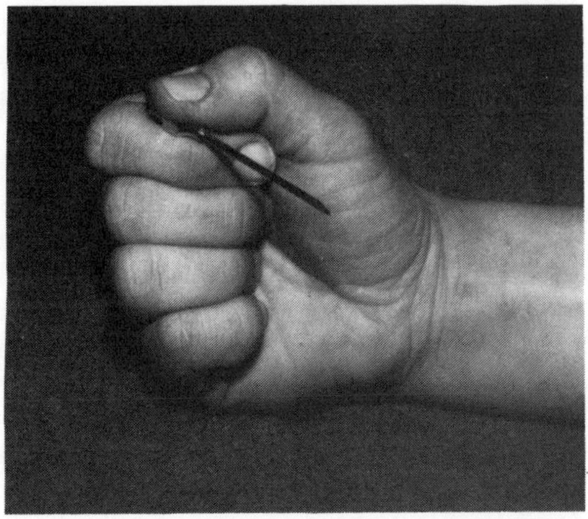

Fig 4. Correct positioning of the needle for jugular venipuncture.

back of the hand holding the needle. These warning strokes may upset the animal more than the insertion of the needle. Gradually increasing the intensity of the strokes often prevents this. After 2-3 warning strokes, flip the hand over and thrust the needle through the skin at a 45-90° angle to the vessel, with the needle directed toward the heart. Keep the jugular vein occluded to observe for blood flow from the needle, indicating proper placement.

If the vein was entered on the initial attempt and a steady flow of blood exits the needle, lay the needle parallel to the skin and advance it further caudad into the vein (Fig 5). The needle may be directed toward the head for administration of small volumes, but larger volumes should be given with the needle directed toward the heart. If the needle slips out of the vein during insertion, retract it until blood steadily flows from it; then attempt to rethread it.

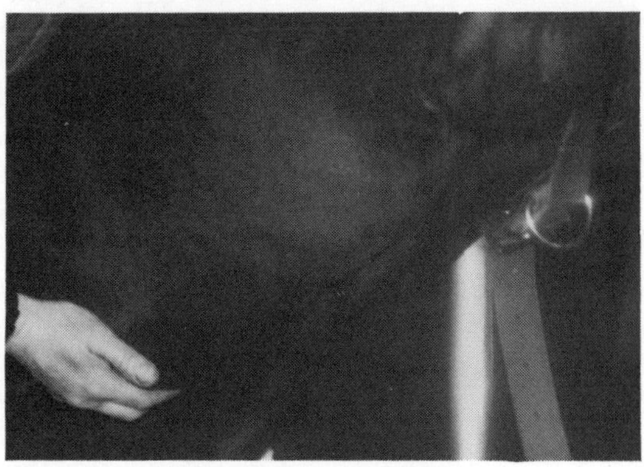

Fig 5. The needle is threaded into the vein up to its hub while the jugular vein is occluded.

Occasionally, the needle does not enter the vein, but only penetrates the skin. When this occurs, relocate the vein and thrust the needle into it without withdrawing it from the skin. Redirection of the needle may be necessary to find the vein. Once a steady flow of blood is present, the needle should be threaded to its hub. If the needle has been inserted too deeply and has penetrated entirely through the vessel, pull the needle back slowly until blood flows freely from the hub; at this point the needle can be threaded. Apposition of the bevel of the needle against the vessel wall may also occlude it. This may be corrected by slightly rotating the needle. Care must be taken when redirecting the needle to prevent laceration of the vein and consequent hematoma formation.

Small-gauge, disposable hypodermic needles may be inserted as are large-bore needles. However, it is not necessary to use as much force to insert these needles or to strike the animal before insertion, as they are very sharp and easily penetrate the skin. The needle is introduced into the vein at a 30-45° angle, with or without a syringe attached. The needle may be correctly positioned by attaching a syringe and aspirating blood.

When the needle is correctly threaded, the syringe or simplex is attached. Aspirate (slightly withdraw syringe barrel) and inject the medication. If a bottle is used, it should be held in an inverted position (Fig 2). A steady bubbling in the bottle indicates that the medication is flowing into the vein and is being replaced by air in the bottle. If the bubbling becomes irregular or stops, the needle may be occluded or out of the vein. In such cases, lower the bottle, check the needle for correct positioning and make the appropriate adjustments. Whether using a simplex or a syringe to administer fluid, observe the jugular furrow for gradual swelling around the needle. This may indicate that medication is flowing into the perivascular space (outside the vein). Correct the needle's position and continue. After IV injection is complete, remove the needle and apply digital (finger) pressure for 15-30 seconds over the venipuncture site to prevent a hematoma.

Correct and sanitary venipuncture technic must be used to prevent formation of hematomas and thrombi. If phlebitis or thrombosis develops, the routes for IV administration become severely limited. Perivascular injection of caustic or hypertonic solutions may produce tissue damage. Perivascular injection of a hypertonic solution, such as 50% dextrose, results in localized edema. This not only provides a medium for growth of bacteria and may develop into an abscess, but it also looks unprofessional.

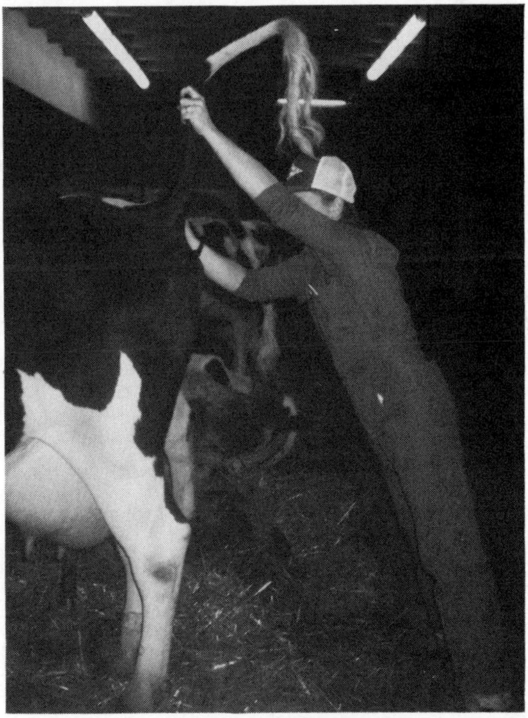

Fig 6. A proper "tail jack" is required for coccygeal venipuncture.

Coccygeal Venipuncture

For smaller volumes of medication, the coccygeal (tail) vein is often used rather than the jugular vein. Cattle usually become less agitated when the tail is used for venipuncture. This method also usually requires less restraint than when the jugular vein is used.

Limited restraint is needed for coccygeal venipuncture. Dairy cattle require a halter or stanchion and a "tail jack" (Fig 6). Beef cattle generally are more fractious and may require restraint in a chute. A tail jack must be used for coccygeal venipuncture, as it is impossible if the tail is not held in a vertical position. Holding the tail in this manner also simultaneously serves as restraint.

An 18- or 20-ga, 1½-inch needle and a 3-, 5- or 10-ml syringe are appropriate for coccygeal venipuncture. A needle larger than 18 ga is too large for the coccygeal vein. A 20-ga needle is most commonly used.

To locate the correct sites for injection, one must know the position of the coccygeal vein in the tail (Fig 7). The middle coccygeal vein

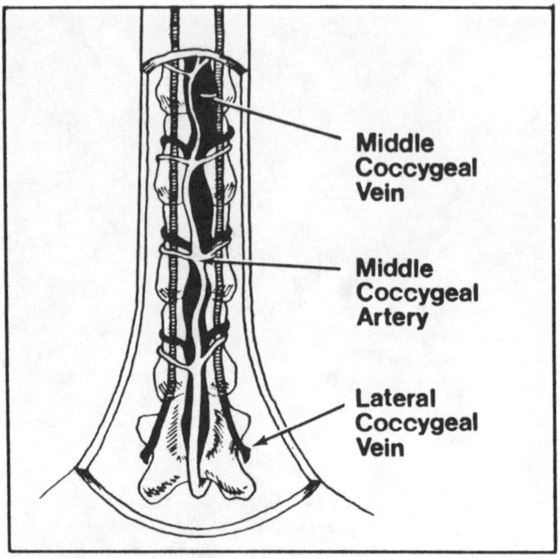

Fig 7. Ventral view of coccygeal vessels at the base of the tail.

and artery run together along the ventral midline between the hemal arches of the coccygeal vertebrae. As the vein and artery course caudad along the tail, their size decreases; therefore, the first 3 coccygeal vertebrae (near the tail base) are the sites for coccygeal venipuncture.

To locate the correct site, apply a tail jack and clean the ventral surface of the tail to remove gross contamination (Fig 8). Palpate the tail for the bony protrusions (hemal arches) of the vertebrae (Fig 9). About midway between 2 hemal arches, insert the needle, while gently aspirating, directly on the midline at a 45° angle to the tail (Fig 10).

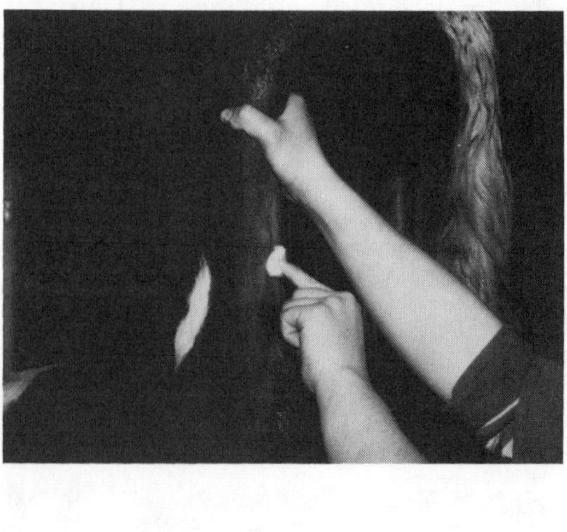

Fig 8. Coccygeal venipuncture sites should be cleaned with an alcohol swab.

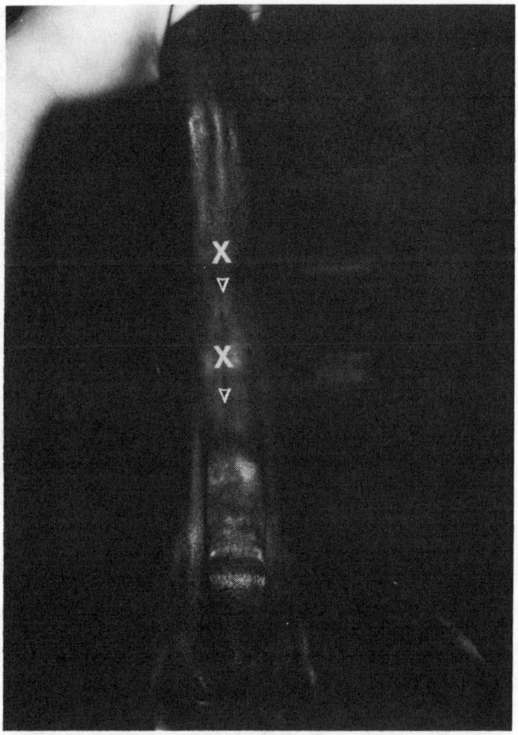

Fig 9. Location of the hemal arches (X) and venipuncture sites (arrowheads) on the ventral aspect of the bovine tail.

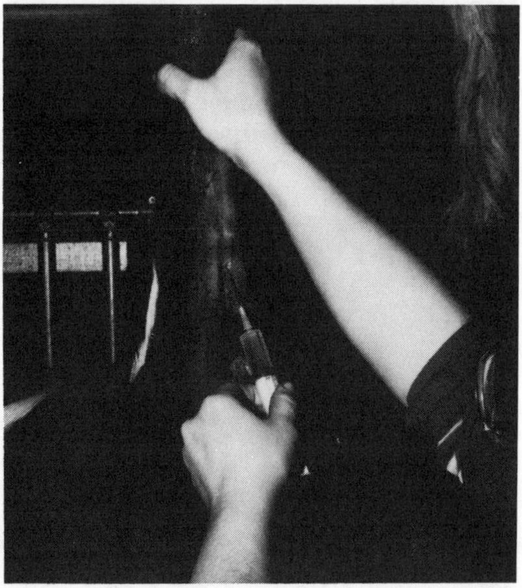

Fig 10. Correct positioning of the needle for coccygeal venipunçture.

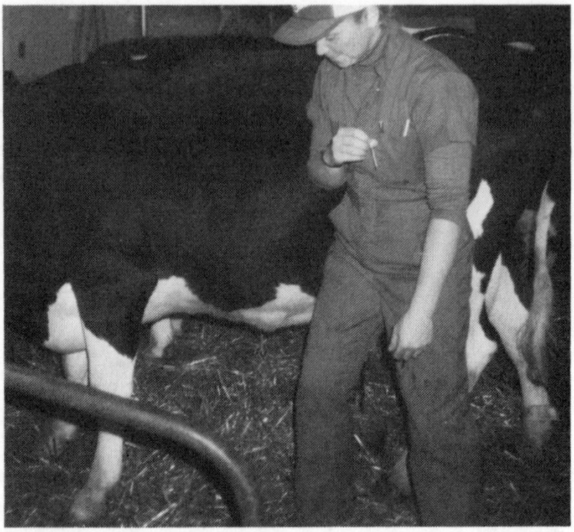

Fig 11. The correct and safest position for subcutaneous abdominal venipuncture.

If blood is not withdrawn into the syringe, check the needle for the correct angle and position. It may be necessary to advance or retract the needle to locate the vein. Remove the needle and redirect it if necessary. Inject the medication when the needle is correctly positioned. Periodically aspirate blood into the syringe and reinject this to clear the needle of residual medication. Either the coccygeal artery or vein may be used for injection. After the injection is completed, remove the needle, lower the tail and apply digital pressure for 10-15 seconds. Hematoma formation is usually not a problem, though digital pressure should be applied if the artery was punctured.

Subcutaneous Abdominal Venipuncture

The milk veins are used when the jugular veins cannot be raised or are inaccessible for other reasons. These veins should be used for ad-

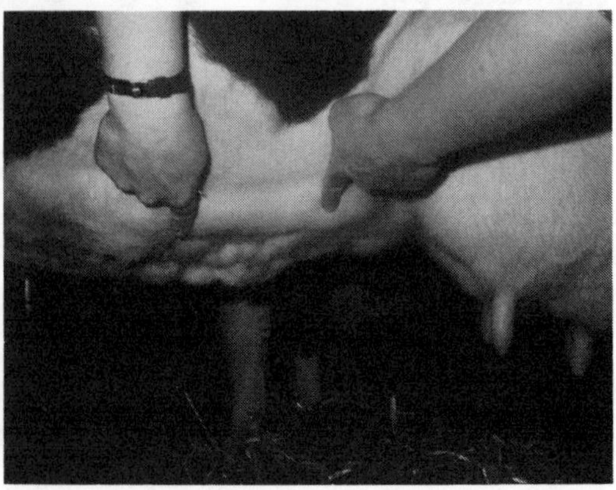

Fig 12. Segment of the subcutaneous abdominal vein most commonly used for venipuncture.

ministration of large volumes of medication only. It is too dangerous to obtain routine blood samples from them.

The animal should be tied securely or restrained in a stanchion. Stand close to the cow's flank, facing the same direction as the cow (Fig 11). One should not face the cow's rear, since the cow may kick.

A 14-ga, 2- to 3-inch needle is used for venipuncture. A syringe may be used to inject medication; however, a simplex system is frequently used. Because blood flows slowly in this vein, administration through a simplex may require more time than anticipated.

It is not necessary to occlude the milk vein before puncturing it, as it is normally distended (Fig 12). The preferred venipuncture site is immediately caudal to the point where the vessel enters the abdomen; this section of the vein is the most stable (Fig 12). As with jugular venipuncture it takes some force to introduce the needle through the skin. The needle should be inserted caudad and threaded into the vein (Fig 13). If blood does not flow freely from the needle, check the position of the needle and redirect it. Exercise caution when redirecting the needle, for it is easy to create hematomas in this area. Observe the area for perivascular infiltration during administration. When the injection has been completed, remove the needle and apply digital pressure for several minutes. Even with digital pressure, hematomas form easily.

Swine

The vein used in pigs for IV injections is the caudal auricular vein (ear vein). The jugular veins are too deep to be used. A surgical cutdown may be performed if necessary, but this is rarely done for routine injections. The volume injected into the ear vein is limited due to its small size. Catheterization of the vein is possible, but this is difficult unless general anesthesia is used. Fortunately, most injections in swine are given by other routes.

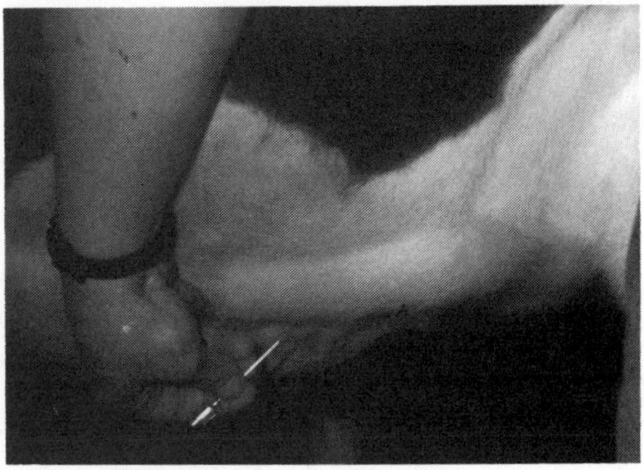

Fig 13. The correct angle and direction of the needle for subcutaneous abdominal venipuncture.

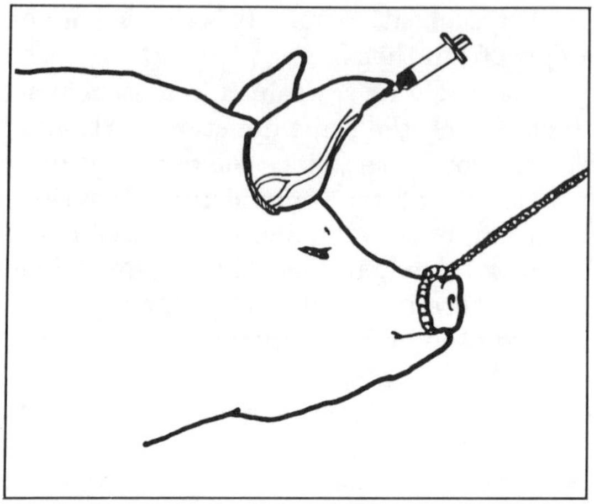

Fig 14. Auricular venipuncture in swine.

Pigs are restrained with a hog snare or noose (see Chapter 2). They may be backed into a corner or pinned against a wall. A 20- to 22-ga, 1½-inch needle and a 3- to 5-ml syringe are appropriate. A rubber band placed around the base of the ear or rubber tubing pulled tightly around the ear and clamped with hemostats distends the vein for venipuncture (Fig 14). Venous distention can be hastened by slapping or rubbing the ear. Clean the injection site with an antiseptic. The thumb may be placed beside the vein to prevent it from rolling. The needle should be inserted, bevel up, into the distal portion of the vein (near the ear tip) and threaded into the vein to the hub. Aspirate to check for correct needle placement. Aspirate gently, for even a little negative pressure may collapse the vein. Before injecting the medication, release the rubber band. Observe the vein for perivascular infiltration as the medication is injected. If the medication is injected perivascularly or a hematoma forms, remove the needle, apply pressure to the site, and attempt another venipuncture closer to the base of the ear.

Goats and Sheep

Intravenous medication is almost always given in the jugular veins in goats and sheep. The cephalic and femoral veins are used only if both jugular veins are thrombosed.

Jugular Venipuncture

For jugular venipuncture, sheep and goats should be restrained as are calves. The head is elevated and turned slightly to one side by an assistant. Sheep may also be "thrown" into a sitting position. A single person can perform venipuncture on a sheep in this manner.

An antiseptic is applied to the jugular furrow. Sheep may require clipping in the jugular area to increase visibility of the vein. A 16-, 18- or 20-ga, 1½-inch needle should be used on adults; a 20- or 22-ga, 1½-inch needle is good for lambs and kids.

The vein is held off about two-thirds of the way down (caudal on) the neck at the jugular furrow, or at the thoracic inlet. Stroking the vein with a finger helps raise it. The needle is inserted at a 30-45° angle, with or without the syringe attached. The vein seems deeper in unshorn sheep due to the thickness of overlying wool. Thread the needle into the vein and aspirate to check its location. If the needle position is correct, inject the medication. Remove the needle while applying digital pressure.

Cephalic and Femoral Venipuncture

The technics for venipuncture of these veins are similar to those used in large dogs. When choosing the type of restraint, remember that most goats and sheep are not pets and therefore are not as docile.

INTRAVENOUS CATHETERIZATION

Intravenous catheterization is primarily used for prolonged fluid therapy, but is also used for administration of injectable anesthetics or repeated IV injections. The jugular vein is most often chosen for IV catheterization in cattle, sheep and goats. The caudal auricular vein can be catheterized in swine, though this vein is used mainly for injection of small volumes of medication. It is difficult to secure a catheter in the ear vein for an extended period because of its location.

A 10- to 14-ga catheter is used for adult cattle. Calves, goats and sheep require a smaller-gauge catheter (14-, 16- or 18-ga). An 18- to 22-ga, 1½-inch catheter is adequate for kids and lambs. A butterfly catheter or a 22-ga, 1½-inch catheter is used to catheterize the ear vein of pigs.

Restraint required for IV catheterization is identical to that described for IV injection. The site should be clipped and surgically scrubbed. Local anesthesia is not required for most food animals. An antiseptic is applied to complete skin preparation. Because of the skin's thickness, attempts to introduce a catheter through it may bend the catheter or damage the tip. To help introduce a catheter, a disposable needle of the same gauge is used to puncture the skin. This enables the catheter to pass through the skin with ease.

Cattle, Sheep, Goats

The catheterization procedure for cattle, sheep and goats is similar to that used in horses (see Chapter 5).

Swine

A rubber band placed around the base of the ear distends the vein. Introduce the catheter at the distal section of the vein (near the ear's tip) at a 30-45° angle. When blood enters the catheter, advance it into the vein to the hub. Remove the stylet if using an over-the-needle catheter, attach a syringe and aspirate. Blood should flow easily through the catheter. Place an injection cap or an IV extension set onto the catheter's hub. Remove the rubber band, then flush the catheter with heparinized saline and observe the site for perivascular infiltration. Dry the ear before attempting to secure the catheter. A ½-inch strip of adhesive tape is placed around the catheter's hub and wrapped around the entire ear.

It is important to use aseptic technic when inserting a catheter to minimize the chances of such complications as hematomas, phlebitis, thrombosis, and catheter breakage.

INTRAMUSCULAR INJECTIONS

Intramuscular (IM) injections are commonly used in cattle and swine. Other routes are preferred in sheep and goats due to their small muscle masses.

Cattle

Several large muscle masses are available for IM injections in cattle, including the gluteals, semimembranosus, semitendinosus and the lateral cervical muscles. The gluteals are located on the dorsal aspect of the rear legs. The semimembranosus and semitendinosus are located in the rear limbs, between the stifle joint and ischium. The lateral cervical muscles are cranial to the scapula, dorsal to the cervical vertebrae and ventral to the ligamentum nuchae.

The needle selected for IM injection depends on the viscosity of the medication to be administered and the size of the muscle mass selected. A 16-, 18- or 20-ga, 1½-inch needle is commonly used for adults. A smaller-gauge needle is used for calves (18-, 20- or 22-ga).

Gluteal Muscle Injection

The gluteal muscles may be injected with minimal restraint; securing the animal's head is usually adequate. The site is swabbed with an antiseptic solution and allowed to dry. One should stand close to the cow's flank, cranial to the stifle, facing the opposite direction as the cow (Fig 15). The needle can be inserted into the muscle mass nearer the technician or into the muscles of the opposite hip (Fig 16). Because an animal usually kicks on the same side where the pain is felt, the needle should be inserted into the opposite side to reduce the chances of being kicked.

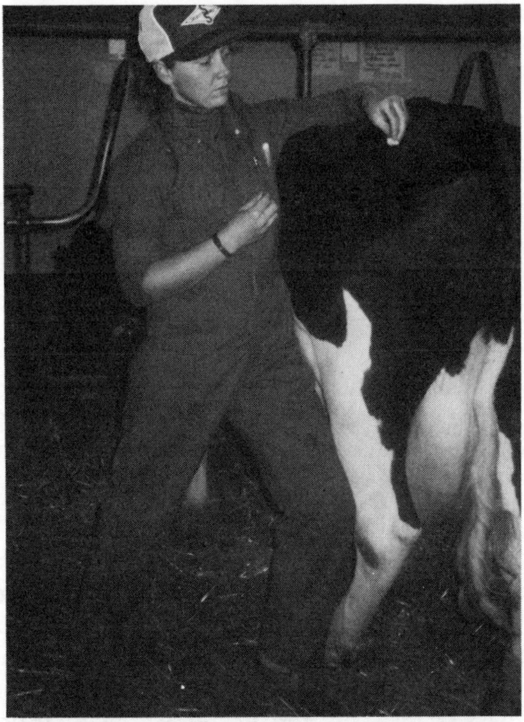

Fig 15. Correct position for IM injection into the gluteal muscle mass.

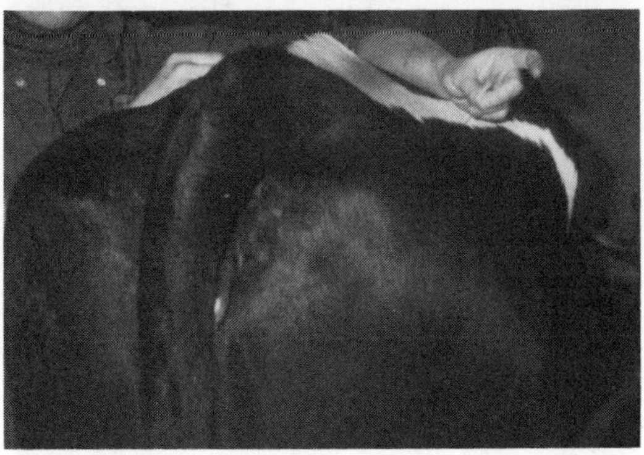

Fig 16. Insertion of the needle into the muscle mass on the cow's opposite side.

The needle is removed from the syringe before insertion and held by its hub, between the thumb and forefinger (Fig 17). Strike the animal several times with the back of the hand holding the needle. Keeping the same rhythm, flip the hand over and insert the needle into the muscle. The preliminary strokes are used to warn the animal of the impending injection. Attach the syringe and aspirate. If blood is withdrawn into the syringe, withdraw the needle and repeat the pro-

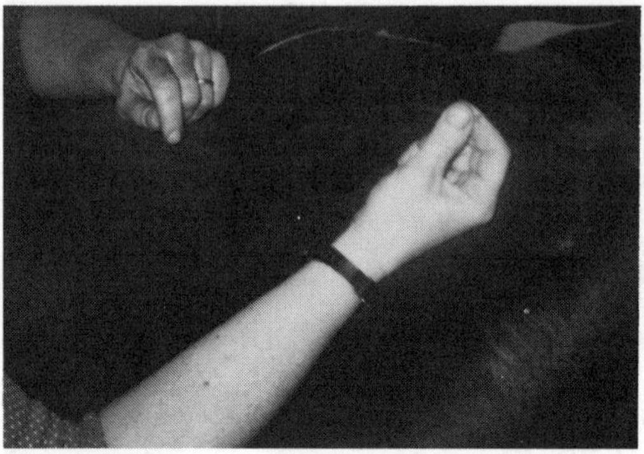

Fig 17. Grasping the needle for IM insertion.

cedure at another site. Once it is certain the needle has not entered a vessel, the medication may be injected. The site may require digital pressure after withdrawing the needle to prevent leakage of medication from the site.

Semimembranosus/Semitendinosus Injection

The restraint, equipment and site preparation for semimembranosus or semitendinosus injections are the same as for the gluteals. As with the gluteals, medication can be injected into the opposite muscle mass or into that nearer the technician (Fig 18). The needle is inserted and medication injected in the same manner as previously described for the gluteals.

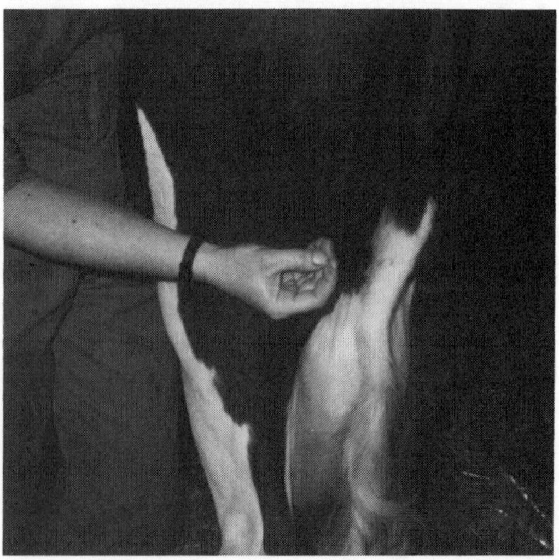

Fig 18. Correct position and proper insertion site for IM injection into the semimembranosus and semitendinosus muscles.

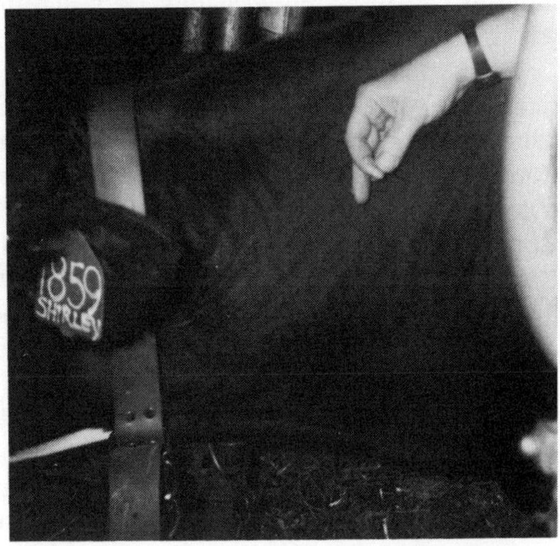

Fig 19. Correct site for IM injections into the cervical muscles.

Lateral Cervical Muscles

The neck muscles may be used for IM injections, though the muscles of the rear legs are preferred (Fig 19). In general, cows are "head shy" and react more to injections into the neck than at other sites.

Restrain the animal and prepare the site with an antiseptic. It is best if the neck region is not struck before inserting the needle for the animal may become "head shy." Attach the syringe, aspirate and inject the medication. Withdraw the needle and apply digital pressure to the site to prevent leakage of medication.

The maximum volume of medication that can be deposited per IM site in adult cattle is 15-20 ml. Up to 10-15 ml can be injected per site in calves, depending on their muscle mass. For numerous injections, injection sites should be rotated to prevent soreness and local inflammation in one particular muscle.

Swine

The sites for IM injections in swine are limited, as drug residue in various muscles may decrease the animal's market value. The gluteal, semimembranosus and semitendinosus muscles can be used, but are avoided in market-bound swine. The dorsolateral muscles of the neck, directly caudal to the ear, are best for IM injections in swine.

The animal should be adequately restrained before IM injection. When a number of swine are to be injected, it helps to crowd them into a pen. The technician then injects each animal as he or she walks among the pigs. Piglets may be restrained by holding them up by their rear legs.

A disposable 18- to 20-ga, 1½-inch needle is appropriate for IM injections in adult pigs. Piglets require a smaller-gauge needle. Wipe the site with an antiseptic and remove the needle from the syringe before insertion. Striking the animal before inserting the needle is not necessary, as it may excite the animal. Insert the needle with a quick thrust and attach the syringe. If no blood is present upon aspiration, inject the medication. The needle and syringe are removed and digital pressure is applied briefly to the site. A maximum of 10-15 ml may be injected per site, depending on the size of the muscle mass.

Sheep and Goats

The semimembranosus and semitendinosus muscles are commonly used for IM injections in sheep and goats. The gluteals and triceps may be used, but have such a small muscle mass that only minimal amounts may be injected at these sites. Injection into the cervical muscles generally is not recommended, as the animals become too sore. This is important in young animals, as they may refuse to nurse if they become too sore to lift their head.

Sheep and goats are easily restrained by an assistant or by confinement to a small area. The injection site is prepared with an antiseptic solution. An 18- to 20-ga, 1½-inch needle is recommended for use in adult sheep and goats. Young animals require a 20- to 22-ga needle.

Insert the needle at a 90° angle to the muscle, with or without the syringe attached. After aspirating, inject the medication. Apply digital pressure to the site after withdrawing the needle. The maximum volume that may be injected is 15 ml, with an average of 5-10 ml. Care must be taken in kids, lambs or thin animals to avoid hitting the sciatic nerve, running down the caudomedial aspect of the rear legs.

SUBCUTANEOUS INJECTIONS

Subcutaneous (SC) injections are given anywhere loose skin can be raised. In cattle and goats, this is easily done on the lateral aspect of the neck and thorax, the axillary region, the fold of the flank and the brisket. The sites chosen in sheep should be free of wool, such as on the axillary region and flank folds. Subcutaneous injections are not commonly used in swine because of the difficulty in raising loose skin. Possible sites for SC injections in swine are the axillary and inguinal areas. The area just caudal to the base of the ear also may be used.

Subcutaneous injections generally require minimal restraint. Swine, sheep, goats and calves can be cornered in a small area. Small pigs can be held by the rear limbs for injections into the fold of the flank. Adult cattle should have a halter applied and be placed in a headgate or stanchion. Aggressive animals may require a chute.

An 18-, 20- or 22-ga, 1½-inch needle is used for SC injections in goats, sheep, calves and swine. A 14-, 16- or 18-ga, 1½-inch needle is used for cattle. The needle size selected depends on the viscosity of the drug and the thickness of the skin. A syringe is used to inject small quantities. A simplex system may be used to administer larger quantities. The site should be cleaned with an antiseptic, such as 70% alcohol. Pinch the skin and raise it to form a "tent." Insert the needle with a quick thrust into the "tent," taking care not to penetrate the other side. After the needle is positioned, aspirate. If blood is not observed upon aspiration, inject the medication. If there is blood present in the needle, withdraw the needle and attempt the injection at a new site. When the injection is completed, withdraw the needle, release the skin fold and massage the area to enhance spread of the medication and increase its absorption rate.

The volume of medication injected at each SC site varies according to personal preference, the species involved and the animal's size. For cattle, 50-100 ml per site is the recommended maximum, though up to 250 ml may be given SC. When giving large volumes, the needle should be intermittently redirected to prevent depositing large quantities in one site. The amount that can be injected at each SC site for goats, sheep and calves varies from 2 to 30 ml, with a maximum volume of 50 ml. The maximum volume that can be injected SC in swine is about 30 ml.

INTRADERMAL INJECTIONS

Intradermal (ID) injection is directed into the dermis, one of the skin layers. In food animals, ID injections are used mainly to aid in diagnosis of certain diseases. Cattle and goats are tested for tuberculosis using ID injection of bovine tuberculin. Intradermal injections are also used for allergy testing, a procedure usually limited to pets. Local anesthetics are injected ID to anesthetize sites for surgery or other invasive procedures.

The caudal tail fold is the site used most often for ID injections of tuberculin. They may also be given on the lateral aspect of the neck and abdomen. In swine, ID injections are given at the base of the ear.

The restraint required depends on the site chosen, the number of injections to be given and the animal's temperament. Most animals require minimal restraint. The sites must be free of hair before ID injection is attempted. If a diagnostic test is to be performed, the site should not be cleaned with antiseptics, as they might create a skin reaction and interfere with test results. Usually removal of dirt and feces is all that is required for preparation. Antiseptics can be applied to the site if local anesthetics are being deposited before surgery.

For goats, sheep and swine, a 25- or 22-ga, ½-inch to 1-inch needle is used for ID injection. Cattle require a larger needle, such as a 20- to 22-ga, 1½-inch needle, due to their thicker skin. A tuberculin or 3-ml syringe is adequate for injecting small volumes ID.

The needle, with the syringe attached, is placed parallel to the skin. The free hand is used to pinch the skin. This pulls the skin taut and helps stabilize it. With the bevel directed up, gently insert the needle into the dermis of the skin. Aspirate if the injection is for local anesthesia over a vessel. A raised area ("bleb") should be visualized as the drug is deposited. If a bleb does not form, the needle is too deep; retract it a small distance and inject the drug. It is not necessary to massage the site, for the object is to keep the drug localized.

INTRAPERITONEAL INJECTION

Use of intraperitoneal (IP) injections is not recommended for routine injection of medication. This technic is used when IV administration is impossible or in local treatment of peritonitis.

Cattle

In adult cattle, IP injections are given in the paralumbar fossa. The rumen may be punctured if the injection is given on the left side. Injections into the right paralumbar fossa may puncture loops of intestines or dilated organs, such as the cecum or a displaced abomasum.

With the cow securely restrained, the site is clipped and surgically scrubbed, and local anesthesia is administered.

A 14-ga, 2-inch needle is commonly attached to a 20- to 50-ml syringe for IP injections. A simplex system may be used to deliver large volumes. The needle is gently inserted into the peritoneum. Air may be heard escaping through the needle as the peritoneum is punctured. If the rumen or intestines have been inadvertently punctured, a distinct gas odor can be detected. A syringe can be attached and aspirated to check for gastrointestinal contents. As the medication is injected, it should run in freely if the needle is correctly placed in the peritoneum.

Calves, Goats, Sheep and Swine

The caudoventral abdominal wall is best for IP injections performed on calves, goats, sheep and swine. The animal is restrained in dorsal recumbency, with the rear limbs elevated. The site is prepped as for IP injections in adult cattle.

A 16- or 18-ga, 1½-inch needle and a 10-, 20- or 50-ml syringe are used. The needle is inserted and directed caudad. To avoid puncturing the bladder, or in males, injuring the penis, insert the needle slightly off midline. Aspirate and inject the medication.

Several complications may occur with IP injections. Puncturing the gastrointestinal tract or other vital organs may result in peritonitis. Inadequate site preparation and poor technic may also result in peritonitis or an abscess.

INTRAMAMMARY INFUSION

Veterinarians and dairy farmers often employ intramammary infusions to treat mastitis or to infuse quarters when cows are dry. The best time to infuse the udder is after the last milking of the day, which allows the medication to remain in the udder overnight. The udder should not be infused before milking because the beneficial effect of the medication would be lost. Because intramammary antibiotic therapy affects the results of milk culture, milk samples from mastitic quarters must be obtained before treatment.

Minimal restraint is required for intramammary infusion. Tail restraint may be used for nervous animals or those in pain. A chute may be necessary for fractious cows. Care must be taken with beef cows, especially if they have been separated from their calves, as they are usually very aggressive.

Crouch beside the udder to work; never sit down or kneel. This makes it easier to avoid injury from kicking. The udder should be thoroughly cleaned before treatment, using warm water and antiseptic soap. A separate cloth or paper towel should be used to wash each teat so as to decrease the spread of microorganisms among the quarters. Dry each teat with a separate towel to remove contaminated water droplets. The teat orifice is wiped with an alcohol swab and allowed to air dry. If all 4 quarters are to be infused, swab the far teats before swabbing the near ones, so as to prevent contamination when reaching past the near teats.

Empty the quarter by manually "stripping" out the milk before infusing medication, as residual milk mixes with the medication and dilutes it. Collect the discarded milk in a bucket to prevent contamination of the environment by the bacteria in the milk. After the teat is prepared, grasp it near the base and insert a teat cannula or sterile,

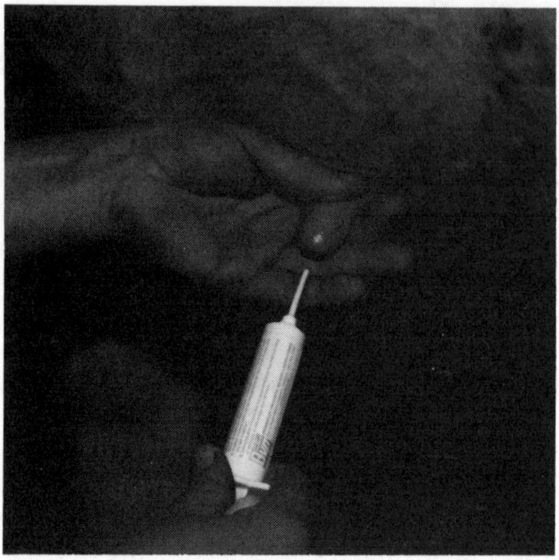

Fig 20. After proper preparation of the teat, a teat cannula or cannula on an intramammary treatment tube is inserted into the teat's orifice.

disposable mammary infusion cannula into the teat orifice. More commonly, commercially prepared, disposable syringes with an attached cannula are used (Fig 20). Advance the cannula to the hub and inject the medication slowly. As little as 10-20 ml or as much as 250 ml may be infused into a quarter. Remove the cannula and massage the teat and quarter to disseminate the medication. When the procedure is completed, dip the teat in teat dip to prevent invasion of microbes (Fig 21). If the weather is extremely cold (0 C or less), do not let the cow outside until the udder is dry, so as to prevent chapping and frostbite. Mark the cows that were treated so their milk can be discarded.

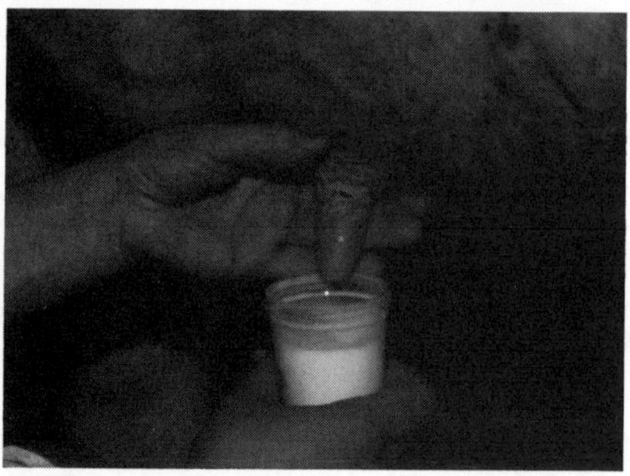

Fig 21. The teat should be dipped after intramammary treatment.

Always use sanitary technics when manipulating the udder, as mastitis can be transferred to unaffected quarters in cows with mastitis or to other cows in the barn.

The veterinarian is responsible for informing the client of withdrawal times for any drug given to a food animal. Most pharmaceutical companies furnish drug withdrawal times on the labels of their products.

Of the food animal species, only cows and goats are milked on a routine basis. Intramammary infusion technics, as described for dairy cows, also apply to treatment of goats.

INTRANASAL INSUFFLATION

The intranasal route is most commonly used to administer vaccines and local anesthetics. As of this writing, intranasal vaccines have been approved only for infectious bovine rhinotracheitis (IBR) and parainfluenza-3 (PI_3) infection. Vaccines not designed for intranasal use are not effective when given by this route. Intranasal anesthetics may be given before potentially painful procedures on the nasal cavity, such as nasogastric intubation, bronchoalveolar lavage and endoscopy.

Restraint of the head is a necessity. Calves may be manually restrained, while adults should be secured with a halter and headgate. Nasal secretions should be wiped from the nostril with moist cotton before medication administration. A 3- to 5-ml syringe is filled with the vaccine or local anesthetic, with a disposable, blunt tip attached to inject the drug, though the syringe alone may be used (Fig 22). Facing the same direction as the animal, one hand is placed over the head, pulling it close to your body. The head must be slightly elevated

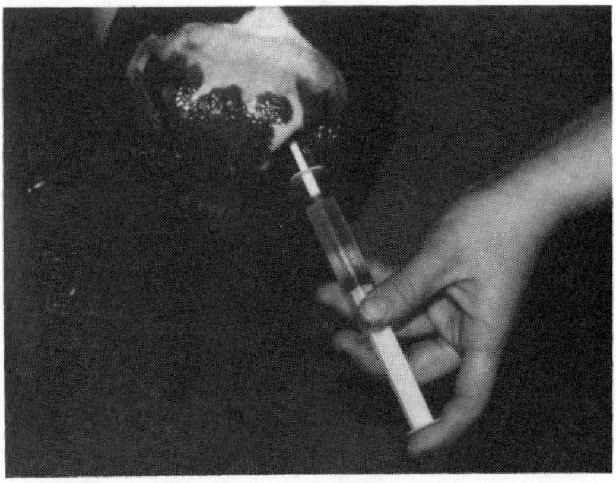

Fig 22. A syringe and a blunt-tipped cannula are often used for intranasal injection.

to prevent the medication from running out of the nostril. The free hand is used to insert the syringe into the nostril (Fig 22). When the injection is completed, elevate the head for 10-15 seconds before releasing it.

OCULAR MEDICATION

Ocular medication technics are used to locally treat ocular disorders with ointments and solutions. The technics for application of ocular medication are similar for all species. Immobilization of the head is required.

Rest the hand holding the medication on the animal's head, dorsal to (above) the eye. With the free hand, separate the lids and apply the medication. Do not touch the tip of the applicator to the eye, as this may traumatize the cornea and contaminate the applicator. When applying both solutions and ointments to the eye, administer the solution first, as the solution will run off if it is applied on top of an ointment.

INTRAUTERINE MEDICATION

Medication is placed in the uterus to locally treat metritis. Though this technic may be performed by veterinary technicians, they are not routinely instructed in this procedure. It is up to the veterinarian as to whether technicians should perform this procedure.

Uterine medication is available as boluses, capsules and solutions. The form of the drug used depends on the condition of the uterus, the

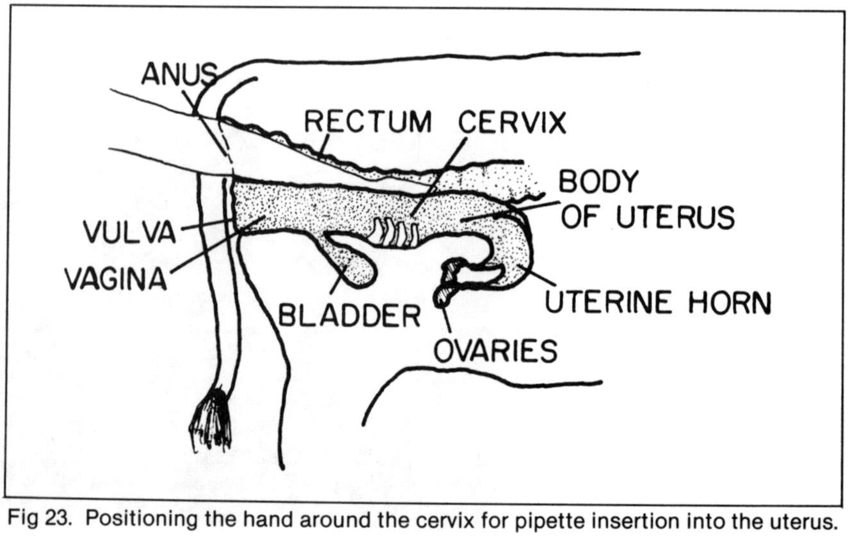

Fig 23. Positioning the hand around the cervix for pipette insertion into the uterus.

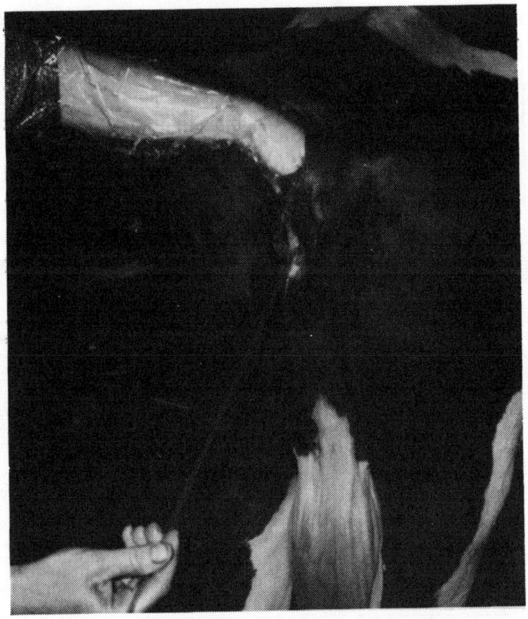

Fig 24. Inserting a sterile pipette without contaminating the tip.

stage of the reproductive cycle, the types of drugs available and personal preference.

Cows require minimal restraint for this procedure. The tail should be secured away from the perianal region. Feces should be "raked" (manually removed) from the rectum before the vulva is cleaned, so as to aid in palpation and prevent contamination of the area and equipment. An antiseptic soap, warm water and cotton are used to wash the vulva and surrounding area. Wipe the vulva, starting at the dorsal commissure of the labia and progressing down to the ventral commissure. The soap should be rinsed off before treatment.

Intrauterine Infusion

A uterine pipette is used to infuse solutions into the uterus, using a syringe to inject the medication through the pipette. An equine nasogastric tube and stomach pump may be used to flush large volumes of medication into the uterus.

To aid passage of the pipette into the uterus, guide it with the opposite hand, placed into the rectum. The cervix, which lies about 3-4 inches cranial to the vulva, is grasped with the left hand (for a right-handed person) so the thumb is dorsal to the cervix and the fingers are located ventrad (Fig 23). The pipette is inserted into the vulva, exercising care to avoid touching the pipette's tip to the labia (Fig 24).

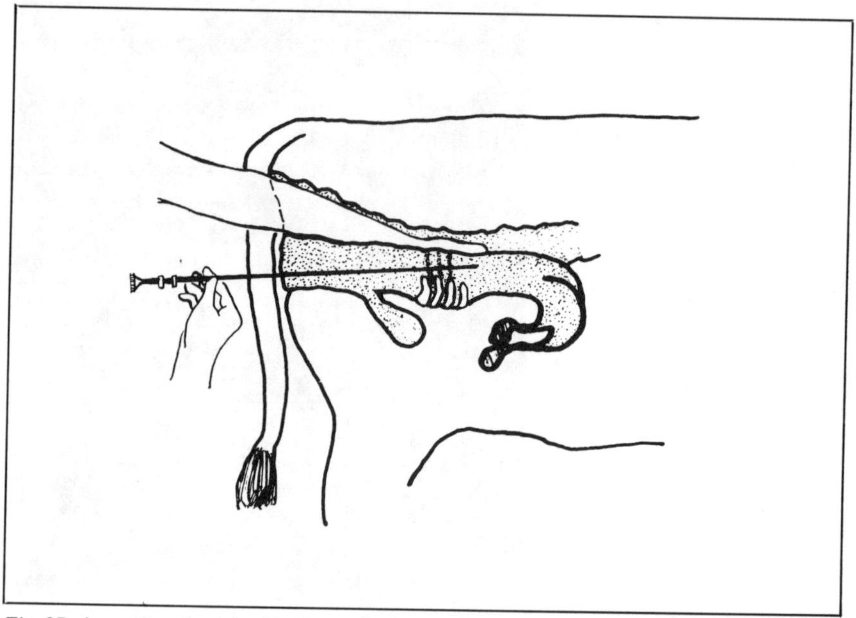

Fig 25. Inserting the pipette through the cervix into the uterus.

The pipette is advanced at a 30-40° angle for 3-4 inches. This prevents the pipette from entering the urethral opening, located on the floor of the vagina. Once past the urethral orifice, the pipette is advanced in a horizontal position. To aid in passage of the pipette, pull the cervix craniad to straighten the folds of the vagina. As the pipette is advanced, it may become caught in a vaginal fold. If this occurs, do not force the pipette craniad, but simply withdraw and redirect it.

Introduce the pipette's tip into the cervical opening, which is usually in the center of the cervix. Gently manipulate the cervix over the pipette. Once the pipette is through the cervix, it slides craniad easily and may be palpated rectally (Fig 25). Beginners commonly deposit the medication in the vagina or cervix, rather than in the uterus. Always make certain the tip has passed into the uterus. Advance the pipette just beyond the cervix into the uterus. The medication is injected and then the pipette is flushed with air to remove residual medication.

Through the entirety of this procedure, it is important never to force the pipette craniad, as this may damage vaginal or cervical tissue. Also, the vaginal and rectal walls may be penetrated if excessive force is used. This could result in such complications as peritonitis, metritis, abscesses and possible reproductive disorders.

Intrauterine Boluses

A sterile sleeve should be worn to insert boluses or capsules into the uterus. Advance the hand into the vulva and vagina until the cervix is located. The hand is formed into a wedge, inserted into the dilated os cervix (cervical orifice) and advanced into the uterus, where the medication is deposited. There are fewer complications with this method of intrauterine medication than with infusion. The primary complication is introduction of bacteria into the uterus by using poor sanitary technics. Rough handling can damage vaginal and cervical tissue.

Many farmers medicate their animals with these methods. They should be carefully instructed in use of the proper technics and informed of possible complications. They should also be informed of drug withdrawal times so meat or milk from treated animals is not immediately sold.

ORAL MEDICATION

Oral medication is available in many forms, including liquids, pastes, powders, tablets, capsules and boluses. Instruments used to deliver the medication include the balling gun, Frick's speculum, dose syringe, drench bottle and stomach tube.

The different methods used for giving oral medication require similar restraint measures. The head is secured in a stanchion or

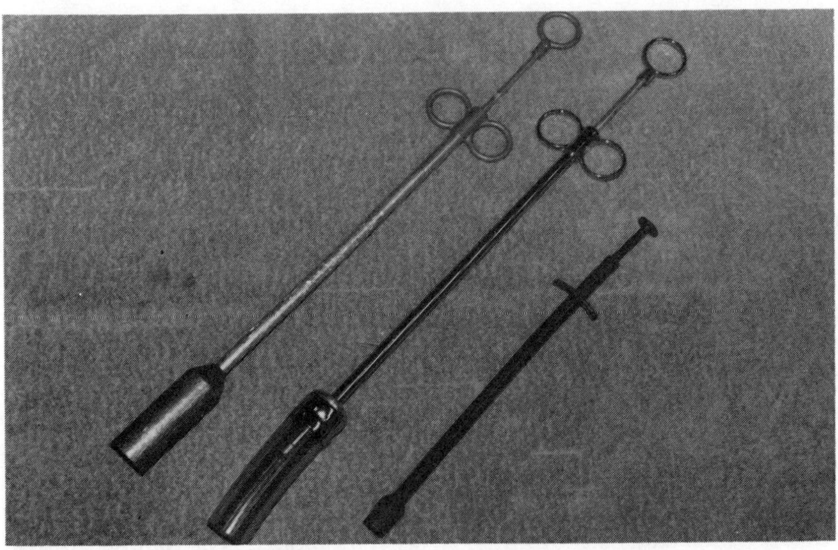

Fig 26. Various sizes of balling guns are available.

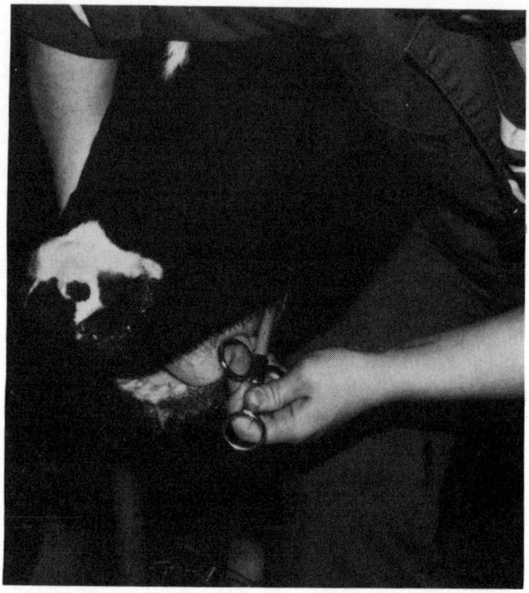

Fig 27. The correct positioning of the head and the insertion of the balling gun.

headgate. Halters are not usually required; if they are used, they should not be applied too tightly over the muzzle so the animal can adequately open its mouth. Swine, sheep and goats may be restrained by backing them into a corner or against a wall.

Balling Gun

Boluses, capsules or magnets may be given *per os* (PO) with a balling gun (Fig 26). This instrument is available in various sizes for use in different species. Cattle require a gun with a large head and long handle, with a metal or flexible plastic head. The plastic head produces less trauma to the pharyngeal tissue than a metal head but is easily damaged by teeth. Small balling guns are manufactured for use in sheep, goats, swine and calves.

The methods of introducing a balling gun, dose syringe, drench bottle or Frick's speculum are similar in all species. Standing cranial to the cow's shoulder and facing the same direction as the animal, place one arm over the animal's head and caudal to the poll, with the animal's head positioned on your hip (Fig 27). This technic may not be possible for people with short arms. In this case, reaching across the bridge of the nose is acceptable. Insert the fingers of this hand into the mouth at the interdental space and apply pressure to the hard palate, which causes the animal to open its mouth. The balling gun, or similar instrument, is inserted at an upward angle at the interdental space, opposite the restraining hand (Fig 27). Direct the instrument caudad and advance it over the base of the tongue. Once it is over the tongue's base, advance the balling gun in a horizontal position until the rings of the handle reach the buccal commissure (corner of the mouth) (Fig 27). This insures that the gun is back far enough in the mouth to deposit the bolus, forcing the cow to swallow and preventing expulsion of the medication. Depress the plunger to eject the bolus and remove the instrument. Observe the cow to be sure the medication was swallowed. It is not necessary to elevate the head until the bolus is swallowed if the bolus was deposited correctly.

Frick's Speculum

A Frick's speculum may be used to give 2 or more boluses to cattle (Fig 28). Insert the speculum in the same manner as the balling gun. Once the speculum is placed over the base of the tongue, the boluses are inserted into the speculum. Allow the boluses to travel down the speculum and into the mouth. Remove the speculum and observe for swallowing. This method is used to save time but has the added danger of aspiration of medication.

Drenching

Giving small volumes of liquids PO is often referred to as "drenching." Drenching is done with a dose syringe or a drench bottle (Fig 29). A 60-ml, catheter-tipped syringe or a bulb syringe may be used as a dose syringe in calves, sheep, swine and goats. The drench bottle, commonly a wine or soft drink bottle, should be made of strong glass and have a long, tapered neck and smooth mouth.

The technic for drenching is similar to that described for the balling gun. Be certain to insert the drench bottle at the interdental space to prevent the cow from breaking it with its molars. The head should

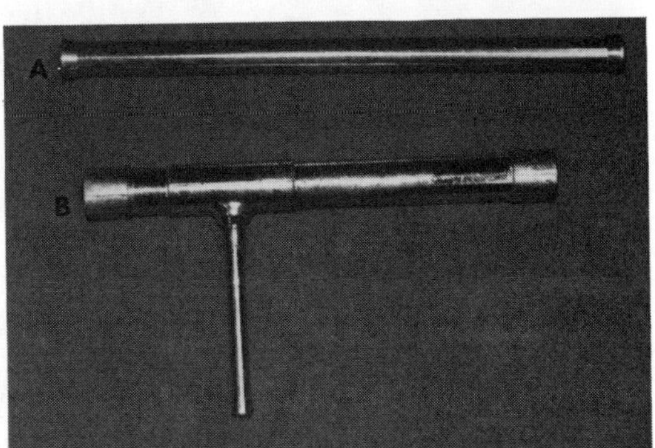

Fig 28. Regular Frick's speculum (A) and a modified Frick's speculum (B).

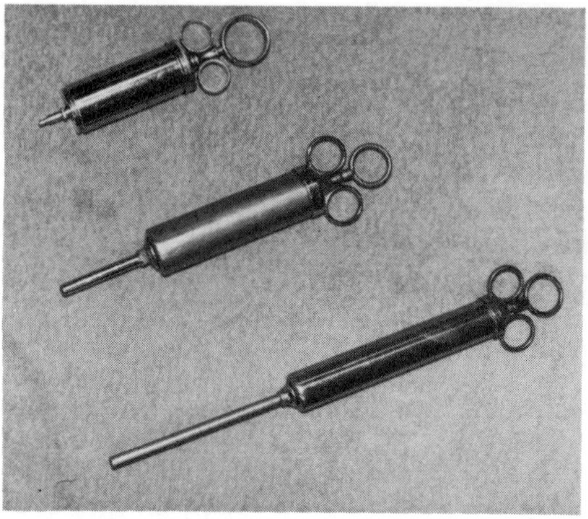

Fig 29. Various sizes of dose syringes.

be held slightly elevated so the nose is level with the animal's eye. If the head is raised excessively, the animal may aspirate some medication. Give the medication slowly, allowing the animal to swallow at its own pace.

Dose syringes are also used to give pastes. Commercially prepared syringes containing medication are available, though these are used more often in horses.

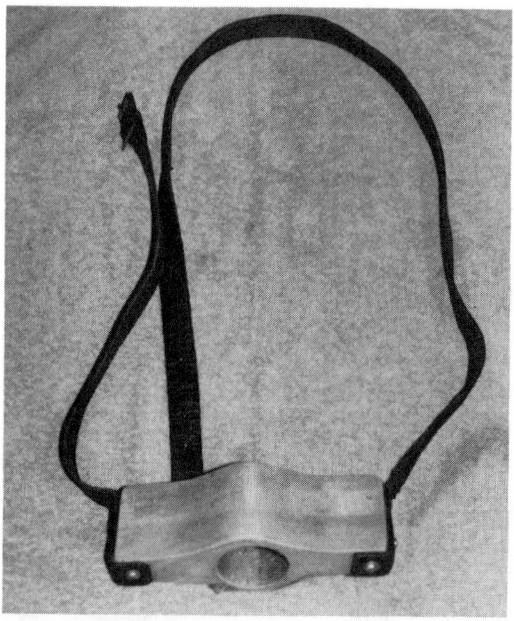

Fig 30. The Colorado bovine speculum is positioned in the animal's mouth, with the straps fastened behind the poll.

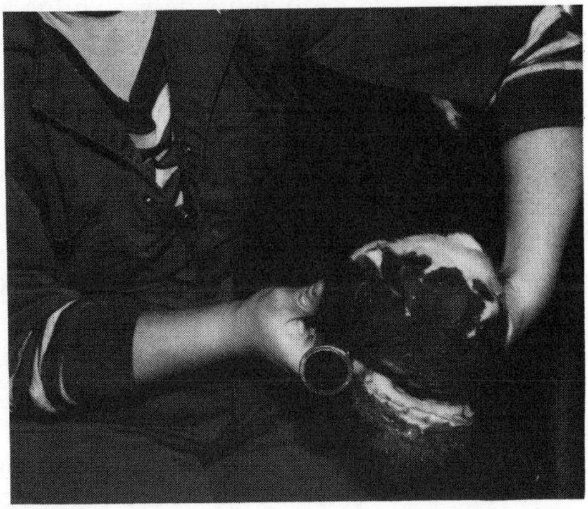

Fig 31. Correct placement of a Frick's speculum for passage of a stomach tube.

Gastric Intubation

"Stomach tubing" is a quick and relatively painless method to deliver large quantities of liquid medication or fluids. A stomach tube may be passed through the nasal cavity, as in horses, but this method is not commonly used in food animals. In food animals, the stomach tube is usually passed through the oral cavity, with the aid of a metal speculum.

Cattle: An oral speculum is required to prevent damage to the soft stomach tube from the animal's teeth. Specula used in cattle are the Frick's speculum (Fig 28) and Colorado bovine speculum (Fig 30). The Frick's speculum is inserted into the mouth and held in place by an assistant. The Colorado bovine speculum, once inserted, is secured behind the poll with straps. Using the Colorado speculum allows one person to complete the intubation procedure, whereas use of the Frick's speculum requires 2 people.

Stomach tubes are available in different lengths and diameters. Choose an appropriately sized tube for the individual animal. A tube with an outside diameter of 5/8-1 inch is the average size used for adult cattle. A foal stomach tube is often used for "tubing" calves. A stomach pump or a funnel can be used to facilitate administration.

Measure the distance externally from the mouth to the rumen and insert the tube approximately this distance. Once this skill has been mastered, the mouth-rumen distance is easily estimated. The first 3 feet of the tube should be lubricated with water, mineral oil or lubricating jelly before intubation. With an assistant holding an oral speculum in place, insert the tube into the speculum and advance it with gentle pressure (Fig 31). Some resistance may be felt when the tube reaches the esophagus. Observe for swallowing, then advance the tube into the esophagus. If passage is difficult, rotate the tube slightly and apply gentle pressure to advance the tube.

After inserting the tube the measured distance, check for correct placement in the rumen. If the stomach tube was inadvertently placed in the trachea, the animal may cough, though this should not be used alone to determine correct placement. If the tube has been inadvertently passed down the trachea, air may be felt exiting the tube upon exhalation. Remove the tube and reintubate. Another test used to check if the tube has been passed into the rumen is to have one person blow air into the end of the tube while another listens with a stethoscope at the rumen. A gurgling sound should be heard as air is blown into the tube. The smell of rumen gas may sometimes be detected exiting the tube. In some lightly muscled animals, the tube can be observed progressing down the esophagus. In these animals, one may also palpate the neck for 2 tubular structures, *ie,* the trachea and the stomach tube within the esophagus.

Once the stomach tube is correctly positioned, the medication can be given. After the medication has been infused, rinse the tube with water to flush out remaining medication. Kink the tube or occlude its end and withdraw it quickly. This prevents any fluid remaining in the tube from entering the trachea upon tube removal.

Swine, Sheep and Goats: A stomach tube with an outside diameter of 3/8-1/2 inch can be used to give liquid medication PO to swine, sheep and goats. A stallion urinary catheter or a small canine stomach tube may be used for kids and lambs.

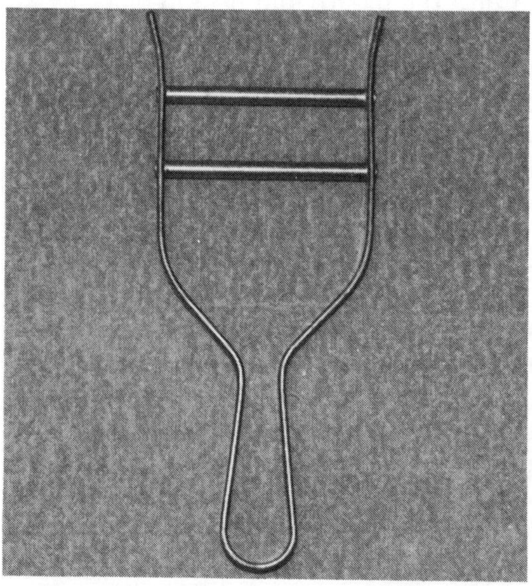

Fig 32. A swine oral speculum may be used on other species.

A swine mouth speculum can be used not only for swine but also for sheep, goats and calves (Fig 32). This instrument is placed into the mouth in a horizontal position (see Chapter 2) and then rotated to a vertical position at the interdental space. A hollow tube, simulating a Frick's speculum, may also be used as an oral speculum.

The technic for stomach intubation used in cattle also applies to sheep, swine and goats. Tests to confirm the tube's position are the same as for cattle. However, it is difficult to palpate a pig's neck or observe tube passage due to the fat and muscle in its neck.

BLOOD COLLECTION

Small volumes (0.5-10 ml) of blood may be collected for various blood tests, such as hematologic examination and serum chemistry analysis, to aid in diagnosing a disease, or to monitor a disease's progression or an animal's recovery. Blood is also collected for transfusion of whole blood or plasma to treat anemic or hypoproteinemic animals.

Collecting Samples

Cattle

The veins most often used to obtain blood samples from cattle are the jugular and coccygeal (tail) veins. Blood can also be collected from the mammary vein, though this is rarely done. The coccygeal vein is easily accessible and blood collection is less traumatic to the cow than with use of the jugular vein. The jugular vein is used for blood collection in calves, as their coccygeal veins are difficult to puncture due to small size.

A syringe and needle combination or a convenient vacuum tube system (Vacutainer) may be used (see Chapter 5). When a syringe is used, the blood must be immediately transferred to a vial containing an anticoagulant to prevent the sample from clotting. A syringe that has been flushed with an anticoagulant, such as heparin, can be used to obtain small volumes (3-5 ml) of blood. Vacuum tubes are available with various anticoagulants or no anticoagulant. Tubes containing an anticoagulant must be inverted several times immediately after blood collection to thoroughly mix the blood and anticoagulant to prevent clot formation.

Jugular Vein: A 22- or 20-ga Vacutainer needle is used to collect blood from calves. Adult cattle require a 20-ga Vacutainer needle for jugular venipuncture. The collection tube chosen depends on the type of tests requested. A 20-ga, 1½-inch injection needle is more suitable for adults.

With the animal properly restrained, cleanse the site with an antiseptic. Distend the vein and insert the needle at a 30-45° angle to the skin, directing it craniad (toward the head). Thread the needle into the vein, observing the hub for blood. Attach the syringe and withdraw the amount required. After removing the needle, apply digital pressure to the venipuncture site.

When using the Vacutainer system, insert the needle as previously described. Observe the needle's end for blood droplets and attach the collection tube to the needle. Blood flows into the tube until the vacuum is gone. After the first collection tube is removed, another may be attached if necessary. A Vacutainer needle holder is available to facilitate attaching the tubes to the needle (see Chapter 5).

Coccygeal Vein: An 18- or 20-ga, 1½-inch needle with an attached 3-, 5- or 10-ml syringe, or a 20-ga Vacutainer needle and collection tubes, can be used to obtain blood from the coccygeal vein. Use of a Vacutainer holder makes this procedure easier for beginners. The technic of coccygeal venipuncture is identical to that described for giving coccygeal vein medication.

Auricular Artery: Samples from this artery are used for blood-gas analysis on anesthetized cattle or those with severe respiratory or metabolic disorders. An 18- to 22-ga, 1½-inch needle and a 3- to 5-ml syringe flushed with an anticoagulant are used to collect the sample.

In animals that are not anesthetized, the head must be restrained for this procedure. The artery is located by palpating the ear for a pulse. The site is shaved and scrubbed with an antiseptic. Insert the needle into the artery, with the bevel directed up. Aspirate slightly to collect the sample. Withdraw the needle and apply digital pressure over the site. Remove all air bubbles from the syringe and quickly cap the end of the tube to prevent air entry into the tube. The blood-gas analysis should be done immediately after sample collection.

Sheep and Goats

The jugular vein is most commonly used to collect blood from sheep and goats, though the cephalic or femoral veins are occasionally used. The venipuncture technic for these veins is similar to that used on dogs (see Chapter 4).

Jugular venipuncture can be accomplished with a 16- to 20-ga, 1½-inch needle for adults and a 22- to 20-ga needle for lambs and kids. Alternatively, a 22- to 20-ga Vacutainer needle and tubes may be used. The technic for jugular venipuncture in sheep and goats is identical to that used in cattle.

Swine

Venipuncture sites are limited in swine by their lack of accessible veins. The caudal auricular (ear) vein may be used to obtain small volumes (3-5 ml) of blood. The cranial vena cava is used for collection

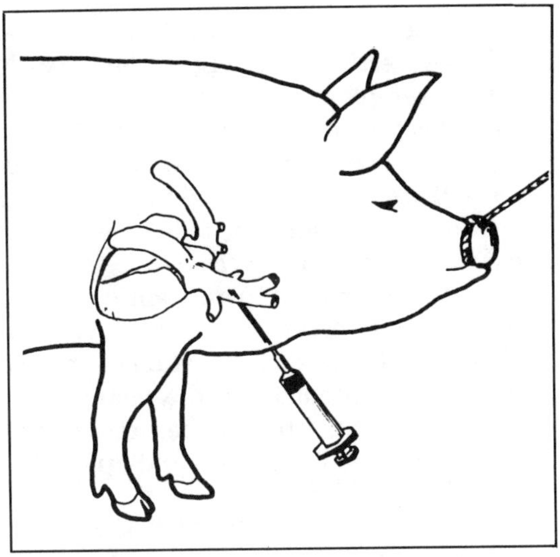

Fig 33. Venipuncture of the cranial vena cava in swine.

of larger blood volumes. This vein is located deep in the thoracic cavity and requires skill and practice for venipuncture.

Cranial Vena Cava: An 18- or 20-ga, 3- to 4-inch needle should be used to collect blood from the cranial vena cava of adult pigs. Large boars may require a 5-inch needle. Small pigs (under 40-50 lb) require a shorter needle (1½-inch needles are usually sufficient).

The cranial vena cava is located by using several landmarks (Fig 33). Adult pigs should be restrained in a standing position for this procedure, though small pigs may be held or placed in dorsal recumbency. The same landmarks are used for all positions.

Palpate the manubrium sternum, a bony projection located on the ventral midline, cranial to the forelegs. Move the hand to the right of the manubrium, where a slight depression should be felt. This may be difficult to feel in large pigs. Pigs are bled from their right side to avoid the phrenic nerve, which is located on the left side.

Insert the needle through the skin in the depression. Use an imaginary line drawn from this depression to the opposite shoulder to direct the needle. It may help to place your free hand on the pig's opposite shoulder and aim the needle toward that hand. Aspirate slightly to create a negative pressure in the syringe and advance the needle with short stabbing movements. When the needle punctures the anterior vena cava, blood immediately enters the syringe. Maintain the needle in this position and withdraw the desired volume of blood. If blood is not obtained at the first attempt, withdraw the needle but do not remove it entirely from the animal. Never redirect the needle when it is deep inside the pig for laceration of the vena cava could result in death from hemorrhage. Before another attempt, check the needle's direction and repeat the procedure. Withdraw the needle once the sample is obtained and apply digital pressure to the site to control hemorrhage from skin vessels.

Caudal Auricular Vein: To collect blood from the auricular (ear) vein, a 22-ga needle attached to a 3- to 5-ml syringe, previously flushed with an anticoagulant, may be used. A rubber band or tubing, applied to the base of the ear, serves as a tourniquet.

Swab the ear with an antiseptic and place the rubber band around the ear's base. Allow time for the vein to become distended. Insert the needle into the distal portion of the vein. Aspirate slightly, as excessive vacuum collapses the vein. After the sample has been collected, place a thumb over the site and withdraw the needle. Immediately release the tourniquet and apply digital pressure.

Collecting Blood for Transfusion

Transfusions are not commonly used in most food animal practices, but are done more frequently in dogs, cats and horses (see Chapters 4, 5).

The needle size depends on the species involved. Adult cattle require a 10-, 12- or 14-ga, 2- to 3-inch needle for blood collection. A 16- or 18-ga, 1½-inch needle is sufficient for sheep, goats and calves.

The jugular vein is almost always used for collecting large volumes of blood. The site should be cleaned with an antiseptic and the needle inserted into the vein toward the heart (see Jugular Venipuncture). A collection line is then connected to the needle. During collection, gently invert the container to mix the blood and anticoagulant. To prevent hemolysis of the sample, avoid excess or rough movement of the bottle. When the desired amount is collected, remove the needle and apply digital pressure to the site.

Transfusions

Many food animal veterinarians do not cross-match donor and recipient blood before transfusion unless the recipient is a valuable animal or has previously received a transfusion.

An IV catheter is placed in the recipient's jugular vein and a blood administration set is connected to the catheter. The transfusion is started at a slow rate, while the animal is observed for possible reactions, such as increased respiration, dyspnea and tremors. Blood administration should be stopped immediately and emergency drugs administered under a veterinarian's supervision to control any adverse reaction during transfusion.

7

theriogenology

S.D. VAN CAMP & J.S. KRISH

Theriogenology is the official term for veterinary obstetrics and gynecology. This name was derived from 2 Greek terms: "therio," which means animal or beast, and "gen," which means coming into being. The suffix "-ology," which means the study of, was then added. Thus theriogenology encompasses the body of knowledge that can influence the *number of animals that come into being.*

To understand theriogenology, one must understand reproductive physiology and how it is affected by management, environment, nutrition and drugs.

NORMAL REPRODUCTIVE PHYSIOLOGY

Nonpregnant Animals

Unlike women and other female primates that have *menstrual cycles,* with variable levels of sexual receptivity, the mammals that we deal with commonly in veterinary medicine have an *estrous cycle,* in which the period of sexual receptivity, "estrus," is concentrated during a short period lasting one to several days. During the rest of the estrous cycle, the female does not accept the male's advances nor allow mating.

The *estrous cycle* is made up of 4 or 5 stages, depending on the species and whether the animal is polyestrous (cycles repeatedly) or is monestrous (cycles only once during the breeding season). These estrual cycle stages are:

Anestrus: This is the period of ovarian inactivity and no behavioral signs of heat or estrus.

Proestrus: Under the influence of gonadotropin-secreting hormone (GnRH) from the hypothalamus, follicle-stimulating hormone (FSH) from the pituitary acts on the ovary to cause initial follicle development on the ovary. These growing follicles produce estrogen, which causes the genital and behavioral changes that attract the male and prepare the female's reproductive tract for mating. The proestrous female does not allow mating.

Estrus: This is the period of true heat, during which the female allows mating. The estrogen levels peak early in estrus and cause the pituitary to release luteinizing hormone (LH), which causes maturation of follicles and results in release of the egg(s) at ovulation.

Metestrus: This is a short stage during which the female may still attract males but no longer allows mating. During this stage, ovulated follicles metamorphose into corpora lutea (CL), which begin to secrete progesterone. Metestrus is so short in some species that it is not even discussed as a separate stage and is included in diestrus.

Diestrus: This is a stage of ovarian activity without signs of heat. The CL develop fully and produce maximum levels of progesterone to ready the uterus for the conceptus and maintain pregnancy.

If pregnancy does not occur, prostaglandins are released from the uterus and destroy the CL and stop progesterone production. The female then either enters anestrus (if it is a monestrous species, such as the dog) or reenters proestrus (if it is a polyestrous species, such as the cow).

When reading about the days of the cycle, it is important to know what the author is calling "day 1." In the menstrual cycle, day 1 is the first day of menstrual bleeding. However, in the estrous cycle, bleeding may or may not occur and occurs at a different stage of the cycle for those species that show bleeding. Therefore, for this text, the first day of standing heat (estrus), when the female accepts the male, will be called day 0. Day 1 will be the day after the female first accepts the male. Some females are still in heat at this time, while females of other species already are out of heat on day 1.

Pregnant Animals

If the female conceives, the embryo signals its presence to the uterus in some manner, which prevents release of prostaglandins from the uterus. Thus, the CL remains active and continues to secrete progesterone throughout pregnancy or until the placenta takes over production of progesterone. The CL is necessary throughout pregnancy in the cow, goat and bitch. The ewe needs it for the first half of

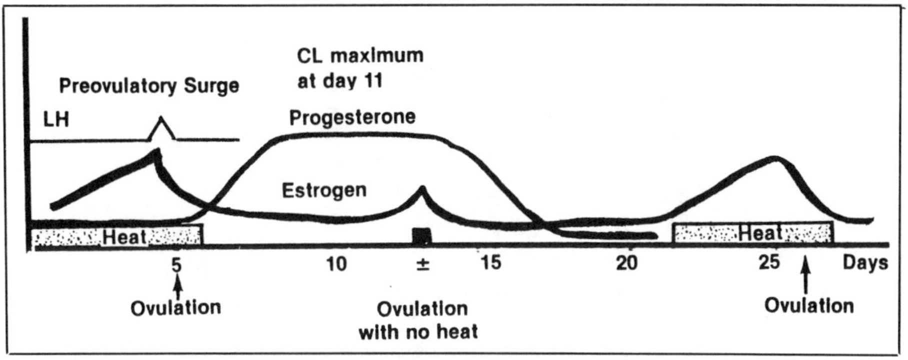

Fig 1. Hormone levels in the estrous cycle of nonpregnant mares.

pregnancy (66 days) and the queen needs it for about 45 days. The mare only needs the CL's progesterone for 100 days of its 330-day gestation. The embryologic signal of pregnancy may be estrone sulfate. As we shall see later, estrone sulfate detection may be a valuable aid for early pregnancy diagnosis in some animals.

Mares have an additional hormone present during part of their pregnancy. Pregnant mare serum gonadotropin (PMSG) is present from about 35 to 120 days of gestation. It acts on the ovaries to stimulate formation of secondary CL, which fortify progesterone levels. PMSG is useful in veterinary medicine because it is the basis of some blood tests for pregnancy diagnosis in mares.

Figure 1 shows the temporal relationships of the hormones during the estrous cycle of the mare. Figure 2 shows the hormonal rela-

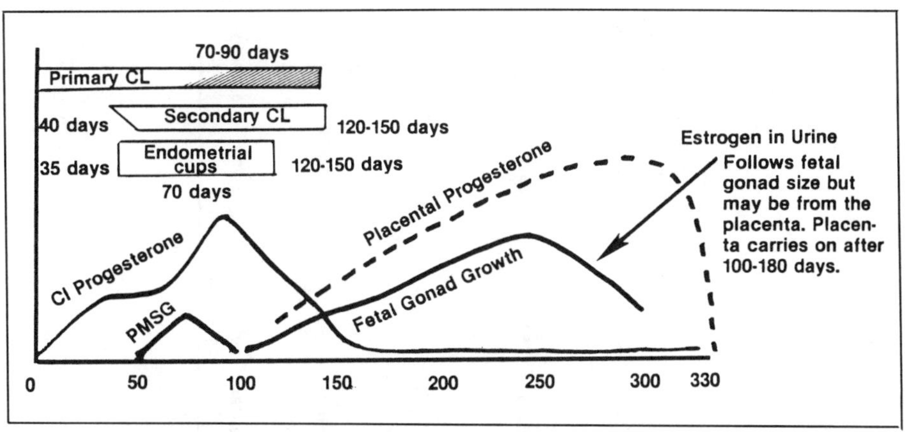

Fig 2. Hormone levels during pregnancy in mares.

Table 1. Reproductive Data for Various Domestic Species

	Cycle Pattern	Cycle Length	Heat Length	Ovulation Time	Time to Breed: Natural	Time to Breed: AI	Gestation Length	Puberty	Age to First Breed
Cow	polyestrous	21 days	18 hours	12-18 hours after heat	heat	12 hours after 1st see heat	280 days	6-16 months	14-22 months
Mare	seasonally polyestrous	21 days	5 days	24-36 hours before end of heat	day 2 and every other day of heat	same as natural	330 days (320-360)	18 months	2-3 years
Sow	polyestrous	21 days	2-3 days	36 hours after onset of heat	daily when in heat	same as natural	115 days	7 months	8-9 months
Bitch	seasonally monestrous	4-7 months	7-9 days	day 2-3	days 1, 3 and 5 of heat	same as natural	63 days	6-12 months	12-18 months
Queen	seasonally polyestrous	21 days	4-10 days	induced	in heat	in heat	63 days	7-12 months	12-18 months

tionships of pregnancy in the mare. With the exception of PMSG, which is only found in mares, these hormonal relationships are representative for most of the animals dealt with in this chapter. The days involved vary with the species.

Reproductive Physiologic Patterns

With the previous generalized review of the estrual cycle in mind, we will now discuss the specifics for various species. This information is summarized in Table 1.

Cows

The normal cow is a polyestrous animal that cycles throughout the year, with a 1-day heat about every 21 days (range 18-23 days) unless pregnant. Heat lasts about 18 hours in cows. The signs of approaching heat in cows include nervousness, vocalization, and attempting to mount and ride other animals. A cow in "true" heat stands to be ridden by other cows. A thick, clear, tenacious string of mucus can often be seen hanging from the vulva of cows in heat. Unlike other animals, cows ovulate about 1-2 hours after going out of heat. Cows that are to be bred artificially should be bred 1-2 hours after heat is first detected, if the herd is watched 20-30 minutes twice daily for estrual animals. Obviously, cows to be bred naturally must still be in standing heat. Cows often show metestrous bleeding in the mucus 1-2 days after they have ovulated. It is too late to breed cows that have evidence of metestrual blood in their mucus.

Mares

The mare is a seasonally polyestrous animal. Most mares stop cycling (become anestrual) during the winter; however, a few mares cycle also during the winter. The mare's natural breeding season is in the late spring and summer. However, breed registration rules force us to breed mares in February and March. During the natural breeding season (May-August), the mare's estrous cycle is about 21 days long. They are in standing heat for about 5 days and then out of heat for 16 days.

Estrual mares (in heat) seek out the stallion. They squat and urinate frequently in the presence of the stallion, raise the tail to the side and evert (wink) the clitoris. Estrual mares stand to be mounted by the stallion. Mares that are not in heat squeal, kick, swish the tail from side to side, pin their ears back, and may bite at a stallion nearby or attempting to breed them.

Mares enter and leave the natural breeding season with very erratic cycles. They often have prolonged heats in the early spring.

These early season erratic periods result in extra labor and ineffective breedings. Rectal examinations by a veterinarian at this time can be used to predict the optimum time for breeding. Mares usually ovulate 24-36 hours before going out of heat. The best time to breed a normally cycling mare is on the second day of heat and every other day until she goes out of heat. In the early spring, when mares have prolonged heats, breeding all mares every other day may exhaust the stallion.

The veterinarian can predict ovulation based upon changes in the follicles, as palpated rectally, and on changes in the cervix. The follicles become large and soft before ovulation and the cervix changes from a dry, firm, tight, pale organ to a very pink, edematous, soft, amorphous mass on the floor of the vagina before ovulation.

Sows

Gilts reach puberty at about 6-7 months of age, though this varies with the breed and time of year they are born. Pigs are nonseasonal polyestrous animals, though in hot, humid climates they may show a reduction in cyclicity during the summer. Pigs are unique in that they show an early postpartum heat but do not ovulate in this heat. Then they undergo a true lactational anestrus in that they do not resume cycles until the litter is weaned. After resumption of cycling, the pig demonstrates heat for 2-3 days every 21 (18-24) days. Heat is recognized in sows by a slightly swollen, reddened vulva. They are restless, seek out the boar, and assume a characteristic braced stance when the boar mounts. This stance is used to detect sows and gilts in heat. A female in heat assumes the same stance if pressed on the back by a person.

Sows ovulate in the last half of heat. They should be bred on the first day of heat and 24 hours later for maximum conception rate and litter size.

Bitches

The bitch is a seasonally monestrous animal with a definite anestrous period between cycles. Most dogs come into season about once every 6-7 months. The heats can be at any time of the year; however, they seem to be concentrated in the spring and fall. Some dogs may cycle only once a year, as in the Basenji. Other individual dogs may cycle every 4 months and still be considered normal.

Bitches reach puberty at 6-24 months of age, with an average of 10-12 months. Small breeds usually reach puberty earlier than large breeds.

The estrous cycle of the bitch has 5 characteristic stages. Vaginal smears can be used to effectively determine the stage of the cycle.

Owners say a bitch has come into heat when they notice attraction of males and dripping of blood from the vulva. This is actually proestrus, not estrus.

Proestrus: This stage is characterized by increased vulvar swelling, a bloody vulvar discharge, attraction to males, and courtship play, such as spinning, crouching in front, nuzzling, and even mounting the male. However, proestrous females do not stand to be mounted by males. The vaginal smear at this stage shows a variable amount of RBC and WBC, and initially predominantly small, round parabasal and small intermediate vaginal cells (Fig 3). Parabasal and small intermediate cells can be recognized by their round shape and relatively large nucleus compared to the amount of cytoplasm.

As the bitch progresses through proestrus, the number of RBC remains variable. The number of WBC declines and vaginal cells con-

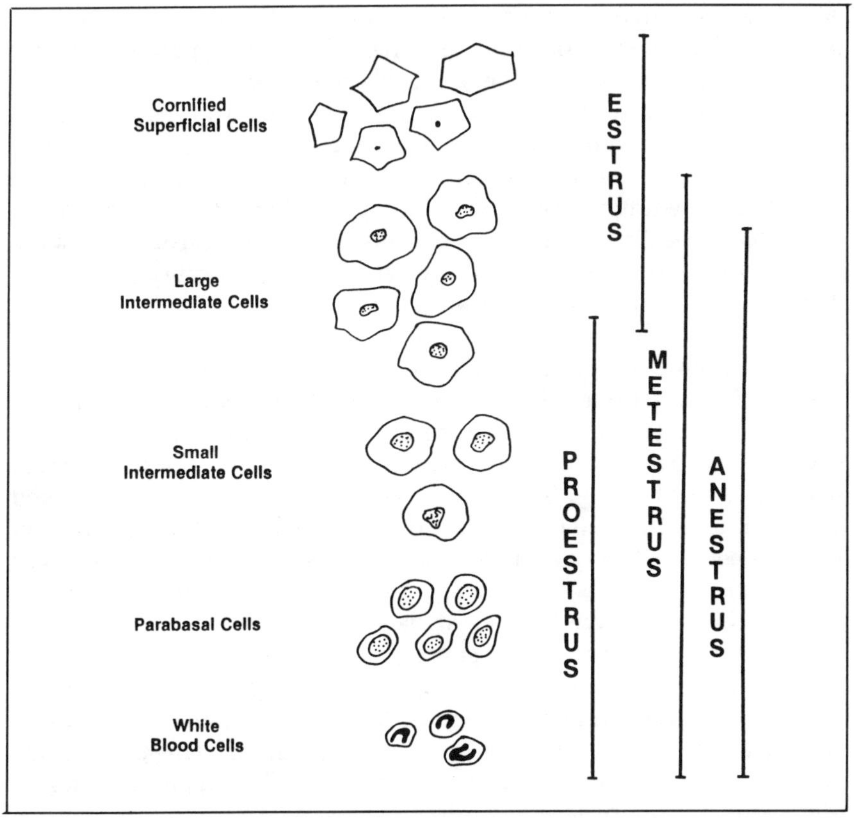

Fig 3. Characteristics of vaginal cells as seen on cytologic examination in the bitch.

sist of large intermediate and superficial cells, which are thin, large and angular, and have small pyknotic (dense) nuclei or no nuclei. The vaginal cells are becoming keratinized or cornified. The vulva is still large and edematous at this stage. Proestrus lasts an average of 9 (range 3-17) days. By the end of proestrus, more than 50% of the vaginal cells are anuclear (no nucleus), keratinized superficial cells (Fig 3).

Estrus: The onset of estrus is marked by the bitch standing to be mounted by the male. Estrus averages 9 days in the bitch but can be as short as 3 or as long as 21 days. During estrus, the bitch lifts the tail and deflects it to the side, arches the back, and elevates the vulva. The vulva is less turgid than in proestrus; this facilitates copulation. The estrual vulvar discharge may remain red or become straw colored. As mentioned earlier, the estrual vaginal smear consists almost entirely of superficial and large intermediate cells, which are very thin and angular, and have small, dark nuclei or no nuclei (Fig 3). The WBC are no longer present in the smear; RBC may or may not be present. The presence or absence of RBC is not a significant finding when trying to determine the stage of the cycle.

Bitches ovulate early in estrus. The best time to breed a bitch is on the first, third and fifth day of standing heat. Breeding bitches on the ninth and eleventh or eleventh and thirteenth day after the onset of vaginal bleeding is less than satisfactory because of the ranges of days that proestrus and estrus can last. Breeding bitches on these predetermined days assumes the owner noticed the first day of vulvar discharge. However, this is often not the case.

During breeding, it is important to be sure that the stud has inserted the penis completely and that the bulbus glandis (enlarged portion of the penis) is completely inserted into the vagina, producing the coital lock or "tie." The tie is important for stimulating contractions that help move the semen into the uterus and up the oviducts. A normal tie can last 15-30 minutes. The dogs should not be disturbed at this time. Efforts to physically separate the bitch and stud may injure the penis or the vagina. At the end of estrus, the bitch no longer accepts the stud dog, even though he continues to show interest in her. The bitch then enters metestrus.

Metestrus: Metestrus is a short stage in the bitch; in fact, some authors do not even discuss it. It is marked by refusal of the male's attentions by the female and reappearance of WBC and noncornified parabasal and small intermediate cells in vaginal smears. Vulvar swelling and vaginal discharge decrease rapidly during this stage. Metestrus rapidly progresses into diestrus.

Diestrus: This is the longest stage of the canine estrous cycle; it lasts about 60 days, which is nearly the same length as a normal pregnancy. There is no vaginal discharge after the first few days of diestrus. The vaginal smear contains predominantly noncornified cells, with a few WBC.

Toward the end of diestrus, about the time a pregnant bitch would be ready to whelp, the nonpregnant bitch often shows *pseudopregnancy* or *false pregnancy.* The abdomen may enlarge and the mammary glands may swell and fill with milk. The bitch may start nest building and even undergo a false first stage of labor. Pseudopregnant bitches often "adopt" socks, stuffed toys or kittens as their surrogate puppies. They may have a behavior change at this time and become aggressive if attempts to remove their "puppies" are made. Pseudopregnant bitches have been known to raise an orphaned litter of kittens. Not all bitches show clinical signs of pseudopregnancy; however, they all undergo the same hormonal changes that could make them exhibit these signs.

Anestrus: After diestrus or pregnancy, the uterus undergoes a period of regeneration or repair during anestrus. Anestrus may last 1-11 months, depending on the breed, 4-5 months being the average. The vaginal smear at this time is mainly comprised of noncornified parabasal and small intermediate cells, with variable numbers of WBC. At some times, WBC can be quite numerous, making it difficult to rule out infection. Anestrous females do not attract males nor do they allow courtship or mating behavior by the stud. After anestrus, the bitch reenters proestrus and the cycle repeats itself.

Queens

The queen is different from other animals that we have discussed so far in that the others are spontaneous ovulators. That is, they release their eggs at a predetermined time in their cycle, after the appropriate hormonal changes. The queen, on the other hand, is an induced ovulator, meaning coitus is necessary to stimulate ovulation. The queen is a seasonally polyestrous animal. Queens have a short anestrous period between October and January, but then cycle regularly the rest of the year if they do not conceive. Since the cat is an induced ovulator, CL are not produced unless coitus has occurred. The cycle lasts about 14 days and is composed of 1-2 days of proestrus 3-6 days of estrus (heat) and about 7 days of metestrus before proestrus occurs again.

Estrus: Estrus in queens is recognized by behavioral changes. They become more affectionate, vocalize and rub up against inanimate objects and people. When petted, they arch their back, elevate the hindquarters and laterally displace the tail. Treading of the hind feet is also often evident at this time.

Queens do not show the vaginal bleeding that dogs do, but they have similar changes in the vaginal smear. Reappearance of WBC in the smear marks the end of estrus and the beginning of metestrus. Natural breeding can successfully take place at any time during estrus, since the eggs are not ovulated until after breeding. Many owners find the recurrent estrous behavior annoying. It can be stopped by inducing ovulation and pseudopregnancy after a sterile mating or false mating using a glass rod (*eg,* a sanitized rectal thermometer) to stimulate the queen's vagina. Ovulation can also be induced by injection of the appropriate luteinizing hormone. Overaggressive probing for a vaginal smear for estrus detection can also stimulate ovulation. Induced ovulation should keep a queen out of heat for 40-60 days or longer if winter is approaching.

Like dogs, cats can also show the clinical signs of pseudopregnancy and experience false labor, lactation and adoption of objects or another animal's litter.

PREGNANCY DIAGNOSIS

One of the cardinal signs of pregnancy in large animals is failure to return to heat after breeding. However, this is not true for dogs and cats. Traditionally, animals are examined for pregnancy by palpation (manual examination) of the uterus through the abdominal wall or by rectal palpation. However, pregnancy diagnosis is becoming more technologically advanced; now various histologic, chemical, electrical, ultrasonic and radiographic technics can be used.

Manual Examination

Bitches

Transabdominal (through the abdominal wall) palpation of the uterus is a valuable aid in the middle and latter part of gestation in bitches and queens. By 18-21 days postbreeding, a string of half-inch swellings can be felt in the uterus. By 45-55 days, these individual swellings coalesce, the uterus feels like a long sausage and the fetuses are difficult to palpate. By 55-63 days, the individual pups can usually be palpated again.

Queens

Fetal bulges in a queen can be felt between 20-30 days of gestation. After 30 days, it is difficult to feel the individual fetuses but the enlarged uterus is quite evident. Late in pregnancy, individual kittens can be palpated.

Mares

Pregnancy may be diagnosed by rectal examination as early as 19-20 days after breeding. The tone of the uterus and the amniotic bulge can be easily identified. Later, the fetus can be palpated. Because the mare's rectum is extremely fragile, this technic should be done only by a veterinarian.

Cows

Palpation of the cow's uterus through the rectum reveals an amniotic vesicle at about 30-35 days. The chorioallantois can be felt as a membrane at 36-90 days. After this, the cotyledons and the fetus can be used to confirm pregnancy. Fremitus (palpable vibration) in the enlarged middle uterine artery is an indication of pregnancy in the middle trimester, when it is difficult to feel the fetus.

Sows

The sow's uterus is not usually palpated; however, it is possible and can be highly accurate. Good tone in the cervix and fremitus in the uterine artery are indications of pregnancy.

Histologic Diagnosis of Pregnancy

The sow is the only animal in which this technic is broadly applied. A vaginal biopsy 20-25 days after breeding is examined microscopically after histologic preparation. The epithelium of the biopsy should be only 2-4 cell layers thick if the sow is pregnant. At 20-25 days postbreeding, a nonpregnant sow that is coming back into heat typically has a very thick vaginal epithelium 10 or more layers thick. A diestrual sow also has a thin epithelium but of intermediate thickness, between that seen in estrus and pregnancy.

Chemical Diagnosis of Pregnancy

Chemical methods of pregnancy diagnosis include immunologic, endocrinologic and biologic technics, in addition to strict chemical tests.

Progesterone Assay

Considering that progesterone levels remain elevated in pregnant animals, a high progesterone level in the blood at about the time of the expected subsequent estrus is an indication of pregnancy. The analysis is conducted between 17 and 23 days in the cow, mare and sow. Progesterone assay is not used in dogs and cats because their CL are retained after estrus and progesterone is secreted for the next 9-11 weeks even if they are not pregnant. Either blood or milk can be analyzed for progesterone. The technic is very accurate for detecting nonpregnant animals, but it produces 5-15% false positives (incorrect diagnoses of pregnancy) because of other conditions that cause the CL to remain active and produce progesterone. Pyometra, a mummified fetus or cystic ovaries can cause false positives in cows. Spontaneous prolonged diestrus can cause a false positive in mares.

Estrogen Assay

Estrone sulfate is produced by the fetus early in pregnancy and can be measured in blood, urine and possibly milk. Estrogen assay is accurate at 18-34 days in sows, after 40 days in mares, and after 70 days in cows.

Estrogen levels are also high in the urine of mares after 5 months of pregnancy (Fig 2). These estrogens can be detected by the Cuboni test. Pregnancy is indicated by a dark-green fluorescence in the bottom of the test tube after urine is mixed with hydrochloric acid, sulfuric acid and benzene.

PMSG Assay

Pregnant mare serum gonadotropin (PMSG) is present in the blood of mares between 35 and 120 days of gestation. Several commercial test kits can detect this hormone. The mare immunologic pregnancy (MIP) test is a hemagglutination-inhibition test for PMSG that detects the lack of agglutination of RBC in the pregnant mare's blood. Biologic tests for PMSG, using female rats or rabbits or male frogs, detect ovulation in females and sperm production in males after PMSG is injected into the animal. Radioimmunoassays (RIA) and enzyme-linked immunosorbant assays (ELISA) are available for PMSG detection at some laboratories.

Electronic Pregnancy Detection

Ultrasonography

Several types of ultrasound machines are used for pregnancy detection. The A-mode or amplitude-depth ultrasound machine bounces sound waves off different tissue layers and records the echoes, received as an audible beep or a set of peaks on an oscilloscope. Ultrasonography is reportedly 98% accurate at 21-90 days in sows and 18-23 days in bitches. Another type of ultrasound is Doppler ultrasound, which detects differences in maternal and fetal pulses by reflection of the sound waves they produce. These pulses are registered as sound or as oscilloscope blips. It is 100% accurate after 40 days of gestation in sows. It is also used in bitches after 30 days of gestation. The third type of ultrasound is B-mode or brightness mode. This type of ultrasound can be used in mares as early as 15 days of pregnancy to detect the amniotic vesicle and fetus. On a screen, it produces a visual image that can be measured and photographed.

Electrocardiography

Fetal electrocardiograms have been used to detect the fetal heart beat in mares and cows.

Radiography

X-rays can be used to diagnose pregnancy in dogs and cats after 45 days of gestation. At this time, the fetal skeletons and skulls are calcified and can be counted. Radiographs can also be used in pigs but are rarely used due to the cost and impracticality.

PREPARTUM CARE

Some special considerations must be observed in preparing the dam for parturition (birth) and nursing offspring. Nutrition is probably the most important of these.

Nutrition

The major amount of fetal growth occurs during the last third of gestation. Up until this time, dietary requirements parallel those of a nonpregnant animal, provided the dam was in good condition at the time of breeding. Nutrition is extremely important in the last trimester (third) for beef cows. The dam's nutritional status at this time affects the size and viability of the calf and also affects the cow's fertility by influencing the interval to return to estrus after calving. In the case of dairy cows, lactation is the major nutritional drain. Pregnancy is an additional stress, especially during the last third of gestation. Special attention must be paid to increased protein and caloric requirements, and calcium and phosphorus balance in the ration. To reduce some of the nutritional stress and allow dairy cows to prepare for calving, they are "dried off" during the last 8 weeks of pregnancy. During this *dry period*, good pasture or well-cured hay and silage with a vitamin-mineral supplement are usually sufficient. An adequate dry period also results in improved fertility in the subsequent lactation. Cows that have lost a lot of condition during lactation may require additional grain during the early dry period.

Bitches in good condition when they get pregnant and that are maintained on a high-quality commercial diet usually do not need special supplementation during pregnancy, except for moderate, gradual increases in total intake during the last half of pregnancy and during heavy lactation. As parturition approaches, a more laxative diet is usually fed in small, frequent feedings to eliminate any digestive discomfort due to the enlarged uterus and fetus. The well-nourished animal must be housed properly to ensure healthy neonates and a postpartum period free of complications for the dam.

Facilities

There are 3 basic requirements for an adequate area in which to give birth. It must be clean, dry and free of drafts; it must be easily observed so that assistance can be given if needed; and, most important, it must be acceptable to the dam. The most "deluxe" whelping box will be abandoned by a bitch that feels more at ease in the bedroom closet. The whelping box should be set up in a warm, draft-free, secluded place a week or so before the bitch is due to whelp, to allow her to become accustomed to it. The size varies with the size of the bitch, but it should be large enough to allow the bitch to lie down and still have plenty of room to nurse all the pups. A queening box is similar to a whelping box. Its sides must be at least 4-6 inches high so that nursing kittens are not dragged out as the queen leaves.

Mares and cows seem to do best if allowed to give birth in a clean, well-drained pasture. Again, it should be in a spot where impending parturition can be easily observed and the dam and offspring protected from predators. If such a pasture is not available, a well-bedded box stall at least 14 ft x 14 ft does nicely.

Sows are usually provided a farrowing crate, which is a narrow stall-like structure with low rails along the sides to prevent the sow from turning around or lying down on the baby pigs. These crates usually have a heat lamp at one end to keep the baby pigs warm. The accepted practice is to house the farrowing sows in a heated barn, thus eliminating the need for bedding. This also allows for easier, more thorough cleaning. These large animals should be introduced to the farrowing (delivery) area several weeks before the due date, if practical, to allow the dam to produce and concentrate antibodies in the colostrum against the organisms to which the neonate will be exposed shortly after birth. Once animals are introduced to their farrowing area, they must be observed regularly for signs of parturition.

Signs of Impending Parturition

As parturition approaches, several physical and behavioral signs are displayed by the dam. The mammary glands usually fill with milk one to several days before parturition, but this can occur up to several weeks ahead in some species. At the same time, the ligaments of the tailhead relax to allow for passage of the young through the birth canal.

"Waxing" of the teats occurs in mares within 24 hours of delivery; however, several false "waxes" may occur. Many times there is a temperature drop from the animal's norm. To check this, daily or twice-daily monitoring is usually necessary for as much as a week before the due date. The temperature decrease is a valuable tool for prediction of parturition in bitches and sows.

About 12-24 hours before parturition, there are often signs of frequent defecation, urination and anorexia due to pressure within the abdomen. The animal becomes restless and may even appear to be looking for her young, hours before they are born. Mares may show intermittent colic. Bitches, queens and sows attempt to build a nest for their young, whereas mares and cows tend to seek out an isolated area of the pasture.

Preparation for Parturition

Before parturition, steps should be taken to be sure that the perineal and mammary areas are washed and any long hair clipped. Sows are often washed completely before entering the farrowing crate. The mare's tail should be wrapped to prevent soiling and tangling with the foal and afterbirth. Mares that have had a Caslick's operation should have their vulvar suture line reopened. This is also the time when you should gather all necessary equipment, such as obstetric chains, 7% iodine, towels, oxygen and other supplies you might need to assist in delivery and care of the neonate.

PARTURITION

After the preparatory changes of late pregnancy, which ready the dam and fetus for birth, parturition begins. Parturition has several common names, depending upon the species involved. *Calving* and

Table 2. Stage of Labor in Various Domestic Species

Stage	Cow	Mare	Sow	Bitch	Queen
I	1-4 hours (longer in heifers); restless; off feed; isolates self; allantois protrudes	1-4 hours; colic; sweats; isolates self; defecates; urinates; placenta ruptures	2-12 hours; 1-2 F drop in rectal temp; builds nest	6-12 hours; 1-2 F drop in rectal temp; builds nest	2-12 hours; 1-2 F drop in rectal temp; builds nest
II	½-4 hours; abdominal straining; amnion ruptures; calf delivered	5-40 minutes; forceful abdominal straining; amnion ruptured; foal delivered	1-5 hours; amnion ruptures; straining; pigs delivered	3-6 hours; amnion ruptures; pups-delivered	3-6 hours; amnion ruptures; kittens delivered
III	½-8 hours; uterine contractions; passes placenta	½-3 hours; rests; uterine contractions; ± mild colic	⅓-4 hours; eats; drinks;	½-1 hour; greenish-black fluid passed	½-1 hour; brownish fluid passed
			---often passes several fetuses prior to passing a placenta---		

foaling are self-explanatory. However, parturition in the sow or gilt is called *farrowing* and in the bitch it is called *whelping*. In the cat it is called *kittening* or *queening*.

Parturition is divided into 3 stages. Stage 1 is preliminary to expulsion of the fetus. During this stage, the uterine muscles undergo rhythmic contractions, which reposition and advance the fetus toward the cervix. In response to these contractions and the pressure of the fetus, the cervix relaxes fully and dilates. The dam in first-stage labor often is anxious and restless, and shows evidence of abdominal cramps. Stage 1 ends with delivery of the fetus into the pelvic canal and rupture of the fetal membranes.

Stage 2 is the stage of expulsion of the fetus from the birth canal. Uterine contractions are stronger and accompanied by abdominal straining to help expel the fetus. The importance of abdominal straining versus uterine contractions in the birth process varies among species. Abdominal pressing is very important in foaling but uterine contractions are relatively more important in farrowing. With successful delivery of the fetus, the dam completes stage 2 and rests during the first part of stage 3.

Stage 3 of parturition is characterized by expulsion of the placenta. Uterine contractions continue but are not as severe as those in stage 2. The uterus begins to shrink toward its nonpregnant size. In polytocous (litter-bearing) species, the cycle of stages 1-3 repeats itself with each fetus. Actually, stages 1 and 2 may occur several times and result in several fetuses being passed before a placenta is actually passed in stage 3 in these species.

After delivery of the fetus, the dam rests and begins to care for the newborn. She licks it dry, which helps stimulate breathing, and licks and chews off any amniotic membrane remaining on the fetus. The bitch and queen usually chew the umbilical cord to sever the placenta. The cord usually ruptures spontaneously during delivery of the calf and during the foal's struggles to get up. The specific signs, events and duration of the various stages of parturition vary among species (Table 2).

Delivery of the fetus by the cow and mare usually occurs with the neonate coming out head and feet first, in a "diving" position. Most pigs, pups and kittens are also delivered head first but frequently 1 or both legs are retracted alongside the body. However, in these small species, rear-end (breech) delivery is common and results in normal, live offspring. Most dams deliver while lying down but occasionally a cow or mare may deliver while standing up. This can be dangerous to the fetus.

It is often difficult to tell when a dam has finished delivering all of its offspring. Twins in mares and cows are uncommon and can be detected by manual exploration of the vagina and uterus. However, because this is not as easily accomplished in sows, bitches and queens, we may have to rely on other signs or tests. The bitch's abdomen may be palpated for more pups or a finger in a sterile glove may be introduced into the vagina to feel for another pup. Radiographs of the abdomen may be necessary. Sows often get up to drink and may eat a little after a period of rest once the last pig is delivered.

One of the most difficult situations encountered in theriogenology is to decide when parturition is not proceeding normally and the dam is in dystocia (difficult birth) and requires assistance. Table 3 contains guidelines that have proven helpful.

MANAGEMENT OF DYSTOCIA

Dystocia means difficult birth and should be promptly corrected if the dam and offspring are to survive without permanent damage. The causes of dystocia can be classified as those due to maternal problems and those caused by fetal problems. Some examples of maternal causes of dystocia are: uterine torsion; healed pelvic fracture restricting birth canal; failure of cervix to dilate; and primary uterine inertia due to hypocalcemia (*eg,* milk fever in cows, eclampsia in bitches). A few fetal causes of dystocia are a single large pup; enlarged head due to hydrocephalus (water on the brain); and forelimbs of a calf retained alongside the body.

These are only a few of the many conditions that can result in dystocia. Consequently, before attempting to manage a case of dystocia, it is important to know the past history of the dam. The following information should be determined: What is the due date? How long has the animal been trying to give birth? Has the animal given birth before? If yes, when? Have any offspring already been delivered this time? Has anyone attempted to assist the animal before you? After this information is obtained and assessed, careful examination of the dam and fetus is in order. The cause of the dystocia must be determined before attempting to deliver the offspring.

The exact procedures involved and the equipment necessary vary with the species, the cause of the dystocia, the condition of the dam and fetus, and the desires of the veterinarian involved. However, certain general principles must be kept in mind:

- Treat life-threatening conditions to keep the dam alive until delivery is completed. Heroic attempts to remove a fetus from a dead dam are usually unsuccessful.

Table 3. Guidelines for Intervention in Dystocia in Various Species

Bitch, Queen
- intense straining that does not produce a pup or kitten in 30 minutes
- weak, intermittent straining that does not produce a pup or kitten in 2-3 hours
- an interval of over 4 hours between pups or kittens, without further labor
- illness in the dam
- a bloody, malodorous or greenish vulvar discharge
- prolonged pregnancy (overdue)
- obvious difficulty in delivering the pup or kitten (*eg*, a pup halfway out)

Sow
- prolonged pregnancy (over 115 days)
- malodorous or bloody vulvar discharge
- expulsion of fetal feces (meconium) without expulsion of a fetus
- weak labor or cessation of labor before delivery of all fetuses
- incomplete expulsion of a fetus

Cow
- first-stage labor lasting more than 6 hours, without abdominal pressing
- second-stage labor, with abdominal pressing, lasting over 2-3 hours without progress
- rupture of the waterbag (amnion) without expulsion of the calf within 2 hours
- fetal malposition (backwards, legs retained, etc)
- fetal monstrosity (malformed fetus)

Mare

Parturition, especially stage 2, in mares is quicker and more violent than in other species. Further, foals seem more susceptible to the adverse effects of dystocia than other neonates. Therefore, differentiation between a normal birth and dystocia is especially important in mares. Delivery should be assisted with:
- appearance of the unruptured placenta at or outside the vulva at the start of second-stage labor, with evident straining
- failure of the clear amnion to appear soon after the start of second-stage labor
- failure to locate the foal's head and legs in the pelvic inlet at the beginning of second-stage labor
- rolling, repeated getting up and down and reversing of the recumbent position by the mare, without progressing through stage 2 of labor and delivering a foal
- repeated straining without delivery of a partially expelled foal
- fetal malposition (backwards, legs retained, etc) or other abnormality in delivery
- fetal fecal (meconium) staining on the foal

- Proper restraint is essential. This may be a squeeze chute or a halter and post for a cow or general anesthesia for difficult foalings and whelpings.

- Obstetric equipment should be in good working order, clean and disinfected.

- Strict attention to sanitation is important. The vulva and perineal area should be scrubbed and rinsed thoroughly. Long-haired bitches should have the hair in this area clipped. Care should be taken to prevent feces from contaminating instruments and hands. The veterinarian should scrub his or her hands and arms thoroughly and don glove and sleeve before introducing the hand and arm into the vagina.
- Gentle, dexterous manipulation is then initiated. Liberal and frequent application of lubricants facilitates manipulation and delivery. Straining during manipulation of the fetus can be suppressed by epidural anesthesia or, in the case of cattle, by passing a stomach tube into the rumen to prevent closure of the glottis.
- After correcting the cause of the dystocia, gentle continuous traction should be applied to the fetus. This may involve the use of leg chains in the case of large animals or forceps for small animals. A calf jack may also be required for large animals. Using a fence stretcher or hooking the chains to a tractor or truck should be avoided. A rule-of-thumb is to use no more traction than can be applied by 2 people. As stated previously, adequate lubrication greatly facilitates delivery with traction. A steady, continuous force is much more effective than short bursts of violent tugging. Constant traction allows the cervix and birth canal to expand as the fetus passes. Violent tugs often tear these tissues and can be detrimental to the fetus.
- After delivery, the dam should be rechecked for additional fetuses and for any injury that may have occurred during delivery.

Occasionally, the fetus cannot be delivered intact through the birth canal. The veterinarian must then decide whether to perform a cesarean section or attempt to dismember the fetus (fetotomy) into parts small enough to be delivered. The condition of the dam, uterus and fetus must be evaluated in making this decision. A live, healthy fetus is usually taken by cesarean section. A dead fetus can be taken by cesarean section but many veterinarians prefer to do a fetotomy on these. Fetotomy is the the method of choice if the fetus is decomposing and the uterus is highly infected.

POSTPARTUM CARE

The Normal Neonate

Owners often become concerned about the condition of the neonate. Consequently, the veterinarian or his staff spend a lot of time reassuring them and answering questions regarding the normality of

Table 4. Characteristics of Normal Neonates of Some Domestic Species

Puppies
- can crawl and right themselves at birth
- open eyelids by 1-3 weeks
- require bitch's stimulation to urinate and defecate for about 2½ weeks
- dried umbilical cord drops off by about 2-3 days
- cannot regulate body temperature in the first few weeks (normal = 94-99 F at 1-2 weeks, 97-100 F at 3-4 weeks, 100-101 F thereafter)
- can shiver by 7 days
- breathe 15-35 times/min at birth
- have a rapid pulse rate (220/min) in the first 2-3 weeks
- suckle shortly after birth
- have ear canals open by 13-17 days of age
- mostly sleep and nurse during the first week

Kittens
- can suckle and right themselves at birth
- open eyelids by 10-14 days; see well by 22-28 days
- ear canals open by 6-14 days
- require queen's stimulation to urinate and defecate for first few weeks
- double weight in first week
- sleep 90% of the time and nurse the rest of the time
- crawl by 18 days and walk by 21 days

Foals
- see, hear and shiver at birth
- breathe rapidly at first (75 breaths/min) and more slowly (35 breaths/min) by 12 hours of age
- have a pulse rate of 40-80/min; left-sided heart murmurs often present during the first few days of life
- attempt to become sternally recumbent (on chest) within 2 minutes of birth
- have a suckling reflex within 5 minutes
- break the umbilical cord by about 8 minutes after birth
- stand within an hour
- nurse within 2 hours
- have a rectal temperature of 99-101 F (37.2-38.3 C)
- pass meconium within 72 hours
- urinate within 6 hours (colts) or 11 hours (fillies)

Calves
- hear, see and shiver at birth
- stand within 1-2 hours
- suckle by 2-5 hours

Piglets
- crawl toward the teats shortly after birth
- have eyes open at birth

the neonate. Table 4 contains a summary of characteristics of normal neonates.

Care of Neonates

A number of steps must be followed to ensure survival of the neonate. The most immediate concern for the newborn is a patent airway. Be sure that the fetal membranes are removed from the head and that no excess fluid is in the upper respiratory tract. In the calf, foal and pig, tickling the nostril with a piece of straw is often used to stimulate a "sneezing" reflex to clear excess fluid from the airways. Often the calf is held up by the rear legs to allow fluid to drain from the nose and trachea. Pups and kittens can also be held head down or gently swung. Rubbing the neonate's back whle drying it off helps stimulate respiration. Licking by the dam also stimulates the neonate's respiration. However, some dams, especially in the case of carnivores, get carried away and begin to cannibalize their young. In such cases, the young must be removed and the dam restrained or tranquilized until it no longer tries to cannibalize or kill the young. This is a particular problem with inexperienced, anxious, first-time dams.

Once respiration is established, examine the newborn for congenital abnormalities. If an abnormality is found, look closer, since these problems often come in multiples. Next, the umbilical cord should be dipped in 7% iodine or other suitable astringent disinfectant to prevent an umbilical infection, which may lead to "navel ill" and infected joints.

The next step is to assure that the neonate finds the udder or teats and nurses to ensure adequate immunization through the dam's colostrum. Some inexperienced or poorly socialized dams may resist the neonate's attempts to nurse, and may have to be restrained or tranquilized until accustomed to nursing. Needle-sharp milk teeth in baby pigs may irritate and lacerate a gilt's teats, which can lead to cessation of nursing after a few days due to pain. Therefore, the ends of these teeth should be clipped with wire cutters at 1-2 days of age. If the dam has little milk or the colostrum has been lost (due to dripping before parturition), an alternate source of colostrum should be given to the neonate within 6 hours of birth before other material is ingested. Colostrum is not as essential to puppies or kittens as to other young because they acquire some of their passive immunity across the placenta.

Another item of concern is defecation and urination by the newborn. Meconium (fetal feces) impaction can cause colic in foals. Also, a ruptured bladder is not uncommon in newborn male foals. In many equine practices, a routine enema is given to every newborn foal, along with tetanus immunization and an injection of vitamins and/or antibiotics. A better idea is to vaccinate the mare with tetanus toxoid 1 month before foaling; this allows time for production of antibodies against tetanus and their concentration in the colostrum. Thus the foal is passively immunized and the mare is protected at foaling.

If the dam does not accept its young, has no milk or dies during birth, the owner must handfeed the offspring. Care must be exercised to prevent over- or underfeeding or feeding the wrong type of milk.

Feeding Orphans: Handfeeding the newborn is a tedious and time-consuming task. A few guidelines can be adapted to all species. Using a stomach tube reduces the time needed to feed young that are not strong enough to have a good suckling reflex. The tube must be measured along the animal's body and marked to estimate the distance to the stomach. Care must be taken not to force passage of the tube, since this can cause irreparable damage to the esophagus. When inserting the tube, check to see that it can be seen or felt next to the trachea as it moves down the esophagus. If the tube is not seen or palpated, it may be in the trachea, which could be fatal if milk were pumped into the lungs. Recently, esophageal feeders have been developed for use in the calf. These feeders have a firm tube with an enlarged end that closes the larynx when introduced into the pharynx and ensures that the fluid goes down the esophagus.

As a rule, calves and foals need 10% of their body weight in milk or milk replacer (formula) a day. Two feedings per day for most healthy calves is quite sufficient, whereas at least 4 feedings are preferred for foals. Puppies and kittens require 25% of their body weight in milk daily. It is most desirable to feed them 6 times per day for the first 2 weeks, with 4 daily feedings thereafter until maturity. Baby pigs should be fed similarly to puppies.

There are various commercial animal milk substitutes on the market. However, these may not be readily available in your area on short notice. Recipes for milk replacers are contained in Table 5. All of the formulas in Table 5 should be well blended and warmed to 95-100 F before feeding. Overheating may denature the proteins in the formula.

Care of the Dam

After an uneventful parturition, the dam should be allowed to rest undisturbed so it can care for and become acquainted with its offspring. The dam should be unobtrusively observed periodically to be sure that it and the offspring are comfortable and happy. The dam should always have access to small amounts of water and feed. The udder or mammary glands should be checked for evidence of mastitis during the first few days. Dairy cows ultimately require milking and should be checked for mastitis.

Table 5. Recipes for Milk Replacers for Kittens, Puppies, Foals and Baby Pigs

Kittens
2/3 cup whole homogenized cow's milk
3 egg yolks
1 tbsp corn oil
1 dropper liquid vitamin supplement
Puppies
2/3 cup whole homogenized cow's milk
3 egg yolks
1 tbsp corn oil
1 dropper liquid vitamin supplement
pinch of salt
Foals
human baby formula can be used temporarily
goat milk also can be used
Baby Pigs
1 qt whole homogenized cow's milk
1 cup half and half (cream and milk)

The uterus should not be entered manually after an unassisted delivery. This usually reduces the incidence of postpartum uterine infection and results in better future fertility. However, after a delivery that involved assistance, one should check the uterus and vagina, digitally or manually, for the presence of another fetus and for indications of injury to the dam. This should be done in a clean and sanitary manner. Cows that have required forced extraction of the fetus should be encouraged to stand shortly after delivery to rule out the possibility of rear-leg paralysis.

The dam should be observed to be sure all fetal membranes are passed. It is often difficult to account for all placentas with the bitch, queen and sow, since they regularly eat them. Cows may eat their placenta also; however, one should attempt to prevent this, since ruminants cannot digest this material and it may cause a digestive upset or obstruction. The bitch, queen and sow usually pass the placentas during parturition between birth of each offspring and after the last. A retained placenta in these animals may lead to severe metritis (uterine infection); toxins from the infected uterus may be passed to the offspring in the milk and make them sick. A foul-smelling vulvar discharge several days after parturition is an indication that examination by a veterinarian is necessary. Normal mares pass the placenta within 1 hour after delivery. It should be saved and filled with water so it can be examined to be sure it is all present. If the entire placenta or a piece of it is retained in the mare, a veterinarian should examine the animal. Retention of the placenta in mares may lead to laminitis (founder) if untreated. Cows usually pass the placenta within 8-12 hours. Those retained longer than 12 hours usually are passed within a week. Unless the cow is sick, one should not try to remove the placenta until at least 3 days after delivery. Earlier attempts may damage the cow's uterus. Manual intrusion into the uterus is not recommended.

During the first few postpartum weeks, the dam should be observed for mastitis, hypocalcemia (milk fever in the cow and eclampsia in the bitch and mare), metritis and agalactia.

BREEDING SOUNDNESS EVALUATION

Evaluation of Females

The reproductive examination often determines the chances of a brood animal carrying a healthy fetus to term without endangering its health. In mares and cows, the methods and equipment used for the routine examination are similar.

Rectal palpation is the most widely used method to examine the reproductive tract of large animals. With the aid of a rubber sleeve and lubricant, the veterinarian can assess the condition of the uterus, activity of the ovaries, and pregnancy status of the animal. With mares, the tail should be wrapped and tied out of the way.

After rectal examination, the vagina is usually evaluated with the aid of a speculum and light. The vulvar area should be cleaned thoroughly with a disinfectant scrub and dried before examination. The speculum should be lubricated with a sterile, water-soluble lubricant and the labia spread to avoid contamination of the speculum as it is introduced. Once the speculum has been introduced, the vaginal walls and floor are examined for color, conformation, inflammation and evidence of a discharge. In mares, the tone and position of the cervix should be noted, since this can help indicate the stage of the estrous cycle.

A uterine culture may be done to detect uterine infection. The optimum time to do this is during estrus. Preparation of the patient for this procedure is the same as for the vaginoscopic exam. A shielded, sterile swab is used to obtain a sample from the uterus. To avoid contamination of the swab in the vulva or vagina, it may be introduced through a speculum or with the aid of a sterile gloved hand. Once collected, the culture swab is transferred to transport medium and sent to the laboratory for culture. Because uterine cultures are difficult to obtain in the bitch, queen and sow, one often must settle for a vaginal culture. The procedures are the same.

Table 6. Semen Evaluation in Some Domestic Species

	Collection Methods							Motility Evaluation		Morphology (maximum % abnormal acceptable)
	manual	electro-ejaculator	artificial vagina	Volume (ml)	Concentration (million/ml)	No/ejaculate (billions)	Scrotal Circumference	gross gross	individual (minimum % acceptable)	
Dog	yes	no	40-42 C	1-25	125 (20-540)	1.25	no	no	70%	20%
Stallion	no	no	41-50 C	70 (30-250)	120 (30-600)	8.4	yes[c]	no	70%	35%
Boar	yes	yes[a]	45-50 C	250 (125-500)	150 (25-1000)	37.5	yes[c]	no	85%	30%
Bull	yes[b]	yes	40-52 C	4 (1-15)	1200 (300-2500)	4.8	yes[d]	yes[e]	yes[e]	yes[e]

a — must be anesthetized
b — by rectal massage of prostate and seminal vesicles
c — measured by caliper
d — measured with tape
e — score based on Society for Theriogenology bull BSE form

Adapted from Roberts: *Veterinary Obstetrics and Genital Diseases.* 2nd ed. Woodstock, VT, 1971.

Uterine biopsy is occasionally done in cows and mares. After preparing the animal as for vaginoscopic examination, the sterilized biopsy punch is introduced with the sterile gloved hand, through the cervix, into the uterus. The punch remains in the uterus while the hand is withdrawn and reinserted into the rectum. Once the jaws of the punch are identified, the wall of the uterus is pressed between the lateral jaws with the flat of the finger and the jaws are closed. The closed biopsy punch is withdrawn and the biopsy sample is placed in 10% formalin or Bouin's fixative for transport to the laboratory.

In small animals, the uterus cannot be palpated per rectum but is palpated through the abdominal wall. It is difficult to discern from loops of intestine. If a bitch is large enough, when a finger is inserted into the rectum, the first loop of tissue below the finger usually is the uterus. The ovaries are not easily identifiable in bitches or queens unless the animal is in heat or the ovaries are abnormal. A vaginoscopic examination can be conducted with the aid of an otoscope, a nasal speculum, or a piece of small-diameter glass tubing.

In the bitch, vaginal cytology is often used to detect estrus and the approximate time of ovulation. A moist, sterile swab is inserted into the vagina and then rolled onto a slide. The smear is then air dried, stained with a hematologic stain, and observed microscopically. When greater than 50% of the cells are cornified, the bitch is most likely in standing heat (Fig 3).

Evaluation of Males

Breeding soundness examination of males is more than just a semen check. It should include a good physical examination, evaluation of the reproductive organs, and examination of the ejaculate's quantity, percentage of motile sperm, and percentage of normally shaped sperm. Procedures used in such examinations vary with the species (Table 6). Semen collection can be conducted by electroejaculation in the bull, tom and anesthetized boar. An artificial vagina can be used in the dog, bull, tom, boar and stallion. Manual stimulation of the penis is effective in producing an ejaculate in the boar and dog. After collection of a semen sample, care must be taken to prevent the sperm from becoming cold or heat shocked, which decreases motility and produces large numbers of secondary abnormalities in the sperm.

Motility is evaluated subjectively as soon after semen collection as possible, using prewarmed slides, preferably on a microscope stage warmed to about 98.6 F (37 C). The motility score for nonruminants is the percentage of individual sperm with rapid progressive motility when examined under high power. Bull sperm is evaluated for motility by examining the gross motility of the sample under low power, examining the individual sperm motility under high power and assigning a score to these based on the system designed by the Society for Theriogenology for semen evaluation of the bull.

After evaluating motility, a smear of the sperm should be stained and evaluated for morphologic abnormalities. A smear for morphologic evaluation can be made by staining the sperm with any number of stains, such as eosin-nigrosin, Cassarett's or fine-grain India ink (positively silhouettes sperm). The stained sample should be smeared onto a slide to produce a thin layer of sperm so that individual cells can be seen in their entirety and counted. Several hundred sperm should be examined and categorized as normal or affected by a primary abnormality or secondary abnormality (Fig 4). The percentage of each type of sperm should be recorded. Acceptable levels of these abnormalities for each of these species is listed in Table 6. Primary abnormalities of sperm occur in the testis, whereas secondary abnormalities are produced in the extratesticular ducts (epididymus) or are artifacts produced by careless semen handling technics.

Primary abnormalities are predominantly abnormalities of the head but include some tail abnormalities (Fig 4).

After the morphologic evaluation, the concentration of sperm in the sample should be evaluated in all species except the bull. In bulls, sperm production is estimated by measuring scrotal circumference. This value is then given a score in accordance with the guidelines established by the Society for Theriogenology. In the other species, the concentration of sperm in the sample is determined by counting the sperm with a hemacytometer, Coulter counter or Spectronic 20, calibrated for sperm. When using a hemacytometer, a WBC pipette or WBC Unopet chamber can be used, but care must be taken to be sure the proper dilution factors are used when calculating the concentration.

Since the volume of preejaculatory fluid can vary with the artificial means we use to collect the semen, a value for the number of sperm per ejaculate is more valuable than the concentration in determining the sperm output. The number per ejaculate is arrived at by multiplying the concentration by the volume of ejaculate collected.

Any physical or behavioral abnormality that prevents effective copulation is grounds for declaring a male unsound for breeding, regardless of the semen quality. Poor semen quality may be a permanent or temporary condition. Reevaluation in 2 months is recommended before the problem can be assumed to be permanent.

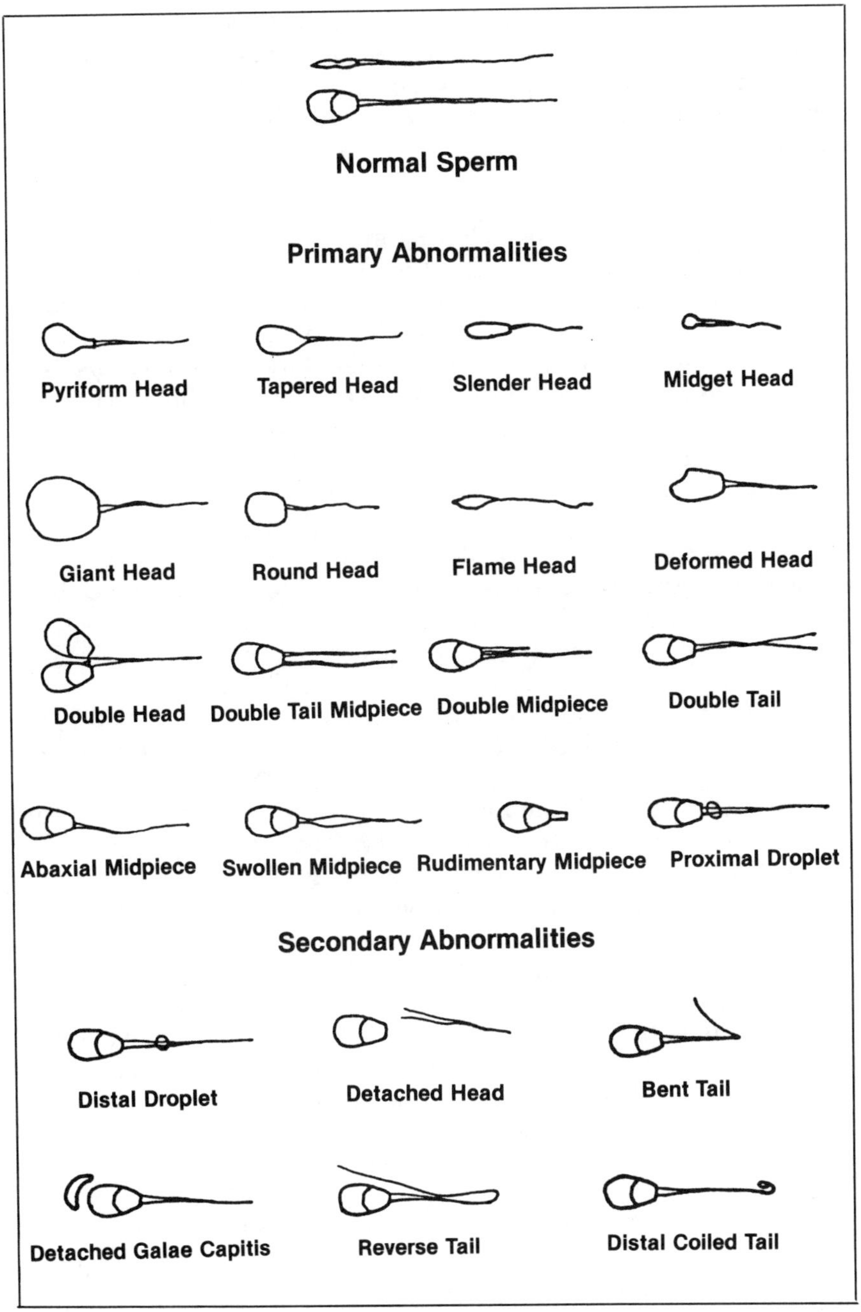

Fig 4. Characteristics of normal and abnormal sperm.

ARTIFICIAL INSEMINATION

Successful artificial insemination (AI) depends upon accurate determination of the appropriate time to breed, use of high-quality semen and careful attention to semen handling and insemination technics.

Cows

Cows are very good about letting everyone know when they are ready to breed. However, it takes time to properly observe their behavior. It is advisable to take at least 30 minutes twice a day, early and late in the day, for observing cows for heat. Cows in heat stand to be mounted by other cows, are usually less interested in eating, act nervous, and vocalize frequently. A long strand of clear mucus is commonly seen draining from the vulva or smeared on the tail or perineum. Though standing heat is the time to breed naturally, AI requires use of the AM/PM rule. That is, cows first seen in heat in the morning should be inseminated that evening and vice versa.

Frozen semen must be handled carefully to avoid killing or damaging the sperm in the straw or ampule. The thawing procedure varies and should be carried out in accordance with the recommendations of the company packaging the semen. In general, ampules are thawed in ice water for 10 minutes. Straws are thawed in warm water (90-95 F) for 45 seconds. Because thawing and refreezing kill the sperm, straws or ampules not being used should not be raised above the "frost line" in the neck of the tank of liquid nitrogen.

Once out of the storage tank, semen should be deposited in the cow within 15 minutes to ensure viability. The straw or ampule must be dried before loading the semen into the gun or pipette, as water kills sperm. Before inseminating the cow, make sure the vulva is wiped clean and dry.

Placing a sleeved hand just inside the rectum, apply ventral (downward) pressure to open the labia. This helps prevent contamination of the pipette and semen during passage into the vagina. Once the pipette is 3-4 inches into the vagina, the hand in the rectum is extended craniad (forward) to identify and grasp the cervix, a firm cylindric structure. The cervix is encircled with the hand or held against the pelvis with the fingers and the vagina is extended to its full length to eliminate any folds in it, which could interfere with passage of the pipette through the cervix. Use your fingers as a guide to make sure the pipette is in the cervix and not in the fornix (along the thinner vaginal wall, beside the cervix).

The pipette must pass through 3-5 constrictions in the cervix. While passing through these "rings," always keep your fingers in contact with the end of the pipette to guide it as well as to protect the uterine wall from being punctured as it enters the uterus. Upon entering the uterus one-quarter inch or so, depress the plunger slowly, depositing the semen. The pipette is then withdrawn and examined for pus or blood.

Mares

Artificial insemination of mares is not as widely practiced as in cows due to breed regulations and the limited availability of frozen equine semen. However, AI may be used in addition to natural breeding to "reinforce" a service in Thoroughbreds and some other breeds. In Quarterhorses, Standardbreds and a few other breeds, AI is used when several mares must be bred at one time and the stallion's ejaculate can be diluted and still have sufficient numbers of viable sperm. Regulations for most breeds that allow AI require that the stallion and the mare be on the same farm at the time of AI. In Hanoverians and some other breeds, freezing and shipping of semen to other locations for AI are permitted. Starting on day 2 of heat and breeding every other day until the mare goes out of heat produces satisfactory results.

Semen is collected with the aid of an artificial vagina. The temperature inside the vagina should be about 105 F at the time of collection. A mare in heat or a "dummy" the stallion is trained to mount is required to collect semen.

Semen samples should be kept as close to 95 F as possible to assure sperm viability. The collection container is often equipped with a filter to assist in separating the gel from the remainder of the semen. Raw semen can be placed in a warm syringe and deposited into the mare's uterus through an infusion pipette, or an extender can be added to the semen if desired.

Extending the semen allows more mares to be inseminated and protects the sperm for a short time until deposition into the uterus. There are several acceptable semen extenders. They often contain antibiotics to help control any bacteria that have contaminated the semen during collection or that may have been introduced into the uterus during insemination. A recipe for an acceptable semen extender is listed in Table 7.

The dry portion of this extender can be mixed and prepackaged by a pharmacist and stored for up to 6 months. It must be kept in dry containers and protected from light. The liquid portions can then be added before use. The extender should be well mixed and warmed to 95 F before adding the semen. The semen can be diluted 1:1 or 1:3

Table 7. Recipe for Equine Semen Extender

Sanalac (instant nonfat dry milk)	2.4 g
gelatin (unflavored, unsweetened)	0.4 g
glucose	4.9 g
gentamicin sulfate (50 mg/ml)	2.0 ml
7½% sodium bicarbonate solution (sterile)	2.0 ml
sterile water for injection (no preservatives)	92.0 ml
total	100.0 ml

with the extender, depending on the sperm concentration in the semen. It is desirable to have 100-500 million live normal sperm per insemination dose.

Sows

Sows can be inseminated with fresh or frozen semen, but AI has not been widely accepted as a practical consideration for commercial swine production. Some reasons for reluctance of the swine industry to extensively use AI are lack of a reliable means of synchronizing heat in gilts and sows, lower conception rates and smaller litter sizes with use of AI, the limited number (6-8) of raw semen doses per ejaculate relative to the amount of time and work involved, and the high level of management required. Heat detection and record keeping technics must be very accurate.

The optimum time to artificially inseminate sows depends on the heat detection technics used. Sows checked for heat once daily should be bred every day they stand, for at least 3 days. If heat detection is used twice daily, sows should be inseminated 12 and 24 hours after the onset of heat.

After estrus is detected, semen is collected in an artificial vagina or directly in a prewarmed thermos by manually massaging the boar's penis. Semen can be collected while the male is mounted on an estrual female or boars can be trained to mount dummies constructed for this purpose. The semen can be extended 1:4 or 1:5. One ejaculate usually contains enough sperm to inseminate 6-8 females. A minimum of 2 billion live normal sperm is needed for adequate conception and large litter sizes. Frozen extended semen is available from at least one commercial source in the US and one in Canada.

When AI is used, relatively large volumes (50-100 ml) of semen are deposited with the aid of a spiral-tipped pipette or an infusion pipette that has the last inch bent at a 30° angle. These pipettes are actually "screwed" into the cervical rings of the sow.

Bitches

AI in the dog is usually carried out with fresh, undiluted semen. However, in the last few years, the American Kennel Club (AKC) has approved registration of litters using frozen dog semen when collection, storage, transfer and insemination are done under very strict rules and regulations. There are now 5-10 AKC-approved locations that freeze and store canine semen.

Canine semen is usually collected by manual massage of the penis. Most dogs do not require an estrual bitch present when this is done; however, some timid males may need teasing by a bitch in heat before collection. The collection should be carried out in a quiet room, with good footing for the dog and no distractions.

The dog ejaculates in 3 fractions. The first fraction is clear, contains no sperm and is discarded. The second fraction, the sperm-rich fraction, should be collected. The third fraction is clear and after a few drops are collected, the rest is discarded. There may be a 15- to 60-second delay between passage of fractions.

The semen is protected from cold and heat shock and transferred to a prewarmed syringe and deposited in the cranial vagina through an infusion rod. The rear of the bitch should be elevated during and for a few minutes after insemination. Some veterinarians prefer to introduce the index finger, covered with a sterile, powder-free glove, into the vagina with the rod. The finger is left in the vagina a few minutes and the dorsum of the vaginal vault is stroked gently to simulate the coital tie between the male and female. It is thought that this induces waves of uterine and vaginal contractions that help the sperm move into the uterus.

Canine sperm is usually not diluted because of a lack of ability to synchronize heats in females. Bitches usually are artificially inseminated because of a lack of ability or desire by the selected male to copulate. Bitches should be inseminated on the first, third and fifth day of standing heat or as determined appropriate by vaginal cytology.

index

index

I

J, K, L, M, N

O, P

U, V, W, X, Y, Z